HEALTH PSYCHOLOGY

Psycho-social Perspective

HEALTH PSYCHOLOGY

Psycho-social Perspective

Edited by
Sunita Malhotra
Promila Batra
Amrita Yadava

Commonwealth

Health Psychology

First Published : 2025

ISBN 81-311-0120-7

Published by :

COMMONWEALTH PUBLISHERS
4831/24, Prahlad Street,
Ansari Road, Darya Ganj,
New Delhi - 110002
Ph. : 23272541, 23257835
Fax : 91- 011- 23257835
e-mail : campusbooks@hotmail.com

Typesetting by :

Arjun Computers
Delhi - 110051

Printed at :
Roshan Offset Printers
Delhi

FOREWORD

The book entitled "Health Psychology : Psycho-social Perspective" is a comprehensive treatise in the area of Health Psychology, both in its conceptual and indigenous Indian aspects. To any eclectical peruser of the book, the book is an informative guide in the area of Health Psychology. The innovative approach adopted in the book covers almost every aspect of the subject. I would strongly recommend the book for prescribed reading for students of subject, as well as to researchers in health psychology for locating the lead or probe areas for the research in this new and upcoming area. I wish the authors all luck and success.

Prof. S.N. Sinha

Professor Emeritus

Formerly Vice-Chancellor & Head
Department of Psychology
University of Rajasthan,
Jaipur-302004 (Rajasthan)
India

Preface

As we enter the 21st century we can look back on the last hundred years as a time of unprecedented change. A person whose life spans across the 20th century, would have seen greater changes in agriculture, manufacturing, transportation and communication than a person born at any other time in human history. Concurrent with these vast developments the concept of disease has also traversed from being conceptualized as caused by demons or punishment for moral to being caused by an unhealthy personality.

The perusal of the factors which resulted in this change brings focus on four causes. Firstly, a new definition of health has emerged where health is considered as a state of complete physical, mental and social well being and not merely the absence of disease. Secondly, the leading causes of death have changed from acute diseases caused by disease pathogens to chronic diseases, causes of which encompass behavioural pathogens as well as changing life styles. Thirdly, the alarming escalation in the cost of medical care and spread of awareness among the masses has spotlighted the benefits of preventive health care. Lastly, health care is no longer an exclusive domain rather the role of health care professionals than medical professionals like clinical psychologists, counselors, social workers and policy-makers is gaining importance.

Before 1970's, health related issues were taken up psychologists under behavioural medicine. The broadening of the concept of Health lead to the creation of a distinct field–Health Psychology in 1978. It had its own goals like study the etiology (psychological, behavioural and social) of diseases, promote development of health enhancing behaviours, prevent and treat illnesses by helping in minimizing risk factors and assisting in adjustment to illness or complying to treatment regimes and promote public health policy and improve health care system.

Recognizing that an individual's health and vulnerability to disease is due to mutual influences among the biological, psychological and social forces, health psychologists work from a biopsychosical perspective. Using a system approach, health illness and medical care are thus viewed as inter-related processes involving interactive changes within the individual and society.

The Organisation of This Book

The present book has been divided into five sections with an attempt to view health from a psychosocial perspective. The concept of health, although more or less same for everyone, varies across cultures and sub-cultures with regard to its meaning, influence and ways of promotion. Realizing the importance of indigenous frameworks in understanding Health in a specific social context a number of articles which reflect upon the conceptual aspects of health have been included in Section-1.

Social ties and relationships with others have always been a source of personal and emotional satisfaction, controlling our behaviour in a variety of ways. The psychological make up of an individual influences his/her social ties and vice-versa. This dual interaction, may in turn have a mute effect on either enhancing maladjustment or lead to effective coping strategies. Likewise environmental influences on health promoting/compromising behaviours are also strong and cannot be denied. Thus, Section II of the book deals with the role of psychosocial factors including cognitions and attributions in health.

The impact of demographic factors such as age, sex, socioeconomic status and typical personality pattern assumes an important dimension when pitted with health related issues. parenting styles, geographical variations in customs and perceptions influence attitudes, personal orientation and behaviour. Section III attempts to understand health from a socio-demographic perspective.

The influence of attitudes on health is not limited to personal or social arena, rather it is carried over to the world of work. Enhancement of competition and career orientation has increased the complexities of work situation. This amplifies the psychological and physical burden of the worker. The articles incorporated in Section IV, unfolds the role of organizational factors such as efficiency, job satisfaction, stress etc. in assessment of Health.

The complexities of the present world, increased stress at both home and work have resulted in an increase in the variety and incidence of health problems. As indicated earlier, today, prevention is major concern for health psychologists. Thus, preventive and coping strategies are receiving a lot of attention. Section V deals with understanding of psychosocial factors underlying various pathologies and the coping strategies used for prevention or cure. Thus, the book attempts to provide a comprehensive insight into the theoretical and applied aspects of Health Psychology from a psychosocial perspective.

This book is a compilation of articles presented at the 8th *International and 39th National Conference of the Indian Academy of Applied Psychology on Positive Health and Well-Being.* Majority of the articles were presented and debated upon during the conference. The Editors are indebted to the Indian Association of Applied Psychology (IAAP) and Department of Psychology, M.D. University, Rohtak for entrusting them with the task of compiling the proceedings of the conference in book form. However, editors regret that due to limitation of the scope of the book to psychosocial perspective of health, a number of articles could not be incorporated. Further, major focus has been kept on empirical contributions in order to provide a data base to researchers and students of Health Psychology to understand the methodological aspects and gain insight into the probable areas for further research.

Editors owe no responsibility for any discrepancy regarding the views and data given in the articles as these are the sole responsibility of the authors. Readers are requested for rejoinder, if any, to write directly to the first author of the articles.

The editors express their heartily thanks to all the contributors and participants whose presence and innovative deliberations made the conference an immemorable event.

Sunita Malhotra
Promila Batra
Amrita Yadava

Contents

SECTION—II

Health in Psycho-social Perspective

SECTION—III

Health in Socio-demographic Perspective

List of Contributors

A.P. Singh, Professor, Department of Psychology, Banaras Hindu University, Varanasi (U.P.).

Abha Singh, Joint-Director, Amity Institute of Behavioural and Allied Sciences, Sector-44, Noida (U.P.).

Abhilasha Singh, Assistant Professor, School of Management Sciences, Varanasi (U.P.).

Abhilasha Singh, Assistant Professor, Department of Psychology, Samastipur College, Samastipur (Bihar).

Akbar Husain, Professor, Department of Psychology, Aligarh Muslim University, Aligarh (U.P.).

Aparna Mehrotra, Research Scholar (Psychology), Department of Humanities and Social Sciences, Indian Institute of Technology, Kanpur (U.P.).

Aradhana Shukla, Head, Department of Psychology, Kumaun University Campus, Almora (Uttaranchal).

Archana Upadhyay, Department of Psychology, Banaras Hindu University, Varanasi (U.P.).

Arvind S. Shah, Lecturer in Psychology, A.S.C. Mahila Arts College, Mehsana.

Bhavneet Kaur Gill, Research Scholar, Department of Psychology, Punjabi University, Patiala (Punjab).

D.J. Bhatt, Professor and Head, Department of Psychology, Saurashtra University, Rajkot (Gujarat).

Dinesh Kataria, Assistant Professor & Head, Department of Psychiatry, Lady Harding Medical College, New Delhi.

Divya Kumar, Department of Psychology, Jamia Millia Islamia, New Delhi.

Farzana Alim, Reader in Home Science, Women's College Aligarh, Muslim University, Aligarh (U.P.).

G. Aruna Mohan, Reader in Psychology, St Joseph's College of Education for Women, Guntur, (A.P).

Geeta Rani Magoo, Lecturer in Psychology, Hindu Girls College, Sonepat (Haryana).

Hempal Punia, Scientist 'B', Defence Institute of Psychological Research, Delhi.

I.S. Muhar, Formerly Professor of Psychology and Director, Distance Education, Maharshi Dayanand University, Rohtak. Present address: #518, Sector: 10-D, Chandigarh.

Jagtar Singh, Ex-Post-Graduate Student, Department of Psychiatry, Post-Graduate Institutes of Medical Sciences, Rohtak (Haryana).

Jitender Dahiya, Counsellor, Distt. Red Cross Society, Rohtak (Haryana).

K. Ramachandran, Science 'E', Defence Institute of Psychological Research, Delhi.

L.R. Yagnik, Professor & Head, Department of Psychology, Sardar Patel University, Vallabh Vidyanagar (Gujrat).

Lalit Kumar Mishra, Project Fellow, Department of Psychology, Banaras Hindu University, Varanasi (U.P.).

Mandeep Kaur, Post-Graduate, Department of Psychology, University of Delhi, Delhi.

Musaddiq Jahan, Senior Lecturer, Women's College, Aligarh Muslim University, Aligarh (U.P.).

N.R. Sharma, Reader, Department of Psychology, M.D. University, Rohtak (Haryana).

Nazirul Hasnain, Professor, Department of Psychology, Jamia Millia Islamia, New Delhi.

Neelam Arya, Research Scholar, Department of Bio-Sciences, Maharshi Dayanand University, Rohtak (Haryana).

Neena Kohli, Department of Psychology, University of Allahabad, Allahabad (U.P.).

N. Pamyaphy, Research Scholar, Jawaharlal Nehru University, Delhi.

Nishat Afroz, Lecturer, Psychology Section, MMV, Banaras Hindu University, Varanasi (U.P.).

Nishi Tripathi, Coordinator of the Counselling Centre, Department of Psychology, University of Allahabad, Allahabad (U.P.).

O.P. Sharma, Assistant Professor, Department of Psychology, University of Rajasthan, Jaipur (Rajasthan).

P.S. Rathore, Associate Professor, University of Rajasthan, Jaipur (Rajasthan).

P.V. Rasal, Reader & Head, Department of Psychology, Niphad College, Nasik (Maharashtra).

Poonam Phogat, Ph.D. Scholar, Department of Psychology, University of Delhi (Delhi).

Prabha Bhatia, Reader, Department of Psychology, M.D. University, Rohtak (Haryana).

Priti Singh, Reader, Department of Psychiatry, Pt. B.D. Sharma Post-Graduate Institute of Medical Sciences, Rohtak (Haryana).

Promila Batra, Professor, Department of Psychology, Maharshi Dayanand University, Rohtak (Haryana).

R. Balakrishnan, Head, Department of Psychology, PSG College of Arts and Science, Coimbatore (Tamil Nadu).

R. Roja Ramani, R. Babu, Post-Graduate Students, Department of Psychology, PSG College of Arts and Science, Coimbatore (Tamil Nadu).

R.K. Bhatia, Department of Physical Education, Kurukshetra University, Kurukshetra (Haryana).

Radheyshyam, Reader, Department of Psychology, Maharshi Dayanand University, Rohtak (Haryana).

Rajbala Singh, Research Scholar (Psychology), Department of Humanities and Social Sciences, Indian Institute of Technology, Kanpur (U.P.).

Rajbir Singh, Professor & Head, Department of Psychology, M.D. University, Rohtak (Haryana).

Rajesh Kumar, Research Scholar, Department of Psychology, M.D. University, Rohtak (Haryana).

Rajesh Nair, Consultant (NGOs), National AIDS Control Organisation (NACO), New Delhi.

Rameshwari Devi, Reader in Physical Education, M.D. University, Rohtak (Haryana).

Ramjee Lal, Department of Applied Psychology, VBS Purvanchal University, Jaunpur (U.P.).

Ranjana Mitra, Reader, Psychology Section, MMV, Banaras Hindu University, Varanasi (U.P.).

Rumki Gupta, Psychologist, Psychology Research Unit, Indian Statistical Institute, Kolkata, (West Bengal).

S.C. Bhargava, Associate Professor & Head, Dept. of Psychiatry, Pt. B.D. Sharma Post-Graduate Institute of Medical Sciences, Rohtak (Haryana).

S.N. Sinha, Emeritus Professor, Psychology & Ex-Vice-Chancellor, University of Rajasthan, Jaipur.

S.S. Kaushi, Professor & Head, Deptt. of Psychology, M.M.V., Banaras Hindu University, Varanasi (U.P.).

Samreen Hasan Khan, Research Scholar, Department of Psychology, Aligarh Muslim University, Aligarh (U.P.).

Sandeep Kumar, Lecturer, Department of Psychology, Banaras Hindu University, Varanasi (U.P.).

Sapna Sachdeva Nair, Consultant, Hindustan Latex Family Planning Promotion Trust (HLFPPT), New Delhi.

Savita Arya, Lecturer, Govt. College of Education, Chandigarh.

Shabu B. Raj, Sc 'B', Defence Institute of Psychological Research, Delhi.

Shikha Dixit, Associate Professor (Psychology), Department of Humanities and Social Sciences, Indian Institute of Technology, Kanpur (U.P.).

Sonika Chhabra, Ex-Student, Department of Psychology, M.D. University, Rohtak (Haryana).

Sudeepa Bose, Department of Psychology, Banaras Hindu University, Varanasi (U.P.).

Sunita Malhotra, Professor, Department. of Psychology, M.D. University, Rohtak (Haryana).

Sunita Siwach, Head, Department of Psychology, Maharani Kishori Devi Jat Kanya Mahavidyalaya, Rohtak (Haryana).

Vandana Sharma, Professor & Head, Department of Psychology, Punjabi University, Patiala (Punjab).

Veenu Tucker, Senior Reader, Gargi College, Delhi.

Vidhu Mohan, Formerly Professor and Chair Person, Department of Psychology, Punjab University, Chandigarh.

SECTION—I

Health in Conceptual Perspective

1

Self in Indian Perspective

Abha Singh* and N.G. Pamyaphy**

While the Greek philosophers were preoccupied with the quest of the World-Stuff, the ancient Indian philosophers were meditating on the Self as is evident when we study the subject. The pre-Socratic philosophy is primarily focused on the world outside, its shift from the universe to man began from Socrates onward. On the other side in the Eastern part of the world, Self was central to the Indian philosophy right from the outset, and it is from therein that it proceeded on the outside embracing the entire universe. Even though the Greek vision had turned towards man it did not really turn inward as life at Athens and perception of man was rational and social. No wonder down the ages in the successive development of thoughts education and science flourished in the West, and India even now is far behind. Though in the absence of science mythological and superstitious roots are certainly stronger in India, it would be an error to state that in Indian system of thoughts science never developed. Vedic science was highly advanced in spite of its subordination to the religious and philosophical thoughts. We have certainly suffered and are still trying to emerge from the mysterious worlds of gods and demons, still the concept of consciousness in Indian psychology is far more profound and transcendental than in the West which is preoccupied with material things and development.

This fact has been aptly presented by Dr. Radhakrishnan and Shri Aurobindo.

According Dr. Radhakrishnan :

"When Greco-Roman civilization was triumphant, it failed to supply its conquered peoples with a religion, and instead was itself conquered by a religion supplied by them. May it not be that today the people of Asia may supply a spiritual orientation to the new world based on science and technology. By its materialistic and political devices, the West is able to provide a secure framework or order within which different civilizations could mingle, and fruitful intercourse between them can take place by which the spiritual poverty of the world can be

*Joint-Director, Amity Institute of Behavioural and Allied Sciences, Sector-44, Noida,

**Research Scholar, JNU, Jawaharlal Nehru University, Delhi.

overcome. Without a spiritual recovery, the scientific achievements threaten to destroy us" (Radhakrishnan, 1954). Thus, there has always been a tendency to overlook the spiritual in the West, the roots of which can be traced to the influence of the Greeks, and exalt merely the intellect bending the mind towards the empirical and the external.

According to Shri Aurobindo :

"The tendency of the normal Western mind is to live from below upward and from out inward.... The average European draws his guiding views not from the philosophic, but from the positive and practical reason.... The West has acquired the religious mind rather than possessed it by nature and it has always worn its acquisition with a certain looseness.... The emphasis of the Western mind is on life, the outer life above all, the things that are grasped, visible, tangible. The inner life is taken only as an intelligent reflection of the outer world, with the reason for a firm putter of things into shape, an intelligent critic, builder, refiner of the external materials offered by Nature" (Aurobindo, 1953). The West has determined the replacement of the syncretic tendency of consciousness by the analytic and separative, parting the spirit and the intellect.

The Cartesian duality is nearly unknown in Indian psychology with individual consciousness as an intimate part of and partial expression of cosmic consciousness. Essentially, the cosmic consciousness and the individual consciousness are united. It is only subjectivity that separates the individual from the cosmic. Consciousness is the ultimate reality out of which mind and matter emerge in every level of existence from minerals to men. Of all the existing bodies that express themselves through behaviour, the human body is the most evolved one. It is capable of self-expression in manifold manners. When consciousness desires expression as an organism it needs a medium and works with the physical body. Beyond the appearances the substratum of your causal, subtle and gross bodies is your real Self.

Although self has been conceptualized as the main focus of existence of man, yet the relation of self with the almighty has been formulated differently. Vedas present incoherent ideas regarding the nature and composition of man but the same becomes clear in the Upanishads. The Taittiriya Upanishad gives an account of the structure of man. During the Upanishadic period distinction between and union of body and spirit, man's physical body and *atman* was stated. Atman is one's real and true self. In Hinduism, the Self is the unified being in which all creation takes a part. This Self (Atman) knows his own nature and knew he was Brahman, and Self became All. The goal in Hinduism is to bring the individual person to the realization that indeed he is not a separate being, but rather a partaker of the great Self. So the saying is "Atman (self, soul) is Brahman." The goal of the individual through yoga and spiritual exercise is to realize and know that he is Brahman (Brhadaranyaka Upanishad I, iv, 10 as one of many examples of this teaching). In this context the idea of losing oneself is to obtain knowledge of the belief that the individual human being should not speak or think of being an individual self and should not act upon the desires and wants of the individual self. The goal in Hinduism is to attain detachment from self-desires and wants, and to become one with the universal Self.

In the teaching of Jesus Christ, the concept of "losing self" is very different. Jesus affirms the individual self as a real and true creature. This individual self is never lost or dissipated into some greater Self, but is a created being with definite personal existence. Jesus teaches that the person will exist as an individual for all eternity in either a state of relationship with God (Heaven) or separation from God (Hell) [John, 5:25-29, Mt, 25:34, 41, 46]. The problem with man is not one of mistaken knowledge. The problem with man according to Jesus is sin, rebellion against God. This happens when a separate and individual creature (man) chooses to live in a manner that does not honour and recognize God (a transcendent and independent being—separate from man). Jesus warned in very strong language against sin and the danger of the individual being consigned to hell for this rebellion (Matthew, 18:8 "If your hand or your foot causes you to sin cut it off and throw it away. It is better for you to enter life maimed or crippled than to have two hands or two feet and be thrown into eternal fire."). The concept that Jesus taught of selflessness was to forsake the desires of a real, independent self that are in rebellion to God's ways. Jesus taught that man has lived in sin and separation from God ever since the fall or rebellion of Adam and Eve (the first man and woman God created). This sin is a part of the very nature of each individual man. To live for the self, according to Jesus, is to live in sin (Matthew, 23:25 "Woe to you, teachers of the law and Pharisees, you hypocrites! You clean the outside of the cup and dish, but inside they are full of greed and self-indulgence."). Jesus said, "If anyone would come after me, he must deny himself and take up his cross daily and follow me" (Luke, 9:23). This means to abandon the sinful self desires that are a part of human nature (Gal, 5:17— For the sinful nature, desires what is contrary to the Spirit, and the Spirit what is contrary to the sinful nature. They are in conflict with each other...). This means to choose as an individual to live for others and for God. In this sense, the selflessness of Jesus' teaching is the virtue of abandoning the sinful and destructive desires of the sinful self and pursue instead God and the good of your neighbour. The virtue of self-denial according to Jesus then is not merely something of knowledge. It is not an enlightenment or realization of being universal Self. It is the individual choosing to deny his real personal desires and to live instead for what God has said is good.

The differences between the two views have been presented in tabular form :

Table 1.1 : Comparison Between Christianity and Hinduism Concept of Self Between the Two Views

Issues	*Christanity*	*Hinduism*
Selflessness	Actual selfless living by individuals.	Realization that we are all Self.
Self desires as evils	Self desires are evil because they are sinful—rebellious to God's ways.	Self desires (individual) are evil because they are not Self-universal (Brahman) desires .
The solution	Repentance, denial of selfish desires and living for God's ways.	Realization and enlightenment that you are Self.
Role of self in selflessness	To deny the self and to live for God.	To turn in to the self to find the Self.

Hindu selflessness is actually an affirmation and strengthening of self in the greater Self. Jesus' teaching is, the self has become corrupt and is living based upon that orientation to corrupted (sinful) self; selflessness is to turn from that self life and to live for God. There is a sense of opposite in this comparison. Hinduism seeks for selflessness through a turning in to the self (Katha Upanishad, IV, 1) to find the Self. Christianity teaches selflessness through denying the self.

Matthew, 16:24 "Then Jesus said to his disciples, "If anyone would come after me, he must deny himself and take up his cross and follow me."

THE NATURE OF MAN ACCORDING TO INDIAN PSYCHOLOGY

To be able to grasp the profound significance of the Indian concept of the divinity of man, we must first review the various prevalent concepts of man.

Biologically, man is an animal with the species name Homo sapiens, whose forebrain or neo-cerebrum is more developed than that of other animals. Consequently man is less governed by his instincts than other animals, which, due to preponderance of the lower brain or paleo-cerebrum are primarily driven by instincts. According to the medical materialists, man is a physiologically driven machine made of complex biochemical molecules. Almost all the non-theological philosophers of the West, each of whom has added his own adjective to the animal-man, have accepted these basic concepts of man. Greek philosophers considered man a rational animal. Aristotle has defined man as a political animal, and the American philosopher Benjamin Franklin calls him homo-faber, or tool-making animal. Man has produced tools as extension of his own body, as it were, and has increased his productivity manifold. He has harnessed energy, like steam energy, electricity, atomic energy, etc. He has produced devices that replace thought itself (automation, cybernetics). Cassier has emphasized that man is a symbol making animal and the most important symbol invented by him is the word through which he can communicate with others.

Of the Western thinkers, special mention must be made of Sigmund Freud and Karl Marx. Freud's outstanding contribution is his discovery of the unconscious. But by laying too great a stress on sex as the most important driving force, he has reduced man into a sexual animal, the homosexuals, with far reaching psychosocial consequences which are too evident in the contemporary society to be mentioned. The whole aim of his system of psychotherapy is to help man attain sexual maturity. Marx believes that man is driven primarily be a desire for economic gains: he is a homo-economicus. However, in *Das Capital*, he has defined man as a social animal. According to him, if man fails to relate himself actively with others and with nature, he loses himself, becomes alienated; his drives lose human qualities and assume animal qualities. He becomes a sick, fragmented, crippled human being. According to Marx man is driven by two sets of drives : fixed or constant and relative. Sex and hunger fall under the first category, while relative drives like hate, avarice etc. owe their origin to certain types of social organizations. This concept, to some extent, resembles the Hindu concept of man: 'Eating, sleeping, fear and sex are common to man as well as animals. In human beings *dharma* (*i.e.* restraint by moral rules) is extra and special. Without *dharma* men are no better than beasts.' *Dharma* is of two types: *pravritti-lakshana* and *nivritti-lakshana*. When one, observing the moral codes of conduct applicable to one's station in life and society performs actions for enjoyment (*kama*) and acquisition of wealth (*artha*), one is said to be following *pravritti dharma*. A time comes, however, when one gets disgusted with sense-enjoyments and acquisition of wealth and aspires for final emancipation (*moksha*). Then one embraces what is called *nivritti dharma*, characterized by renunciation of all worldly desires and selfish actions, and resorting to spiritual practice to attain liberation. Man rises from animal to human level by accepting *pravritti dharma, i.e.* by observing social injunctions. He ascends to godhood and becomes divine by embracing the *nivritti dharma*.

This Hindu concept of liberation, in turn, is based upon another concept of an ever pure, ever free, ever perfect, ever conscious spiritual entity in man called Atman. This Atman is the Real Man as against the body-mind complex, which is only the apparent man. The relation between the real and apparent men has been beautifully described through an allegory in the Katha Upanishad : Know the soul to be the master of the chariot and the body the chariot. Consider the intellect the charioteer, and the mind the reins. The senses, they say, are the horses, and their roads are the sense objects. The wise call Him the enjoyer when He is united with the body, senses and mind.

The Hindus have further elaborated this concept by stating that the real man or Atman is conscious, ever free, blissful and immortal. The apparent man consists of five sheaths, which cover the soul or Atman. These are : (1) the physical body or the physical sheath, (2) the vital sheath or the sheath life force, (3) the mental sheath, (4) the ego sheath, and (5) the Blissful sheath. According to another concept, the real man or the conscious soul or Atman has three bodies : (1) the gross physical body, (2) the subtle mental body and (3) the causal body, which is made up of pure ignorance. At the time of death, the physical body dies, but the subtle mental body and the causal body remain and together with the conscious soul or real man, transmigrate to another physical body to be born again. When we are awake, the gross physical body is active. In sleep, when we are dreaming, the physical body is inactive, but the mental body is active. But when we go into deep sleep and do not even see dreams, at that time even the mental body is not active and only the causal body in the form of ignorance remains covering the pure soul or Atman.

From the above resume it would be evident that the Hindu concepts of the nature of man, his destiny and his drives are far more comprehensive and vastly superior to the western ones. Firstly for western thinkers man is either an animal or a machine but for Hindus he is essentially divine. Secondly, whereas western savants have postulated only three ultimate goals for man, *viz.* sensual enjoyment (*kama*), acquisition of earthly riches (*artha*), and fulfilment of social obligations (*dharma*), the Indian philosophers have postulated a fourth and final goal : liberation (*moksha*), the state of fullest manifestation of innate divinity and perfection. Thirdly, whereas Freud thinks that man must satisfy his passions to remain whole and healthy, Marx states that man cannot truly be a man unless he actively relates with others. However, man is man so long as he is struggling to rise above nature, both internal and external. Finally, Western philosophers say that man's evolution is governed by drives and instincts. But for the Indian sages man's innate perfection is constantly trying to manifest itself and every effort on our part simply acts as a remover of barriers to its manifestation.

Swami Vivekananda laid the greatest stress on the divinity of man because he knew men are divine, and since truth liberates, the only way to be free was to perceive the truth of one's divinity. Secondly, we tend to think and act according to our concept of ourselves. This has profound practical, psychological and social implications. The concepts of man as a sexual, economic, tool-making or social animal may be useful to individual or society to a certain extent, but they are restrictive. If we consider ourselves sexual animals as Freud wants us to believe, sexual shall we become. If we believe we are economically driven machines, we shall run after money. If we think we are social animals, we shall become slaves of society. But if we consider ourselves ever free, blissful divinities, we shall enjoy freedom and bliss. He used to illustrate this truth with the help of the story of a lion cub, which was reared along with a herd of sheep from the very day of its birth. As it grew, it learnt to bleat and eat grass. Then another lion attacked this flock of sheep. He was surprised to find a full-grown lion running away in fear. He caught hold of this younger lion, dragged it to the forest and told it that it was a lion and acting like a sheep did not befit it. To convince it, the older lion showed its reflection in the lake. The young lion was convinced that it was a lion and not a sheep and in a moment gave up its fear.

Once two young sons of a devotee were playing. One was Vivek and another, Shirish. They, for the sake of fun, added '*ananda*' to their names, and became Vivekananda and Shirishananda, and, as their play demanded, started acting according to their new names. Vivek folded his arms and stood erect like Swami Vivekananda with a grave face. Shirish did the same. But then, for some reason, Shirish started weeping. Vivek was surprised, and asked his mother, 'Can Shirishananda weep?' That's it! Weeping does not befit Shirish as long as he is '*ananda*', a dignified monk. If children can temporarily change their behaviour in play according to their assumed identity, can we not change our identity and behaviour permanently?

Normally, we consider ourselves as physical body or a body-mind complex. It is extremely difficult to consider oneself as a conscious soul free from body and mind, and free from the five coverings or three bodies. All the Hindu scriptures are meant to teach this concept of immortal, pure, blissful, eternal soul as man's real nature. This is the central theme of the whole Hindu philosophy and religion, which is taught in various ways through reason, mythology and stories.

MANIFESTATION OF SELF

A great emphasis is laid on ethical discipline in Hinduism. *Yama*—self-restraint—and *Niyama*—religious observances or canons—are the foundations of Yoga and Vedanta. People of the world with average conscience cannot think for themselves and are most of the time deceived by others and things of the world. Hence great sages have laid down rules of conduct. Lord Krishna says in the Gita : "Let the scriptures be thy authority in determining what ought to be done or what ought not to be done. Knowing what hath been declared by the ordinances of the scriptures, thou oughtest to work in this world" (Ch. XVI-24). The Smritis written by Yajnavalkya, Manu and other sages distinctly prescribe the rules of conduct. Since men do not have the power or the time to think of the moral principles and rules given in the scriptures, you can get them from the sages and saints and follow them to the very letter.

The profound basis of Hindu ethics is the one all-pervading Atman in all the things, animate and inanimate. It is the innermost soul of all beings. This is the common, pure consciousness. If you injure your neighbour, you really injure yourself. If you injure any other creature, you really injure yourself, because the whole world is nothing but your own Self. This is Hindu ethics. This is the basic metaphysical truth that underlies all Hindu ethical codes. The Atman or Self is one. One life vibrates in all beings. Life is common in animals, birds and human beings. Existence is common. This is the emphatic declaration of the Upanishads. This primary truth of religion is the foundation of ethics or morality or science of right conduct. From such an ethics flows the unity of all selves. The neighbour is, in truth, the very Self and what separates you from him is mere illusion. One Atman or Self abides in all beings. Universal love is the expression of the unity. Universal brotherhood has its basis in the unity of Self. All human relations exist because of this unity. If you injure another man, you injure yourself. If you help another person, you help yourself. There is one life, one common consciousness in all beings. This is the foundation of right conduct. This is the foundation of ethics.

On the whole the foundation and goal of human life is—*paramapurushartha*—union with God. Soul in the process of union with the Divine should focus on *sadachara* (good conduct), which is displayed in the qualities such as *bhakti, prarthana, dama, niskama karma, pratipaksha bhavana, udyama, shardha* and *mukti*.

Bhakti (Devotion)

Ordinarily three *margas* are taught to attain *parampurushartha* : *karma marga, gyan marga* and *bhakti marga*. Out of the three *margas*, the most suitable *marga* to the *grihasthas* (house holders) is *bhakti*. *Bhakti* is superior to the other two *margas* because it is fundamental to any *margas*. Without *bhakti* all forms of religious practices are shallow and attainment of virtues is not possible. *Bhakti* is the most spiritual act and in-itself fully perfect *dharma—ekantika dharma*.

The etymological meaning of *bhakti* is love as the word is derived from "*bhaj*" which means love. Love, which is so common a human passion, becomes a spiritual devotion man psychologically evolves—individuates—fosters in his heart the sentiment of divine love that not only reaches out to embrace the world but enflames new attachment to God. *Bhakti* is *paranuraktir Isware*, the supreme love and attachment to God. "As one loves me, so do I love him" (Gita, 4.11)

Prarthana (Prayer)

Prayer is mode of communication with the Divine. The love-sentiment, *bhakti*, is best fostered in prayer. A highly psychological process of prayer is taught in the Brihadaranyakopanishad (2.4.5) : *sravana, manana, nididhyasana*.

Sravana means "hearing." Hearing some spiritual discourse—*pravachanam*—or sermon—*upadesh*—, or reading a holy scripture nourishes prayer, which lead to the second step *manana*, *i.e.* reflection or meditation. Without *manana* prayer, a call to God for assistance in life is less effective as the devotee still hold on to *maya* of the earthly pleasures. Mahabharata teaches us "When one reflects (one's heart being purified by such reflection), one comes to know that the things of this world are as valueless as straw" (Shanti Parva, 174.4). It is reflection or meditation that frees man from *kleshas* (afflictions) and the remedy for *avidya* is *vichara, i.e.* reflection.

While *sravana* is the function of the ears or eyes and *manana* is the activity of the mind, *nididhyasana* is the work of the heart. It is a long unbroken contemplative meditation on God. *Samadhi*, contemplation, is both the result of labour of the seeker and a free gift from God.

Dama (Self-Control)

Prayer makes self-control possible. Without self-control all the other virtues are mere ideals. Temptations and passions are not to be considered evil or bad in-themselves if used in accordance to moral principles. Each form of *yoga* necessitates self-control because in the struggle between *sreya* and *preya* (Kathopanishad, 2.1.6) what is pleasurable (*preya*) generally overcomes the beneficial (*sreya*). Those of us who chase the pleasurable live according to the pleasure principle, an epicurean life, and those of us who pursue the beneficial become psychologically healthy and prosperous, and holy. "Restrain the senses first" (Gita, 3.41).

Nishkama Karma (Disinterested Actions)

Kama is "desire" and *nishkama* means "desireless". *Nishkama* primarily refers to non-sensual desires. It denotes desire, which does not emerge from attachment. *Nishkama karma* is precisely offering one's actions to God. "He who works, having given up attachment, resigning his actions to God, is not touched by sin, even as a lotus (is untouched) by water" (Gita, 5.10). Realization of God or higher self within is possible only when one keeps his actions morally undefiled, *nishkama*. "Let not the fruit of action be your motive" (Gita, 2.47). Therefore, without attachment, perform always your duty" (Gita, 3.19). *Nishkama karma* is possible only when every work is offered to God. "Offer up all your works to Me" (Gita, 9.27). "Offer in thought all actions to Me, regard Me as your supreme end" (Gita, 18.57).

Pratipaksha Bhavana (Contrary Sentiment)

To attain union with God in Patanjali's Yoga Sutra (1.33) we find the observance of *pratipaksha bhavana*, which are four social virtues : *maitri* (friendship), *karuna* (mercy), *mudita* (feeling of happiness at the happiness of others) and *upeksha* (disregard for the faults of others). Since many vices spring from our unfriendly attitude towards our neighbours these virtues make us think well of others, inclining us to display love in behaviour towards others, regulate our dealings with fellow brethren. *Pratipaksha bhavana* are positive aspects of *ahimsa*. "Happy at the happiness of others" (Gita, 12.4).

Udyama (Personal Effort)

Realization of God is a free gift. Kathopanishad points out, "By Him alone can He be won, whom He chooses" (1.2.23). However, "*krita-praytna-apekshatu*"—God expects our efforts (Brahma Sutra, 2.3.42). It is one's struggle and perseverance on the path to divinity that counts because "to get oil from seeds, it is not enough to gather them together and gape at them, but one has to put them in the oil-press and crush them" (Hitopadesha, 1.30). Without *udyama*, therefore, every intellectual and spiritual faculty is nothing but potentiality, and though it realization of the spirit comes as a free gift its process of actuality is the road less traveled, *i.e.* hard and tough. "This soul cannot be won by the weak" (Mundakopanishad, 3.2.4).

Shardha (Faith)

Faith is to acknowledge the words of the Shastras as divine in origin and as true, and in the whisperings of the sanctified conscience. It is universal belief of men that God does not intervene in the world of men directly but through manifold ways so men should be vigilant to receive and act in accordance to the divine message. Daivan manushya rupena—God accomplishes His will through men. All that is required is *shardha* in order to be instruments of His will. We should have child-like faith in God. "The man devoid of faith and always doubting perishes" (Gita, 4.40).

Mukti (Liberation/Salvation)

Mukti means attainment of *moksha*. It is a state in which *jivatman* experiences supreme happiness of *Paramatman*. *Mukti* is considered as full possession of the soul's object of its deepest yearning and there can be no return to *samsara* for a liberated soul even as there is no return to one's dream after waking. *Moksha* is *salokya* with Brahman, *i.e.* living in the *Brahmaloka*. *Moksha* is *samipya, i.e.* being near to God, living in Divine Presence. *Moksha* is *sarupya, jivatman* assuming the figure of *Paramatman*. It is being in the image and likeness of God. *Moksha* is *sayujya, i.e.* divine union. *Jivatman* becomes one with *Paramatman*. Gita (14.2) considers *moksha* as *sadharmya*—identity of nature—with *Paramatman*.

Indian psychology is not confined to a religion, its scripture and cult, or to cater to an aspect of our human nature or a part of human expectation rather its purpose is mould the whole of what we are and what we need in life for psychological well-being.

CHANGE OF SELF

For the realization of self, radical transformation through shift of values is indispensably required. The nature of change that is needed for the values to take roots is—

From	To
Ceaseless exteriorization	Periodic interiorization
Complex living	Simple living
Speeding	Stilling
Competitive world	Cooperative world
Greed	Need
Calculative networking	Sincere helping

Keeping this in view, the re-prioritized agenda is—

Priority of	Priority Over
Human values	Professional skills
Silence	Speech
Whole	Fragment
Sacred	Secular
Spirit	Matter
Self	Self

The desire for truth is a seed that is planted deep within every incarnated human being, which when watered with life experience causes the individual to actively pursue the knowledge that will supply this developing life with nourishment. Depending at what point in the evolution of the soul this current personality is made manifest on the material plane, the truth that conforms to that personality may differ from what is accepted as truth by another. It is this truth that develops from within the current personality that leads to the deeper understanding of who we are as individuals. To know the reality of the mechanisms that drive us in this life is to understand the life that we have already lived. God has placed within the Archetype of Humanity a perfect form created in His image and likeness that creates the manifestation of the material plane that is expressed within. As we begin to understand the truth of our own existence, we begin to comprehend how we, as human beings, control the expression of the material universe that we are manifested within.

We are all created with the same elemental substance, no matter what race or ethnic group we may belong to. The development of the human body is dependent on the same need for nourishment provided by those charged with our care. These individuals also provide for us the memories that we one day will base our identity upon; although these memories, stored within our sub-conscious mind, are not valid reflections of the personality that we are or could be. It is only through the development of conscious awareness that we begin to see the reality of who we are.

Through contemplation, prayer and meditation we can begin to examine the mechanisms that have been developed to cope with the reality of life within the material plane. Time spent developing an understanding of the self will lead to a more conscious life experience. By taking the moments before we react to pause and think about our reactions we will allow our words to come from a place of wisdom rather than fear. Fear is what is developing the state of the world that we live in. By continuing to perpetuate the existence of this reactionary emotion, we keep the cycle of hate in control of the human existence. It is only when we begin to think and reason in the way that God has intended that we alter the life experience of all individuals that we come into contact with. The full expression of mind is dependant upon it's understanding of love; not only as an emotional understanding but also as a material force emanated by God.

No matter what religious understandings we may espouse; the basic truth that God is love permeates all teachings put forth. To know God without rational basis through validation is to have no personal realization of God. We must never cease in the work that leads to this realization. God existing in Absolute Beingness creates all principles that are known and unknown to us; and through this, not only manifests the expression of these images but also exists within these images. As the conscious choice is made to alter the current state of being; we invite the reality of God to manifest within our lives; the existence of which demands that the nature of the individual conform to the principles that God created us with, the very basis of which is love.

REFERENCES

Aurobindo, S. (1953). *The Foundations of Indian Culture*, New York : The Greystone Press.

Fromm, E. (1955). *The Sane Society*, London : Routledge.

Radhakrishnan, S. (1954). "*The Ancient Asian View of Man*" in Man's Right to Knowledge, An International Symposium presented in the honour of the Two-Hundredth Anniversary of Columbia University 1754-1954. New York : Columbia University Press.

2

Effect of Yoga on Positive Mental Health

Abhilasha Singh*

The 20th century is observed as the age of stress and anxiety. Scientific studies have shown that there are many factors which predispose to many physical and mental diseases. Also, there are definite factors for the formation of negative attitudes and health. The report of an expert committee convened by WHO indicated life style and behaviour as important catalysts in causing and preventing mental and heart disorders. Stress and strain of life is one of the chief mental factors for poor mental health and happiness. Anxiety, unwanted tensions, negative thoughts are also major factors for the development of negative mental health. Many factors are man-made factors which are preventable. Mental tension, emotional, disturbances anxiety are risk factors for so many heart disorders as well as mental disorders.

Mental peace and stability are the major attributes of sound mental health. When one becomes mentally disturbed, the heart overfunctions. Stress and strain are the number one risk factor for emotional disturbances. Worry of modern life directly affects man's mental health. Sound and positive mental health is possible only in the absence of tension, stress and strain of life, Positive mental health is a treasure. It is characterized by calmness, cheerfulness and happiness. Most of us do not qualify in all attributes of total positive mental health. The practice of yoga-meditation is the strongest foundation for building the base of one's positive mental health. Meditation is a scientific technique to elicit relaxation response to transform life-style. Hence it plays a significant role in the management of positive mental health. Balinet (1970), Chow (1966) and Eccles (1970) claim that meditation is useful to everyone in all situations. It helps to overcome anxiety and strain. It also lowers the respiratory rate, heart rate and blood pressure. Its practice lowers the over activity of sympathetic nervous system. As over function of sympathetic nervous system is reduced, one is able to maintain positive mental health.

A positive healthy mind rests on a healthy body. So before we go in for meditation, the body too should be made to practice simple yogic kriyas (like some asanas, pranayam etc.) so

*Asstt. Professor, Department of Psychology, Samastipur College, Samastipur, Bihar.

that a good and sound physical state induces yoga-meditation (a mental kriya). Just as the yogic kriyas (like asanas, pranayam, surya namaskar etc.) are useful in curing physical ailments like spinal problem, diabetes etc., meditation is also useful for mental health (Aurobindo, 1985).

Numerous scientific studies have proved that psychological stress can have disastrous effect on the physical and mental health. There is also evidence that one can control stress and reestablish mental harmony when one practices Yogic Meditation regularly. This method is known as Raj Yoga Meditation. In simple way, through Raj-yoga, one learns how to detach the mind from its physical connections with the sense organs through brain. In this detached state, the body and the brain are able to relax completely, while his consciousness is centred in his soul.

Raj Yoga Meditation has now been quite well analysed by Yogic studies at the B.K. Spiritual University. Raj Yoga practice produces Delta Waves or Theta waves mixed with Alpha and also many other physiological benefits even after only a week's practice. The subjective correlates of such a brain wave production are serenity, self-confidence and excessive joy leading to positive mental health. People who practice meditation express happiness and calmness. They never feel conflicts within self. They show accommodative intellect. They understand the emotional needs of others. They are considerate and courteous in all dealings. These are the chief characteristics of a mentally healthy person. Thus Yoga-practices are helpful for the management of perfect mental health.

The value of meditation has been documented medically and psychologically. A neuropsychiatrist of California Dr. Fink wrote in this connection—"Relaxation stops the emotions that prod the interbrain and forebrain into misbehaviour. Good mental health depends upon relaxation." Relaxation is a major stage of Yoga practice. It has been reported that stability on mind to a great extent depends upon Yoga Practice. Yoga Practice destroys physical attachments, allows the cortex to remain in its inherent rhythm.

Yoga Meditation is the latest technique to ensure a healthy mind. The practice of Yoga discards waste thought, leads to harmony between mind, intellect and desires. The experience of this peaceful state brings a natural power of concentration.

The purpose of the present study is to observe respiratory rate before and after meditation, performed in order to reduce stress and anxiety.

METHOD

Design

A single group pre-post-design was used.

Sample

Thirty college students who were in pre-examination stress were selected as the subjects of study. They were randomly chosen individuals, both male and female having some experience of yoga-meditation. Their age ranged from 17 to 21 years.

Tools

Raj Yoga Meditation was used.

Procedure

After establishing a rapport with the ss, they were requested to practice Yoga Meditation for 30 minutes daily. Before and after meditation respiratory rate was examined and recorded by trained doctors.

RESULTS AND DISCUSSION

The rate of respiration of each subject is given in Table 2.1 & Table 2.2, indicating mean respiratory rate of each subject before and after meditation with difference per minute. Low and normal rate was between 12 to 16 per minute, which is an indication of positive mental health as it is an expression of normal functioning of the respiratory organs of the subject, who participated with full co-operation in this investigation.

Table 2.1 : Respiratory Rate of Each Subject Before and After Meditation and the Difference

Subject	*Before Meditation*	*After Meditation*	*Difference Per Minute*
1	19	12	07
2	18	13	05
3	18	12	06
4	19	12	07
5	20	13	07
6	19	14	05
7	19	14	05
8	20	15	05
9	19	14	05
10	19	13	06
11	18	14	04
12	20	15	05
13	19	15	04
14	19	14	05
15	20	16	04
16	19	16	03
17	20	14	06
18	21	16	05
19	20	12	08
20	19	12	07
21	20	12	08
22	19	13	06
23	18	15	03
24	19	14	05
25	18	16	02
26	19	16	03
27	19	17	02
28	18	14	04
29	18	14	04
30	19	15	04

Table 2.2 : Mean of Respiratory Rate Both Before and After Meditation

No. of Subject 30	*Before Meditation*	*After Meditation*	*Difference Per Minute*
Total Res. Rate.	572	421	150
Mean	19.07	14.03	5.04
		t-value = 0.79, p <.01	

From the results it is evident that yoga meditation transforms the whole attitude towards mental tension, anxiety and stress. Data shows that the respiratory rate (R.R) in all subjects reduced on an average. The mean R.R. reduced from 19.09 to 14.03 per minute. The reduction of 5.04 per minute in the rate is due to meditation. t-for correlated means was applied to test the significance of difference. The obtained value, *i.e.* 0.79 was found to be significant at 0.01 level. This indicates that the improvement was due to the impact of Yoga only. The reduction in the rate of respiration is useful to one's mental health, happiness and cardio-vascular system. This implies that practice of yoga lowers sympathetic arousal leading to the reduction of R.R. also. The results further imply that practice of yoga meditation is favourable for the control of mental problems. Many studies done in the area and scientific survey of literature concerning meditation also support the idea that, it helps us to produce harmonious alpha waves. Therefore it is a fact that a yogi is able to maintain the tranquility of the electrical activity of brain during normal activities. The over functioning of the sympathetic division of autonomic nervous system is also minimized due to yoga meditation. Consequently one enjoys healthy cardio-vascular parameter.

The practice of meditation lowers the basal metabolic rate and increases organic resistance. The physiological changes are opposite to the fight or flight response. The results clearly advocate yoga meditation, as an auxiliary means to the conventional medicine, so that we can achieve permanent mental balance. So far as the facial expression of the subjects are concerned, they are not dominated by the emotions of worry and fear. They are courteous and considerable in all their dealings.

REFERENCES

Aurobindo, S. (1985). *Bases of Yoga*, Pondicherry : Sri Aurovindo Ashram.

Balinet, M. (1970). *Research in Psychotherapy*, London : Favislocts.

Chow, K.L. (1966). *Clinical Physiology*.

Eccles, J. (1970). *Facing Reality*, New York : Spring Verlag.

3

Subjective Well-Being in Indian Culture

Aradhana Shukla*

There is an increasing interest among psychologists and other social scientists in the context of positive subjective well-being (Warr, 1987, 1993). The people are asked about the psychological well-being and their perceptions and two types of evaluations. The first is related with cognitive states such as satisfaction and contentedness and second type refers to affective states such as the degree to which they experience feelings such as pleasure (Warr, 1987). This distinction between satisfaction and active states has also been made by Warr (1987, 1989, 1990, 1993). Enumerating the role of mental health in life, he advocates three principle axis for the measurement of affective well-being : the pleasure axis (measuring displeasure to pleasure), the anxiety-contentment axis, and depressed-enthusiasm axis. The need to recognize the multifaceted nature of subjective well-being has also been advocated by Brief, Butcher, George, and Link (1993) who claim that different facets of subjective well-being can be affected variably by personality factors, situational circumstances, and their interaction.

Various authors have reviewed researches indicating that the subjective feeling of being in control can contribute to a person's appearance of well-being (Langer, 1983; Strickland, 1989; Jahoda, 2005). Control can refer among the things, to mastery competence (White, 1959), casual explanations and personal agency (De Charms, 1968). Subjective well-being (SWB) is synonymous with one meaning of the lay term "happiness" The term subjective well-being, however, is preferred because happiness has several different meanings in popular usage. It can mean a pleasant momentary mood ("I am happy on payday") or the cause of such moods (*e.g.*, "Happiness in a 3-day weekend"). Happiness can refer to life satisfaction (*e.g.*, "I am happy with my life"), to long-term pleasant affect (*e.g.* "I have been happy since I changed my job last year") or to a predisposition to pleasant affect (*e.g.*, "She has a happy personality"). Because of these diverse meanings, researchers prefer the term subjective well-being to refer to the global state of evaluating one's life in a positive way.

Subjective well-being (SWB) refers to how people evaluate their lives, and includes variables such as life satisfaction and marital satisfaction, lack of depression and anxiety, and positive

---

*Head, Department of Psychology, Kumaun University Campus, Almora.

moods and emotions. The idea of SWB or happiness has intrigued thinkers for millennia, although it is since a very short period that it has been measured and studied in a systematic way. A person's evaluation of his or her life may be in the form of cognitions *e.g.*, when a person gives conscious evaluative judgments about his or her satisfaction with life as a whole, or evaluative judgments about specific aspects of his life such as recreation. However, an evaluation of one's life also may be in the form of affect, *e.g.*, people experiencing unpleasant or pleasant moods and emotions in reaction to their lives. Thus, a person is said to have high SWB if she or he experiences life satisfaction and frequent joy, and only infrequently experiences unpleasant emotions such as sadness and anger. On the other hand, a person is said to have low SWB if he or she is dissatisfied with life, experiences little joy and affection, and frequently feels negative emotions such as anger or anxiety. The cognitive and affective components of SWB are highly interrelated.

People constantly evaluate what is happening to them so that they are usually able to offer judgments about their lives. Furthermore, people virtually always experience moods and emotions, which have a hedonic component that is pleasant, signaling a positive reaction, or unpleasant, signaling a negative reaction. Thus, SWB refers to a person's perceptions of his well-being that are based on both affective and cognitive appraisal. The cognitive and affective components of SWB are highly interwined.

Is SWB a necessary condition for mental health? It appears that some people function well in many aspects of their lives, but are not particularly happy. Examples come to mind of individuals who are dysphonic, but who make significant contributions to society. Some might argue, however, that SWB is a necessary condition for mental health because a person cannot be functioning well if he or she is depressed for prolonged periods of time, or is suffering from debilitating anxiety. However, the level of SWB that is optimal for mental health and good functioning, is yet to be determined.

Subjective well-being is an aspect of psychological well-being. Nevertheless, the subjective frame of reference implicit in the concept of SWB has the strength of being based on the respondent's own internal perspective, and thus, gives priority and respect to people's own views of their lives. Rather than a standard imposed by a mental health professional, SWB is related to importance of the experiences of people. The focus on an internal perspective means that other criteria of well-being recognized by the community, philosophers, or by mental health professionals may not be met by every individual who has high SWB.

Since ancient times, humans have wondered about what makes a good life. Scientists, who study subjective well-being, assume that an essential ingredient of the good life is, what the person likes for him. These evaluations include emotional reactions to events as well as cognitive judgments of satisfaction and fulfillment. Thus, subjective well-being is a broad concept that includes experiencing pleasant emotions, low levels of negative moods, and high level of life satisfaction. The positive expenses embodied in higher order subjective well-being are a core concept of positive psychology because they make life rewarding.

Hallmarks of Subjective Well-being

There are several cardinal characteristics in the study of SWB (Diener, Larson and Emmons, 1984). First, the field covers the entire range of well-being from agony to ecstasy. It does not focus only on undesirable states such as depression or hopelessness. Instead, individual differences in levels of positive well-being are also considered important. Thus, the field of SWB includes the undesirable states that are treated by clinical psychologists, but is not limited to the study of these undesirable states. In other words, the field is concerned not just with the causes of depression and anxiety, but also with the factors that differentiate slightly happy people from moderately happy and extremely happy people.

Second, SWB is defined in terms of the internal experience of the respondent. An external frame of reference is not imposed when assessing SWB. Although many criteria of mental health are dictated from outside by researchers and practitioners (*e.g.*, maturity, autonomy, realism), SWB is measured from the individual's own perspective. If a woman thinks her life is going well, then it is going well within this framework. Again, this characteristic focuses on the respondent's point of view and differentiates the field of SWB from traditional clinical psychology. In the later field, weight is given to people's own perceptions of their lives, but often, people are seen to have a problem even if they themselves do not realize it. In the field of SWB, a person's beliefs, feelings of his or her own well-being are the perspectives of paramount importance. Naturally, this approach has both advantages and disadvantages. Although it gives ultimate authority to the respondents, it also means that SWB cannot be a consummate definition of mental health because people may be disordered even if they are happy. Thus, a psychologist will usually consider measures in addition to SWB in evaluating a person's mental health.

A final Hallmark of SWB is that the field focuses on longer-term states, not just momentary moods. Although a person's moods are likely to fluctuate with each new event, the SWB researcher is most interested in the person's moods over time. Often, what leads to happiness at the moment may not be the same as what produces long-term SWB. Thus, we are interested in relatively enduring feelings of well-being, and not just in fleeting emotions.

Is SWB Necessary for Mental Health?

Subjective well-being is not synonymous with mental health or psychological health. A person suffering from delusion might be happy and satisfied with his life, and yet we would not say that he possesses mental health. A person who is out of touch with her own motives and emotions might say she is happy, but we would not consider her to possess complete psychological health. Thus, SWB is not a sufficient condition for psychological well-being. Ryff (1989) has outlined additional characteristics beyond SWB *e.g.*, environmental mastery, personal growth, and purpose in life that are important to mental health. Therefore, although we believe that SWB is important, it is not identical to psychological or mental health.

Throughout history, philosophers and religious leaders have suggested the diverse characteristics, such as love, wisdom, and nonattachment, as the cardinal elements of a fulfilled existence. Utilitarian like Jeremy Bentham, however, argued that the presence of pleasure and the absence of pain are the defining characteristics of a good life. Thus, the utilitarians were the intellectual forerunners of subjective well-being researchers, focusing on the emotional, mental, and physical pleasures and pains that individuals experience. Although there are other desirable personal characteristics beyond which a person is happy, the individual with abundant joy has one key ingredient of a good life.

Components of Subjective Well-being

There are three primary components of SWB. They are satisfaction, pleasant affect, and low levels of unpleasant affect. Subjective well-being is structured such that these three components form a global factor of interrelated variables. Each of the three major facets of SWB can in turn be broken into subdivisions. Global satisfaction can be divided into satisfaction with the various domains of life such as recreation, love, marriage, friendship, and so forth, and these domains can in turn be divided into facets. Pleasant affect can be divided into specific emotions such as joy, affection, and pride. Finally, unpleasant affect can be separated into specific emotions and moods such as shame, guilt, sadness, anger, and anxiety. Each of the subdivisions of affect can be subdivided even further. Subjective well-being can be assessed at the most global level, or at progressively narrower levels, depending on one's purposes. For example, one researcher might study life satisfaction, whereas another might study the narrower topic of marital satisfaction. The justification for studying more global levels rather than just focusing on the most molecular concepts is that, the narrower levels tend to co-occur. In other words, there is a tendency for people to experience similar levels of well-being across different aspects of their lives, and the study of molar levels can help us understand the general influences on SWB that cause these covariations. A justification for studying narrower definitions of SWB is that we can gain a greater understanding of specific conditions that might influence well-being in particular domains. Further, narrower types of measures are often more sensitive to causal variables.

Many theories of happiness have been proposed since Aristotle's brilliant insights. These theories can be categorized into three groups :

1. Need and Goal

The first constellation of theories centers around the idea that the reduction of tensions (*e.g.*, the elimination of pain and the satisfaction of biological and psychological needs) leads to happiness. Freud's (1976) pleasure principle and Maslow's (1970) hierarchical needs model represent this approach. In support of this view, Omodei and Wearing (1990) found that the degree to which individual needs were met was positively associated with the degree of their life satisfaction.

Goal theorists argue that individuals attain subjective well-being when they move toward an ideal state or accomplish a valued aim.

One implication of tension-reduction theories is that happiness occurs after needs are met and goals are fulfilled. In other words, happiness is a desired end state toward which all activity is directed. These theories can be compared with models of happiness in which engagement in an activity itself provides happiness. Most notably, it is suggested that people are happiest when they are engaged in interesting activities that match their level of skill. He called the state of mind that results from this matching of challenges and skill "flow," and argued that people who often experience flow tend to be very happy. For instance, Harlow and Cantor (1996) found that social participation was a strong predictor of life satisfaction for retired elders. Goal researchers (*e.g.*, Emmons, 1986) agree that having important goals and pursuing them are reliable indicators of well-being, and therefore, goal theories can combine the elements of tension reduction and pleasurable activity in explaining subjective well-being. People who have important goals tend to be more energetic, experience more positive emotions, and feel that life is meaningful.

2. Processor Activity Theories

Both need theorists and activities theorists argue that subjective well-being will change with the conditions in people's lives. When individuals are approaching their goals or are engaged in interesting activities, they should experience positive well-being. However, other theorists argue that there is an element of stability in people's levels of well-being that cannot be explained by the stability in the conditions of people's lives. These theorists argue that subjective well-being is strongly influenced by stable personality dispositions.

Subjective well-being judgments reflect cognitive and emotional reactions to life circumstances. Because circumstances can be short lived and changeable or relatively stable, researchers study both momentary and long term subjective well-being. Not surprisingly, momentary levels of affect, fluctuate quite a bit. For example, Diener *et al.* (1984) found that when people's emotions were sampled at random times through the day, people react to changing circumstances, and these reactions are reflected in momentary reports of subjective well-being.

3. Genetic and Personality Theories

Differences in subjective well-being also result form stable individual difference in how people think about the world. Differences in the accessibility of pleasant versus unpleasant informations, as well as the accuracy and efficiency with which people process pleasant versus unpleasant information influence subjective well-being. Certain people attend to and recall the pleasant aspects of life more than others. Similarly, certain cognitive dispositions such as hope (Snyder, Irving and Anderson, 1991), dispositional optimism and expectancy for control (Grob, Stetsenko, Sabatier, Botcheva, and Macek, 1999) appear to influence subjective well-being.

Self-esteem, for example, is less strongly associated with life satisfaction (Diener, Diener and Diener, 1995), and extraversion is less strongly associated with pleasant affect (Lucas, Diener, Grob, Suh, and Sha, 2000) in collectivist cultures rather than in individualist cultures. Similarly, Suh (1999) found that there are cultural differences in the importance of personality congruence. Personality congruence reflects the extent to which a person's behaviours are consistent across situations and with the person's inner feelings.

At a theoretical level, wealth should predict higher SWB because high income confers higher status. In terms of the goals provided by Maslow's (1954) hierarchy of needs, income conferes advantages in terms of basic physical needs, security, and the actualization of one's abilities (due to the greater freedom of action afforded by increased income). It appears that possessing a high income is the goal of a large number of people throughout the world. Because goal success is a predictor of SWB (Emmons, 1986), it seems likely that those with greater incomes will possess greater SWB.

One of the most progressive avenues in this area carries researches on religious factors in QOL that focuses upon spiritual health rather than upon religion *per se*. Much religiosity is centered across goals and manifestations, but spiritual well-being (SWB) are of religious insulations. Even more important, however, is the fact that SWB covers to the ultimate goals of religious institutions than most other indicators of religiosity.

Culture and Subjective Well-being

In recent years, cultural differences in subjective well-being (Diener & Suh, 2000) have been explored with a realization that there are significant differences in what makes people happy. Although the importance of personality congruence is often emphasized in Western psychology, it is not universally important. Suh (1999) found that collectivists are less congruent than individualists, and that congruence is less strongly related to subjective well-being among collectivists. Suh, Diener, Oishi and Triandis (1998) also found that among collectivists, the extent to which one's life accords with the wishes of significant others is more important than the emotions that the persons feel in predicting their life satisfaction.

By examining between-nation differences in wealth and subjective well-being, researchers have arrived at a more complete understanding of the relation between income and happiness.

Easterlin (1974) argued that people compare their incomes to those around them, and therefore, difference of income between nations does not produce difference in SWB. He reasoned that income only makes a difference relative to what nearby others have because people tend to compare their incomes to the wealth of others, thereby causing differences in SWB. Thus, although there are psychological arguments as to why income should increase SWB and relativistic models predict income should be related to SWB.

Diener, Diener, and Diener (1995) found that even when levels of basic needs were controlled, income had a significant and moderate effect on national subjective well-being. Thus, people in the wealthiest nations tend to be the happiest. This might be because they possess more material goods, but it also could be because the wealthiest nations experience higher levels of human rights, greater longevity, and more equality. However, some argue that wealth leads to higher subjective well-being only within the poorest nations. According to this idea, wealth influences subjective well-being when basic needs are in danger of not being met. (Joshi, 2005; Kakkar, 2005)

Because demographic variables have different consequences in different cultures, these correlates can vary in importance. For example, marriage is an important demographic correlate of subjective well-being. Diener, Gohm, Suh, and Oishi, (2000), found that unmarried individuals who lived together were happier than married or single individuals in individualist cultures (Suggesting that in these cultures companionship is more important than social approval), but unmarried partners who lived together were less happy than married or single individuals in collectivist cultures, suggesting that in these cultures social approval is an important benefit of marriage.

Concept of Well-being in Indian Context : Swasti Ki Avadharana

The pattern of subjective well-being also differs in ascendance with cultural diversity in India. (Shukla; in press). It was found that the magnitude of well-being was highly different among general Kumauni and tribal women. Moreover, it was also found that well-being was adversely related with emotional disturbance and positively related with better temperament. Dealing with the search of happiness and satisfaction in life Kumari (2005) pointed out that rural women evinced more satisfaction with life and higher sense of well-being than urban women. She criticized the existing situation of urban population and stated that the concept of "निन्यानबे का फेर" is highly prevailed in urban culture. In spite of having every sort of levishment they are not satisfied and want to gain something more. In urban society it is also seen that people don't care about the cultivation of personal relations and all the time they engage in the enhancement of their financial height. In contrast, rural people, still in these days are surrounded with "we feeling". They love sharing and mix easily with others. Similarly, tribal society when lives in its own surroundings, evinces the sense of well-being and "we" feeling more as compared to the time of living alone.

Thus, cultural norms can change the correlates of subjective well-being.

The concept and ethics of well-being in Indian context were entirely different. It varied in definitions from time to time. The reason behind this was only the experience of happiness and means of achieving goal. In ancient time spiritual well-being was in practice and it was synonym of Yoga and religiosity. Dharma, Artha, Kama and Moksha were considered as the essence of meaningful life and the people were not supposed to think beyond them. In general, the people of that time had a sense of social welfare in more magnitude as compared to personal self :

सर्वे भवन्तु सुखिन: सर्वे सन्तु निरामया:।
सर्वे भद्राणि पश्यन्तु, माकश्चित् दुख भाग्भवंत्।

(Wish all to be in pleasure, all to be free from illness, all see the good and nobody be the victim of sorrows).

Their self was satisfied or they were supposed to be happy when they used to see some body happy. That is a person having higher sense of well-being may image himself in others or in other sense he absorbs the pain of others (आत्मवत् सर्वभूतेश य: प यति स: प यति). It produces sensitivity in him. In addition, a person who is altruistic (Seva Bhav), sensitive for others' pain (Pardukh katarta) and practices pronelessness, detachment with others' wealth, others' success and failure (Nisprihata), less attachment with others (Asampriktata) was considered as having higher sense of well-being in him. These attributes were exhibited not only by saints but also by the common mass of Indian society. In the Vanparva of Mahabharata, well-being was defined as a condition in which a person has no debt, has satisfaction in himself and resides with his family.

पंचमेऽहनि शश्ठे वा शाकं पचति स्वे गृहे

अनृणी चाप्रवासी च स वारिचर मोदते।

(महाभारत, वनपर्व, 115)

In that era Yasha, Satya, Dam, Shauch, Saralata, Lajja, Achunchanlata, Dan, Tap, Brahmcharya, Ahimsa, Shanti, Daya, Nirbhayata were considered as the components of well-being and direct channel for Moksha As Dharmaraj—the God Justice has told.

यश: सत्यम् दम: शौचमार्जवं ह्रीरपालनम्
दानं तपो ब्रह्मचर्यमित्येतास्तनवो मम

XXXXXX

अहिंसा समता शानितरानृशंस्यममत्सर:
द्वाराण्येतानि में विद्धि प्रियो ह्यसि सदामन

(महाभारत, वनपर्व 7 and 8)

As Dharmraj says—glory, truthfulness, suppression of evil thoughts, cleanliness, simplicity, behavioural constancy charity, meditation, control over ideas and bodily activities, nonviolence, sense of equality, peacefulness, kindness and lack of jealousy are the milestones of the ways following which one can reach me.

Not only in Mahabharata, but also in Gita the concept of well-being has been discussed. In Gita well-being is discussed in terms of others' welfare (concept of Yogakshema). Lord Krishna has told.

अनन्याश्चिन्त्यन्तोमा ये जनाः पर्युपासते,
तेषां नित्यभियुक्तानां योगक्षेममू वहाम्यहम्।

In ancient age future was not so complicated and insecure as it appears in present. In addition, level of aspiration was not so high and people lagged competitive attitude. Moreover, honesty, loyality, sharing responsibility and sense of cultural affinity were the attitudes of prominence following which people form a sense of well-being in them. But now the meaning of well-being is entirely changed. Materialism with higher magnitude has taken the place of spirituality. People use scientific and technological means of advancement as the formula of their life. Failure in achievement causes depression in them.

Interventions to Increase Well-being

Interventions to increase subjective well-being are important not only because it feels good to be happy but also because happy people tend to volunteer more, are more positive in work behaviour, and exhibit other desirable characteristics. Because of the roots of the field of subjective well-being in survey research, only a few direct intervention efforts have been implemented. However, Fordyce (1977, 1983) published several studies in which he evaluated a programme designed to boost people's happiness. The programme is based on the idea that people's subjective well-being can be increased if they learn to imitate the traits of happy people such as being organized, keeping busy, spending more time socializing, developing a positive outlook and working on a healthy personality. Fordyce found that the programme produced increases in happiness as compared with a placebo control.

Seligman, Reivich, Jaycox, and Gillham (1995) performed an experimental study with children in which the treatment groups were exposed to optimism training. Through cognitive training and social-problem solving, elementary school children who were at risk for depression, were taught to see the bright side of events. After the intervention, the treatment groups were found significantly less depressed than the control group, and this effect grew over the period of the study of longitudinal perspective.

Clearly, more efforts to enhance subjective well-being are needed, along with rigorous sample, more diverse dependent variables and measuring instruments. The positive benefits of the few existing experiments, however, suggest that programmes designed to enhance subjective well-being can be quite effective.

To conclude, in terms of measurement and research methods, many researchers, have relied solely on global retrospective self-reports. Studies showing construct validation (Sandvik *et al.*, 1993; Lucas *et al.*, 1996; Lucas *et al.*, 2000; Diener, Larson, Levine and Emmons in press;) illustrated that global self-reports have a degree of validity. However, it is still unclear that to what extent individual and cultural differences found in global reports are accurate reflections of differences in on-line experiences or are manifestations of processes related to global ways peoples see themselves. What is needed is a battery of subjective well-being measures based on experience, informant reports, biological pleasures, and cognitive measures that assess accessibility of positive events in memory. In addition to better measures, we need many more longitudinal studies. Moreover, in terms of substantive areas, more attention could be paid to developmental processes in having subjective well-being.

REFERENCES

Brief, A.P., Butcher, A.H., George J.M., & Link, K.E. (1993). Integrating bottom–up and top-down theories of subjective well being : The case of health, *Journal of Personality and Social Psychology*, *64*, 646-653.

DeCharms, R. (1968). *Personal Causation*, New York, Academic.

Diener, E., Larsen, R. J., & Emmons, R.A. (1984). Person X Situations interactions : Choice of situations and congruence response models, *Journal of Personality and Social Psychology*, *47*, 580-592.

Diener, E., Larsen, R.J., Levine, S., & Emmons, R.A. Frequency and intensity : The underlying dimensions of positive and negative affect, *Journal of Personality and Social Psychology*.

Diener, E., Diener, M., & Diener, C. (1995). Factors predicting the subjective well-being of nations, *Journal of Personality and Social Psychology*, *69*, 851-864.

Diener, E., & Suh, E.M. (2000). *Subjective Well-being Across Cultures*, Cambridge, MIT Press.

Emmons, R.A.(1986). Personal striving : An approach to personal and subjective well-being, *Journal of Personality and Social Psychology*, *51*, 1058-1068.

Fordyce, M.W. (1977). Development of a programme to increase personal happiness, *Journal of Counseling Psychology*, *24*, 511-520.

Fordyce, M.W. (1983). The happiness measures : A sixty second index of emotional well being and mental health, *Unpublished Manuscript*, Edison Community College, Ft. Myers, FL.

Freud, S. (1976). New Introductory Lectures on Psychoanalysis. In J. Strachey (Ed. and Trans.), *The Complete Psychological Works*, New York, Norton.

Grob, A., Stetsenko, A., Sabatier, C., Botcheva, L., & Macek, P., (1999). A cross-national model of subjective well-being in adolescence. In F.D. Alsquer, & A. Flammer (Eds). *The Adolescent Experiences : European and American Adolescents in the 1990s. Research Monographs in Adolescence*, pp. 115-130. Mahawah, NJ : Erlbaum.

Harlow, R.E., & Cantor, N. (1996). Still participation in latter life, *Journal of Personality and Social Psychology*, *71*, 1235-1249.

Jahoda, M. (2005). *Current Concepts of Positive Mental Health*, New York : Basic Books.

Joshi, K. (2005). A study of daily hassels and well being in Kumaunies women of varying SES, *Doctoral Work in Progress*, Deptt. of Psychology, Kumaun University, Nainital.

Kakkar, R. (2005). *A Study of Emotional Disturbance and Well being as Affected by Gender Age and Varying SES*. Ph.D. Thesis submitted, Deptt. of Psychology, Kumaun University, Nainital.

Kumari, K. (2005). *A Study of Life Satisfaction, Tempramont and Emotional Disturbance in Kumauni Women as Affected by Age, Martial Status and Varying SES*, Ph.D Thesis submitted, Deptt. of Psychology, Kumaun University, Nainital.

Langer, E.I. (1983). *The Psychology of Control*, Beverley Hills : Sage.

Lucas, R.E., Diener, E., Grob, A., Suh, E.M., & Sha, O.L. (2000). Cross cultural evidence for the fundamental features of extraversion. *Journal of Personality and Social Psychology*, *79*, 452-468.

Lucas, R.E., Diener, E., & Suh, E.M. (1996). Discriminant validity of well being measures, *Journal of Personality and Social Psychology, 71*, 616-628.

Maslow, A.H. (1954). *Motivation and Personality,* New York : Harper and Row.

Maslow, A.H. (1970). *Motivation and Personality,* Princeton : Van Nostrand.

Omodei, M.M., & Wearing, A.J. (1990). Need, satisfaction and involvement in personal projects : towards an integrative model of subjective well-being, *Journal of Personality and Social Psychology, 59*, 762-769.

Ryff, C.D. (1989). Happiness is Everything or is it? Explorations on the meaning of psychological well being, *Journal of Personality and Social Psychology, 57*, 1069-1081.

Ryff, C.D. (1995). The structure of psychological well being : Revisited, *Journal of Personality and Social Psychology, 69*, 719-727.

Shukla, A. (2005). Mental health of Kumauni women : towards cross-cultural perspective, *Indian Journal of Community Psychology.*

Snyder, C.R. (1994). *The Psychology of Hope : You can Get there from,* New York : Free Press.

Snyder, C.R., Irving, I.M., & Anderson, J.R. (1991). Hope and health. In C.R. Snyder & D.R. Forsyth (Eds.), *Handbook of Social and Clinical Psychology : The Health Perspective*, pp. 288-305. Elmsford : Pergamon.

Strickland, B.R. (1989). Internal external control expectancies : from contingency to creativity, *American Psychologist, 44*, 1-12.

Suh, E.M. (1999). Culture, identity, consistency and subjective well being, *Unpublished Ph. D. thesis.*, University of Illinois, Urbana-champian.

Suh, E., Diener, E., Oishi, S., & Triandis, H. (1998). The shifting basis of life satisfaction judgments across cultures : emotions versus norms, *Journal of Personality and Social Psychology, 74*, 482-493.

Warr, P.B. (1987). *Work, Unemployment and Mental Health,* Oxford : Clarendon.

Warr, P.B. (1987). Job characteristics and mental health. In P.B. Warr (Ed.) *Psychology at Work,* London : Penguin.

Warr, P.B. (1989). *The Measurement of Well being and other Aspects of Mental Health,* MRC/ESRC Social and Applied Psychology Unit, Memorandum, University of Sheffield, Sheffield, U.K.

Warr, P.B. (1990). The measurement of well-being and other aspects of mental health, *Journal of Occupational, Psychology, 63*, 193-210.

Warr, P. B. (1993). Work and health, a general model. In F. LaFeria and L. Levi (Eds.), *A Healthier Work Environment,* pp. 12-30, Copenhagen Denmark : World Health Organization.

White, R. (1959). Motivation reconsidered : The concept of competence, *Psychological Review, 66*, 297-333.

4

Health in Meeting Life with the Mind Free of Conditioning : J. Krishnamurti's Perspective

G. Aruna Mohan*

Life is always in movement, never static, yet our minds are static, conditioned, held, gethered to dogma and irrational beliefs. We are habituated to deal with day to day relationships as we deal with physical facts. We meet life with a psychologically, socially and religiously conditioned mind. Life is in constant movement with swiftly changing problems, and therefore, requires fresh approaches but not conditioned responses. There is a constant struggle where we meet life with the mind that is conditioned and static due to images about ourselves or about others, due to expectations, fears, greed and so on. We push ourselves into being, becoming something which is not natural, thus leading to conflict. Hence our living turns strainsome and hypocritical J. Krishnamurti proposes that our problem lies not in how to meet life but how the mind can be free of all its conditioning to live happily, fully and healthily in our relationships to the material world, humankind and to the unknown.

The significance of life is in living happily, harmoniously and healthily. Life is a relationship. Life is action in relationship. Life cannot be without relationship. It is not an abstract thing. It implies everyday thought, everyday feeling and everyday action in relationship. Every other form of understanding is merely an abstraction. We are not abstract entities, therefore, we have to study and understand ourselves in actuality—as we are, not as we wish to be. Understanding is not merely an intellectual process. Acquisition of knowledge about the outer world of things *i.e.*, knowledge of maths or knowledge of science or learning a language and remember it is a necessity. But in the psychological field of relationship we need not accumulate knowledge and remember it. If we are conditioned to the accumulated knowledge in relationship it becomes a burden, turns mind sorrowful and results in reactionary life. Learning about ourselves is to meet life afresh free from the past.

The objective of the present paper is to understand well-being from J. Krishnamurti's perspective.

---

* Reader in Psychology, St. Joseph's College of Education for Women, Guntur, A.P.

Fact only Drives the Person in Right Direction

Man is conditioned to use all kinds of theories, hopes and beliefs to disguise the facts. Beliefs isolate the human being further, create barriers, dependence and illusions. Beliefs are controlled by ideas, seek guidance, kill the flame of love and affection, generosity and sympathy. When we are ambitious, greedy, acquisitive, we are outwardly and collectively aggressive, violent and destructive. As we have evolved from the animals we have also inherited aggressive violence and hatred. Out of that animal conditioning we respond when we have territorial rights over a piece of land or sexual rights.

We are compelled by the society, in which we live to be aggressive. Society expects that we must be aggressive and fight in order to survive. Thus we are socially conditioned to inbibe what we face or find in society. We have been conditioned by caste, class, religion, language, climate, food, art, literature, family, friends, customs, conventions, propaganda etc. for centuries. Therefore, our responses to every problem are conditioned. We always react inadequately to all challenges. We are not aware of our conditioning at all, if every thing around us goes well. If there is any disturbance the whole violence of our nature comes out. If we get used to disturbance our minds become dull, indifferent, hard and callous or we escape from actual facts. We translate facts according to our conditioning, but the fact only drives the person in right direction.

Ignorance of the Inner World of Self Causes Inability to Discriminate Between Fact and Non-Fact

Learning about ourselves is different from acquiring knowledge about ourselves. Learning implies a great sensitivity. Sensitivity cannot be developed if we have to respond through an idea which originates from the past, dominating the present. We must observe ourselves, know all about nature, structure and movement of our mind and heart. In order to observe the whole movement of our mind and heart, of our whole being we must have a free mind. However, we build images about ourselves, think we are something, build images about others out of our experiences, make generalisations about ourselves and others and act according to them. The relationships are thus between images rather than between the human beings. If we can understand the cruelty, the brutality, the visciousness and the ugliness of these images, we will never build images but be simple and direct in our relationships, thereby becoming free of the conditioned images. Simplicity is looking directly at ourselves without fear. We need a great deal of humility in order to understand ourselves and our fears.

Factual fears are rather rare while imagined fears are many. Fear of fire is a fact. We are to be at a distance from it to be safe. Likewise, body dies only once is a fact, but this fact conditions the mind to be fearful. If there is no thought of death there is no fear of death. Such imaginary fears, which are non-facts, are many in our minds. For instance, we were ill and had pain due to it. This is a fact. Later we think of illness and are afraid that we may get it again. This pain is a non-fact, an idea. The mind with the conditioning about illness and remembrance of pain reacts out its thought of illness. It wants to be safe, free of illness. Thus the mind weaves a network of the past experiences and future projections which are non facts.

What is Psychologically Hurt is an Image

We are to understand what our pain, grief and sorrow are. We have seen that they are physiological as well as psychological in nature. We can get rid of physical pain medically.

Apart from that we can observe pain with a mind that is not attached, with a mind that can observe bodily pain as though from outside. One can observe one's pain without becoming involved emotionally and psychologically in it. If we are involved, the pain becomes more, we become terribly anxious and fearful. *The key is to be aware of the biological pain, and in that, awareness not to get involved with it psychologically.*

Krishnamurti says that, to keep the psychological factor entirely out, one requires a great deal of awareness, a certain quality of aloofness and unattached observation. Then that pain does not bring about neurotic activity of the mind and does not even distort the activities of the mind. When there is a great deal of pain, when the mind is unable to resolve it, the mind gets involved with the pain and the whole outlook of life is distorted. If this whole movement of pain is observed intelligently, the pain can be reasonably dealt with. Psychological pain is more complex and requires clearer examination, closer observation and penetration. From childhood we have experienced many scars, injuries and pains consciously or unconsciously. We shed tears quietly or openly. Out of those hurtful events we want to hurt others, which is a form of violence. Being hurt we resist, we build a wall around ourselves in order not to be hurt in future. But we are going to be more hurt, as we might have stored up the earlier hurts by comparing with others and conforming to society. Our responses might then be based on these hurts. This problem of being hurt will not be solved by the whole machinery of thinking. As long as the thought process is active there is no way of dissolving the hurt. What is hurt is the image we have about us and about others and that image has no reality now. It is a verbal structure fed by thought. When the energy of thought is not active, then the image is not there and only then there is a possibility of not being hurt.

Not Meeting Hate by Hate but Understanding this Phenomenon

If we use violent methods to suppress anger in ourselves then we are using wrong means to the right end. When we fight we too become 'anger'. We become 'that' which the other is. If he is an evil and we fight him with evil means then we also become evil, however righteous we may feel. If we are brutal and if the other person uses brutal methods to overcome us then he becomes brutal. In this there is neither understanding nor transcending anger. Anger is to be studied tolerantly to understand it, but not to be overcome through violent means. We have ideas, and images about ourselves of what we should be or should not be. If the ideas about ourselves are attacked anger is awakened in us. Our idea about ourselves is our escape from the fact of what we are. When we are observing the actual fact of what we are, no one can hurt us. Then if one is a liar and is told that one is a liar, it does not mean that one is hurt, it is a fact.

Understanding is the liberating factor, not the things stored up in the mind. Life is something to understand from moment to moment, without accumulating experiences. One of our unfortunate weaknesses is that we want somebody else to act for us and change the course of our lives. We remain inactive until we are assured of the outcome. So, we wait for others to revolt and build a new situation. Thus understanding and action according to that is creative while memory is static.

Living with 'What is' is the Highest Form of Sensitivity

Krishnamurti questions—*why not be that*—? for instance if we are bored why not be bored? if we are in sorrow be sorrowful. One need not try to find a way out of it. We are conditioned to try to escape from boredom. The mischief is much greater when we escape than when we are what we are and remain with it. If we are really exhausted we can take rest, be quiet. Let the mind gain strength by itself. The mind wants to do something all the time. So, it is very difficult to allow the mind to be quiet. We are interested in that which pleases us, gratifies us. There is sustained interest as long as we are acquiring. Every acquisition is a form of boredom. There is pleasure in acquisition, in knowledge, in fame. As soon as we acquire anything we lose interest. In trying to possess we are alert and interested. But pursuit of more is only a movement towards boredom. When we observe it, learn about it, and all its intricacies, then with the understanding there is a freedom from it.

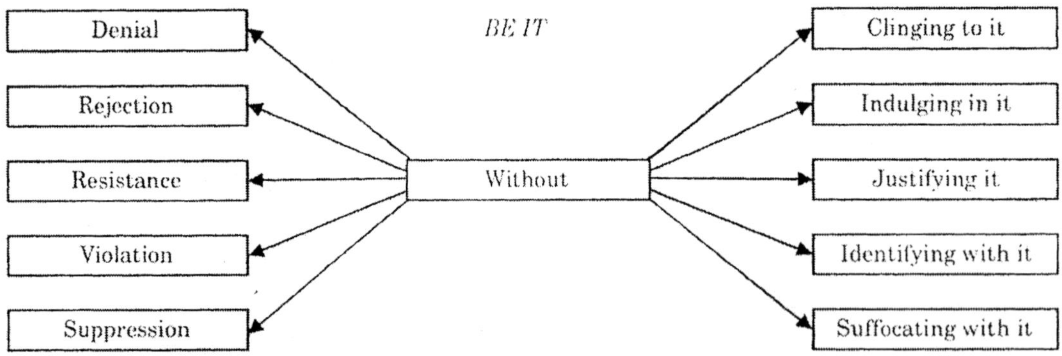

The mind has been conditioned through centuries in its demand for security, self-centered activity, *i.e.* my family, my job and my possession, which results in isolation. Thus, the very nature of the "me", "the self", "the ego" is isolation. The self-centered activities produce a state of emptiness in us. Emptiness is thus a result, a consequence. We make every kind of effort to fill this void, which again is being self centered and this emptiness becomes wider and deeper. Then we suddenly realise that we cannot do anything. The mind itself realises that it can not do anything about it, that thought can not touch it because the moment thought touches it, it breeds emptiness again. The mind sees how absurd it is to dissipate energy in many ways. Seeing this whole process we do not waste energy to fill this emptiness. Thought becomes quiet, the mind becomes completely still, because it has seen the whole process. So there is silence. When there is complete silence of the mind there is beauty and love.

Without Understanding the Mind in Relationship We can't Find what Love is

To live requires a great deal of love, a great feeling for silence, a great simplicity with an abundance of experience. It requires a mind that is capable of thinking very clearly, that is not bound by prejudice or superstition. Freedom is essential for love. Without love and right thinking oppression and cruelty will ever be on the increase. Because of the greatest role of pleasure and desire in our lives love has no place. So the world becomes barren. Without love there is ugliness and poverty in our hearts and minds. We know intellectually that the unity of mankind is essential and that love is the only way. If we do not have it in abundance, if we are not filled with love, it will lead to disaster. However, love is not the product of thought which is the past. Thought cannot possibly cultivate love. Love is not hedged about and caught in jealously, for jealously is of the past. Jealousy contains pain, anxiety, hate and violence. Love is always actively present. It is not "I will love" or "I have loved". If we know love, we will not follow any body. Love does not obey. When we love we are not afraid to do anything and we don't dominate. Love is not dependence or self pity or mere sex alone. Self pity makes us hard, encloses us, makes us dull and stupid. Thus, Love is not the opposite of hate.

We cannot love when we are thinking about ourselves. Love is a feeling in which there is gentleness, tenderness and consideration. The more we look after things, the more sensitive we become. The feeling of care is the beginning of affection. So there has to be affection which is not dependent on environment, circumstance or people. If there is affection one thinks less and less about one self, which is one of the most difficult things in life. Love is the most practical thing in life, in the world. To love, to be kind, not to be greedy, not to be ambitious, not to be dependent but to think for ourselves what is right and what to do—all these are very practical things and these will bring about a happy practical society. If there is love there will be inward and outward refinement that is expressed outwardly in consideration for others, in the way we treat our parents, our neighbours, our children, our servants, or our gardener. We do things because we love. Love is expressed in doing gardening, carpentary, painting, handicrafts and through the senses as seeing the trees, the mountains, the richness of the earth, the poverty we have created among ourselves and in learning music, listening to the song of birds, the murmur of running waters and so on. One of the odd things about love is that whatever we do will be correct if we love. When there is love, action is always right in all circumstances.

Spiritual Health is, when there is Love

When there is that quality of love there is compassion. Compassion means passion for all. *Krishnamurti* finds that "compassion has its own extraordinary limitless intelligence." When there is love, there is beauty. Love and compassion with their intelligence lead to endless truth. Such a love is not limited to time, it is both personal and impersonal; is both for the one and many. Love is something that is new, fresh and alive. *Krishnamurti* says that only the innocent mind can live in the world which is not innocent. There must be love to answer to the whole, to be responsible to the whole of man kind, to nature, to answer globally to children, to neighbour, to all the movement that man has created in his endeavour to live rightly. Real love is when we understand the responsibility to the whole. When thought can understand itself and come to an end naturally, in that inward silence, there is whole, and there is no self or the center, then there is love. Love can bring about the understanding of another. When there is love, there is instantaneous communion with the other on the same level at the same time. The efficiency inspired by love goes far beyond the efficiency out of ambition.

REFERENCES

Krishnamurti, J. (1993). '*A Timeless Spring*', Chennai : Krishnamurti Foundation India.

Krishnamurti, J. (1998). '*Krishnamurti's Journal*', Chennai : Krishnamurti Foundation India.

Krishnamurti, J. (1998). '*Krishnamurti to Himself*', Chennai : Krishnamurti Foundation India.

Krishnamurti, J. (1998). '*On self knowledge*', Chennai : Krishnamurti Foundation India.

Krishnamurti, J. (1999). '*Freedom from the known*', Chennai : Krishnamurti Foundation India.

Krishnamurti, J. (2000). '*On Love and Loneliness*' (p. 97); Chennai ; Krishnamurti Foundation India.

Krishnamurti, J. (2000). '*The First and Last Freedom*', Chennai : Krishnamurti Foundation India.

Krishnamurti, J. (2001). '*The Nature of the New Mind*', Chennai : Krishnamurti Foundation India.

Krishnamurti, J. (2003). '*What are you doing with life*', Chennai : Krishnamurti Foundation India.

5

Moral Development of Children Through Gurmat

Mandeep Kaur[*]

With the boons of technology, curses of egocentrism, individualism and immoral acts are also insidiously proliferating within an individual in this society. Josephson and Rosa (1998) conducted a survey that showed that the percentage of high school students exhibiting cheating acts in exams had risen from 64% to 70% from 1996 to 1998. He concluded that the hole in the moral ozone is getting bigger in the youth. There was also significant increase in percentage of students who lie to their parents or would be willing to lie to get a good job. This is hindering the development of moral values and judgment of the child too.

Several psychologists (Piaget, 1965; Kohlberg, 1966; Varma, 1982) proved that the evolution of moral values along with the ability to make judgment appears from the early years of the child development. The moral values evolve gradually with a progressive change in the capacity of the child to distinguish between right and wrong based on the principles and standard of conduct (Verma & Tripathi, 1998). Earlier researches on moral development have focused on the development of affective, behavioural and cognitive components within a moral being. The psychoanalytic theory emphasizes affective aspect of morality, whereas, social learning theories have conducted researches to demonstrate how children learn to resist temptations and behave morally. The cognitive development theories by Piaget (1965) and Kohlberg (1966, 1984) highlighted the capacity to judge whether and why one is right or wrong. Thereafter, innumerable psychologists (Guerra, 1990; Van & David, 2000) critiqued Kohlberg's theory and his instruments (DIT, 1974; Rest, 1979 & SRM-SF) and questioned the extent to which the theory is universalized. Instruments were observed to be specifically developed for western, Anglo, male Culture. Subsequently, Turiel (1979), Gilligan (1982) and Shweder (1990) propounded theories, which took different philosophical and conceptual stands to explain morality. Shweder (1990) took a cultural perspective and questioned whether morality exists universally in the context.

Some of the researches in Indian context (Sinha & Varma, 1972; Varma & Sinha, 1972; Varma, 1982) focussed on development of knowledge of basic moral values from eclectical

[*]M.A. Psychology, Dept. of Psychology, University of Delhi, Delhi.

perspective. They observed that the basic values get organized in Indian children around the age of nine years. One of such study (Sinha, 1964) revealed that the knowledge of moral values and ability to make moral judgment increases between 6-12 years. The moral knowledge of young children is more concrete in nature in the beginning and gradually becomes abstract, as they get older. Older children understand the basic idea and principles underlying moral concept. Current researches (Miller & Bersoff, 1991) compared Indian and American adults and children's reasoning about moral dilemmas. Results exhibited that most Indians gave priority to the interpersonal expectation whereas American gave importance to the justice orientation.

Subsequent researches exhibited (Josephson & Rosa 1998; Bruggeman, Leistler & Hart, 1996) that instead of moral values, the regard for immoral values is increasing within the innocent mind of a child. Children in their formative years if denied the vital direction that they need, may develop an undisciplined, arbitrary attitude and lack of respect for positive values and acts. Consequentially psychologists have enquired as to how one can curtail the adversarial immoral acts and forge positive acts.

One of the comprehensive solutions for the given problem can be teaching of a religion. The virtues and ethics includes in its purview not only influence actions but also intentions, dispositions, attitudes etc. and offer many insights into how to help the child in developing the capacity to make moral decision (Martone, 1998). A religion teacher (Durka, 2000) can in some amount transform the socially toxic environment of home and neighbourhood into places of " caring community". Considerable researches (Hirschberg, 1955,1956; Manwell & Sophia, 1951) indicate that religions attitudes and understanding can help in healthy emotional growth of children. The development of religion beliefs and function is traced through the stages of childhood. One of the recent research (Kothari, 1994) displayed that the students belonging to Hindu, Islam, Christian and Jain religious group did not differ significantly in discrimination between good and bad, respect, honesty and moral scores. Sizeable researches (Wright, 1993; Carotta, 1999) manifested curriculum, which includes religious education, is effective towards inculcating the moral values in the psyche of a child.

Gurmat (teaching of Sikhism) identifies the main problem for morality as egocentrism, which is inherent in an individual and leads to a limited point of view. The teachings of Sikhism can be one of the ways to make a child realize that social instincts should have preference over selfish ones. Some of Sikh rituals include *Shabad* (holy rhymes sung in raag and taal), *Sakhis* (Narratives), *Sewa* (to serve others), *Langar* (people of any caste creed or colour sitting together and having food), *Path* (inscribed prayers recited from *Guru Granth Sahib*), *and Simran* (focusing and remembering the God-meditation). Within the musical nodes of *Simran* and *Shabad*, the positive moral message underlying both of them expedite the mental well being of an individual. Studies show that music and meditation helps to increase concentration and relax the mind. Langar/Sewa helps to create oneness in the people. The work in Sewa and food in langar is shared without any bias of caste creed or colour. These acts decrease individualism within a person. *Path* inscribed in the *Guru Granth Sahib* has a moral lesson within. This teaches everyone about the way one can achieve balance even in up's and down's of their lives. *Sakhis* (narratives) of lives of *Gurus* is one of the effective tool which leads to the moral development in an individual. These stories help the child to understand about philosophies, which empowers them to fight against bad deeds inherent within each individual. Narratives are disembodied texts known to be creating their own socializations. Spees (2002) found that the moral meaning could also be therapeutic when the child gets hurt. Current researches (Diessner, 1991; Narvaez 1998; Tappan, 1990, 1991, 1997) illuminated that the narrative is the key to understand the narrator's life. Hence, moral aspects are illuminated effectively as a person focuses on the dialogical nature of the moral self.

Hence, in these vicissitudes of life, *Gurmat* (teaching of Sikhism) seems to offer an integrated approach in the development of self. The presence study basically deals with the assessment of the effectiveness of *Gurmat* (teaching of Sikhism) on the moral development of children (8-12 years). The following hypotheses were formulated :

1. There will be a significant difference between the control group and the experimental group on the scores of Moral judgment test (MJTC).
2. There will be a significant difference between the control group and the experimental group on the scores of *gurmat* checklist.

METHOD

Sample

The sample comprised of 28 females (8-12 yrs) who were randomly selected from west part of Delhi (Patel Nagar). The sample was subdivided into two groups of control group and experimental group. Control group involved 14 females (8-12 years) who were not exposed to any teaching of Sikhism while experimental group consisted of 14 females (8-12 years) who were exposed to intervention programme. These groups were matched on various criterions such as socio-economic status (middle class), religion and linguistic background (8 Punjabi, 2 Hindus, 1 Bengali, 1 Muslim, 2 Sikhs children in each group), no previous exposure to teaching of Sikhism and hours of exposure (1 hour).

Tools

For quantitative analysis two tools were used. Moral Judgment Test for children (MJTC) developed by Varma and Sinha (1971) and *Gurmat* Checklist (GC) developed by Kaur (2001). MJTC has been constructed on the model of a general intelligence test in which items on reasoning, discrimination, analogies and best answer etc. have been included but the variation is that all items have moral connotation. The items in MJTC test were especially designed to explore the fourteen cardinal values prevalent in Indian culture. The fourteen values were : 'Ahimsa', 'Duty', 'Betrayal of Faith', 'Purity', 'Forgiveness', 'Greed', 'Anger', 'Punnya (Virtue)', 'Lie', 'Revenge', 'Stealing', 'Truth', 'Sin'. GC consisted of 24 items, which covered the morals underlying the teaching of Sikhism. The test had significant criterion related validity with MJTC at .01 which level proves the strong relation between the two instruments. This indicates that the checklist covers the 14 values that were taken in MJCT.

For Qualitative analysis verbal feedback in the form of unstructured interview from the family members, peer group were taken from the experimental group. The schedule of the interviews included two main areas : the changes they could see throughout the month when the intervention was conducted and the reasons which family members attributed for these changes in behaviour. The data were analyzed by the method of content analysis.

Procedure

The intervention was conducted regularly for 28 days for one hour on weekdays. The content of the intervention programme was disguised from the parents. The first two days were spent on rapport formation. Rest of the days experimental group was regularly exposed to teaching of Sikhism which included *(Simran, Sakhis, Shabad, Rehras Sahib)*, lesson from the book. While control group was instructed to complete their homework silently without any interaction for an hour each day. The two tests, MJTC and GD were administered to the subjects of the two groups, before and after the intervention. An unstructured interview of the family members and peers of the subjects of the experimental group was conducted at the termination of the intervention programme. The specific time foı the various activities for the experimental group was an follows :

Table 5.1 : Details of Curriculum Taught to the Experimental Group

Time		*Activity*	*Description*
From	*To*		
5:00	5:15	*Simran*	The relaxation exercise was given, where the child focused on the *mantra* of "*waheguru*" for 10 minutes. After that problems faced during the exercise were discussed.
5:15	5:25	*Shabad*	Six *Shabad* from Guru Granth Sahib were recited in class, which was repeated 2-3 times during the whole programme.
5:25	5:45	*Sakhis/Rehras Sahib*	Both of them were read alternatively. Seven narratives chosen from the book "ethics of Sikhs". The group recited *rehras sahib from the Nitnem* (a holy book in Sikh religion)
5:45	6:00	Lessons	The lessons were taken from the book "The basic principles of Sikh religion". They were taught 19 lessons from the book.

RESULTS AND DISCUSSION

Results were quantitatively analyzed and interpreted in terms of Independent 't' test (pre-post tests) between experimental and control group. Verbal feedback was qualitatively analyzed and interpreted in terms of content analysis of the interview given by the family members and peer group of the experimental group. Although the two groups (Ex Gr and C Gr) were matched on many variables, it is realized that there are many unknown extraneous variables within these subjects, which were uncontrollable and could confound the result obtained. To reduce the variability, which can be due to organism variability and environmental factors, the difference of pre-test of the test (MJTC, GC) and post-test of the test (MJTC, GC) of each subject in experimental and control group were taken as an independent score. This procedure helped to decrease the effect of unknown extraneous variables, which appeared in the post-test. Now, the individual score of each subject is the measure, which reflects by and large the effectiveness of the curriculum taught.

Table 5.2 : Mean, S. D., t Test After Taking the Difference Between Pretest and Posttest of Control Group and Experimental Group for Moral Judgment Test

Group	*Sample*	*Mean*	*S.D.*	*df*	*t*
Control	14	13.29	6.707	26	1.65*
Experimental	14	17	5.114		

* P >.05.

Table 5.2 indicates that the mean score of control group and experimental group was 13.28 and 17.00 respectively. The standard deviation obtained in control group was 6.707 while in experimental group it was 5.114. The "t" obtained was 1.65, which was, less than "t" value at both .01 and .05 the levels. This indicates that there is no significant difference in the total sores obtained by experimental and control group in the moral judgment test of children (MJTC).

Table 5.3 : Mean, S.D., t Test After Taking the Difference Between Pretest and Posttest of Control Group and Experimental Group for Gurmat Checklist

Group	*Sample*	*Mean*	*S.D.*	*df*	*t*
Control	14	4.143	3.134	26	2.55**
Experimental	14	6.85	2.445		

* P <.01.

Table 5.3 indicates that mean score of control group and experimental group was 4.142 and 6.857 respectively. The standard deviation obtained in control group was 3.134 while in experimental group it was 2.445. The "t" obtained was 2.55 which was more than "t" critical at 0.01 level. This indicates that there is significant difference in the total sores obtained by the experimental and the control group in the gurmat checklist at both .05 and.01 level.

Table 5.4 : Frequency of Changes Reported by the Family Members on the Several Dimensions

Sr. No.	*Dimensions*	*Frequency*
1.	Going to Gurudwara everyday	3
2.	Reading of Prayers and *Shabad*	8
3.	Increase in Concentration through *Simran*	3
4.	Positive impact on studies	5
5.	Controlling anger	2
6.	Increase in compliance towards family member	4
7.	Increase in sense of responsibility	1
8.	No change in behaviour	1

Table 5.4 shows areas in which the family members, peer group, reported changes. These areas were–studies (concentration, capacity); personality (anger management, compliance, responsibility) and spiritual (visiting gurudwara, increase in prayers, *simran* etc.). Only one of the parents reported no improvement.

Table 5.5 : Numbers of Reasons which Family Members Attributed for the Changes in Behaviour

Sr. No.	*Reasons attributed for the change in behaviour*	*Frequency of response*
1.	Due to curriculum	13
2.	Socialization in the class	1
3.	Impact of teacher in class	1
4.	Age related maturity	1
5.	Minimal change	1

Table 5.5 indicates the reasons attributed by parents, peer group for the changes observed in experimental group throughout the intervention phase. Around thirteen of parents reported that changes had occurred due to curriculum. One of them also reported socialization, teacher's impact, or age related maturity, can be plausible reasons for the positive change. One of the parent reported that the change was too minimal.

The results on MJTC test reflects that there was no significant difference in the score obtained between the experimental and control group. One possible reason can be that the test was purely based on Kohlbergian justice model. Recent research (Guerre, 1990; Van & David, 2000) critiqued the understanding of the morality by traditional Kohlbergian perspective. They suggested that Kohlberg's theory is not universal. It appears to have an ethnocentric bias. It is culturally and religiously insensitive. Additional research (Miller & Bersoff, 1991) examined that Indians base their moral understanding on interpersonal perspective while western on justice. Hence, the test was not able to capture the changes occurred due to curriculum.

The significant difference obtained between two groups shows that curriculum had increased the *gurmat* understanding, which had lead to moral development in children. Considerable researches (Wright, 1993; Carrota, 1999) had claimed that these kind of curriculum and environment lead to the development of the moral self in the child.

The content analysis displayed the improvements in the spiritual, personal and cognitive self. The reasons attributed for the development was attributed to the curriculum have also given to the children. Hirshberg (1955, 1956) Manwell and Sophia (1955) and Kothari (1994) commented that religions attitudes and understanding help in healthy emotional growth of children.

Hence, the results of the present study indicate that *Gurmat* (teaching of Sikhism) is one of the effective ways of improving the moral judgment in the child.

REFERENCES

Bruggeman, E.L., & Kathleen J.H. (1996). Cheating, Lying, and Moral Reasoning by Religious and Secular High School Students, *Journal of Educational Research*, 89, 340-344.

Carotta, M. (1999). *Teaching for Spiritual Growth : Doorways to the Heart and Soul of Young People*. Thesis, Spalding University.

Diessner, R. (1991). Kohlbergian narratives : Comment on Vitz, *American-Psychologist, 46*, 168-169.

Durka, G. (2000). Teaching Youth in a Socially Toxic Environment, *Religious Education, 95*, 443-452.

Gilligan, C. (1982). *In a Different Voice : Psychological Theory and Women's Development*, Cambridge, Mass : Harvard University Press.

Guerra, L.R. (1990). *Acculturation and Measurement of Moral Development in Hispanic Adolescent Males*, Ph.D. Thesis, California School of Professional Psychology, Los Angeles.

Josephson, M., & Rosa, M. (1998). *1998 Report Card on the Ethics of American Youth*, Josephson Institute of Ethics, Marina del Rey, CA.

Hirschberg, J. C. (1955). Some Comments on Religion and Childhood, *Bulletin of the Menninger Clinic*, *19*, 227-228.

Hirschberg, J. C. (1956). Comments on Religion and Childhood, *Menninger Quarterly*, *10*, 22-24.

Kaur, M. (2000). *Gurmat Checklist*, Unpublished manuscript.

Kohlberg, L. (1966). Stage and sequence : the cognitive development approach to socialization. In D.A. Goslin (Eds.), *Handbook of socialization theory and research*, Chicago : Rand McNally.

Kohlberg, L. (1984). *Essays on Moral Development, The Psychology of Moral Development*, San Francisco : Harper & Row.

Kothari, S. (1994). Impact of Religion Upon Development of Concepts, *Psycho Lingua*, *24*, 65-72.

Manwell, E. M., & Sophia A. F. (1951). *Consider the Children, How They Grow*, Boston : Beacon Press.

Martone, M. (1998). A Developing virtuous children : A theological perspective, *Journal of Social-Distress and the Homeless*, *7*, 107-119.

Miller, J.G., & Bersoff, D.M., (1992). Culture and Moral Judgment : How are conflicts between justice and interpersonal responsibilities resolved, *Journal of Personality and Social Psychology*, *62*, 1-14.

Narvaez, D. (1998). The influence of moral schemas on the reconstruction of moral narratives in eighth graders and college students, *Journal of Educational Psychology 90*, 13-24.

Piaget, J. (1965). *The Moral Judgment of the Child*, New York : Free Press.

Shweder, R.A., Mahapatra, M., & Miller, J.G. (1990). Culture and moral development. In J. Stigler; R.A. Shweder; & G. Herdt (*Eds.*), *Cultural Psychology : Essays on Comparitive Human Development*, New York : Cambridge University Press.

Sinha, D., & Varma, M. (1972). Knowledge of moral values in children, *Psychological Studies*, *17*, 1-6.

Spees, E.K. (2002). Word movies : Strategy and resources for therapeutic storytelling with children and adolescents. *Annuals of the American Psychotherapy Assn*, *5*, 14-21.

Tappan, M.B. (1990). Hermeneutics and moral development : Interpreting narrative representations of moral experience, *Developmental Review*, *10*, 239-265.

Tappan, M.B. (1991). New directions for child development. In Packer, M.J. (Ed.) Narrative and storytelling, *Implications for Understanding Moral Development*, San Francisco, CA, US : Jossey-Bass Inc.

Tappan, M.B. (1997). Analyzing stories of moral experience : Narrative, voice, and the dialogical self, *Journal of Narrative and Life History*, 7, 379-386.

Tappan, M. B., Brown, L.M., & Witherell, C. (1991) Stories lives tell : Narrative and dialogue in education. In Noddings, N. (Ed.) *Toward a Narrative Approach to Moral Development and Moral Education*, New York, NY, US : Teachers College Press.

Turiel, E. (1979). Distinct Conceptual and Development Domains: Social-convention and morality. C.B. Keasy, ed., Nebraska Symposium.

Varma, M. (1976). *Moral Development in Children*, India, Allahabad : Chugh Publications.

Varma, M. (1982). Development of knowledge of moral values in Indian children, *Proceedings of 2nd Asian Workshop on Child and Adolescent Development*, Bangkok, Thailand.

Varma, M. & Sinha, D. (1972). Pattern of moral values in children, *Psychological Studies, 17*, 42-50.

Van, S., & David. A. (2000). "The Relationship between Religiousness and Moral Development : A Critique and Refinement of the Sociomoral Reflection Measure Short-Form of Gibbs, Basinger, and Fuller (John C. Gibbs, Karen S. Basinger, Dick Fuller)." Ed. D. Thesis, Clark University.

Verma, M., & Tripathi, R.C. (1998). Personality Development. In Srivastava, A.K. (Ed.) Child Development : The Indian Perspective, India : Delhi : NCERT.

Wright, D. (1983). Religious Education from the Perspective of Moral Education, *Journal of Moral Education, 12*, 111-115.

6

Buddhist Approach to Promotion of Psychological Well-being and Behaviour Change

*Ramjee Lal**

Buddhism emerged as a religion in India and spread across to the world. Buddhism has evolved in innumerable forms during its long history. Codes of conduct, guidelines for communal life, rituals, meditative practices, modes of teaching, images, fables, and philosophies have varied greatly over time and place. There are many ways in which people of different times and different cultures have approached Buddhism. Currently, there are at least five forms of Buddhism. The first form is the traditional Buddhism. It is the education of the Buddha's teachings. This original form is rarely seen today. The second form is religious Buddhism. Although originally not a religion, it has become one in the past few hundred years. The external form of Buddhism today is indeed that of a religion. The lessons include listening to lectures and discussions. The cultivation session includes either Buddha name chanting or sitting meditation. Now-a-days these places have become a place for blessings and to conduct memorial services. Third form is philosophical or academic Buddhism often found as a course in universities and colleges. It is reduced to merely a philosophical discipline. The fourth and most recent deviation is Buddhism as a show. It consists of a few hours of music, singing and dancing with a short talk in between. The fifth form is a deviation that has gone too far, that of the distortion of Buddhism into a cult.

Buddhism has awakened considerable interest in the west, and there are many persons who enjoy positions of some note in western society who are either Buddhist or sympathetic to Buddhism. In Europe and America, Buddhism is generally believed to be more than the usual advancement in its thought, rigorously rational, and sophisticated. Buddhism is intended not only for people in the west but also for people in traditionally Buddhist communities who may have become estranged from the religion for a variety of social and cultural reasons.

Buddhism addresses a practical problem. It is not interested in academic questions and metaphysical theories. The Buddhist approach is to identify a real problem and deal with it in

*Department of Applied Psychology, Purvanchal University, Jaunpur (U.P.).

a practical way. In the context of contemporary western culture, scientists, psychologists, and philosophers have found in Buddhism a tradition in harmony with some of the most basic principles of western thought. In addition, they find Buddhism particularly interesting because, although the principal methods and conclusions of the western scientific tradition often closely resemble those of Buddhism, western science has thus far suggested no practical way of achieving an inner transformation, whereas in Buddhism such a way is clearly indicated. While science has taught us to build better cities, expressways, factories and forms, it has not taught us to build better people. Therefore people in the contemporary world are turning to Buddhism, an ancient philosophy that has many features in common with the western scientific tradition but that goes beyond the materialism of the west, beyond the limits of practical science as we have known it thus far.

The Concept of 'Unconscious' in the Framework of Buddhist System

The "Unconscious' has been much discussed subject in connection with psychotherapy and psychology. It is almost a universally accepted theory that man's actions, words, deeds and thoughts, spring from his own mind, which consists of three layers, namely, : the 'conscious', 'the preconscious' and the 'unconscious' (Freud, 1956). Broadly speaking, the mind can be understood in terms of 'the conscious' and 'the unconscious'. Freud maintains that the repressed memories of past experiences, impulses, traumas, latent tendencies, unfulfilled desires and fears, are stored in the 'unconscious'. The unconscious is the realm of that which cannot thus be brought into consciousness. A preconscious idea or memory can become conscious without much difficulty. An unconscious idea or memory is hard to recall because the resistance is greater. Freud has given several characteristics of the unconscious, such as, that it is repressed, it is associated with the "id"; it is not brought into the consciousness; it exerts influence over behaviour, it provides a link between a person's present and his infancy. Though there can be varying degrees of unconsciousness, a special technique is necessary to uncover the deeper levels of the unconscious process.

Buddhism has thrown light on the phenomenon of unconscious. Early Buddhist texts describe the phenomenon of dynamic mental dispositions (*Mano-Sankhara*). Some of them are under the process of being aware (in the 'conscious mind') and some others are not (in the 'unconscious') (*Sampajana mano sankhara and asampjana mano-sankhara*) (Anguttar Nikaya) The Buddha speaks of latent tendencies (*anusaya*) or biases which lie dormant and influence one's actions. There are seven such tendencies : Greed (*Kama-raga*), repugnance (*Patigha*), speculative opinion (*Ditthi*), Skeptical doubt (*vicikiccha*), conceit (*Mana*) craving for existence (*Bhava-raga*), ignorance (*Avijja*), The existence of these tendencies of biases is not known to the person concerned, which means that he is unconscious of their existence in himself. The other characteristic of these tendencies is that they are dormant and influence thoughts, words and deeds of the person concerned. According to all the schools of Buddhism, life is a continuous process. As a result, one inherits the "*kamma*" of one's own previous lives. Therefore, according to Buddhism, in the storehouse called "unconscious", there are residues of past actions or *kammas* committed in one's previous chain of lives, lived even in the far distant past. These previous lives' *kammas* exist along with the *kammas* accumulated within the course of this life. The psychoanalytical schools of therapy use various techniques-catharsis, free association etc.—to dig into the unconscious of the patient and expose to the causes. The Buddhist meditation technique Vipassana focuses on the absolute interconnection between mind and body, that can be experienced directly by disciplines attention to the physical sensations that form the life of body, and that continuously interconnect and condition the life of the mind. The unconscious mind is actually not in conscious, as at all times it remains in contact with this body And with this contact of the body a sensation keeps arising, because every chemical flow in the body generates a particular type of sensation. We feel a sensation—pleasant, unpleasant, or neutral, whatever it is—and with the feeling of this sensation, we keep reacting. At the depth of our mind we keep reacting with craving, with aversion, with craving, with aversion. We keep on generating different types of Sankharas, different types of negativities, different types of impurities, and the process of multiplication continues. We cannot stop it because there is such a big barrier between the conscious and the unconscious mind. When we practice Vipassana we break this barrier and without this barrier remains.

Vipassana Meditation Technique

Vipassana is one of India's most ancient meditation techniques. It was rediscovered 2500 years ago by Lord Buddha and is the essence of what he practiced and taught during his forty-five-year ministry. Five centuries after Buddha, the noble heritage of Vipassana had disappeared from India. The purity of the teaching was lost elsewhere as well. In the country of Burma, however, a chain of devoted teachers preserved it. From generation to generation, over two thousand years, this dedicated lineage transmitted the technique in its pristine purity. In our time, Vipassana has been reintroduced by Sri S.N. Goenka. Vipassana courses were started in India in 1969.

Vipassana meditation, functions as a universal remedy for universal ills. Vipassana is a practical method of mental purification through self-observation. Vipassana means to see things as they really are, to explore the reality within. This process of self-observation purifies the mind of the impurities of illusions and delusions. Vipassana enables us to experience peace and harmony by purifying the mind, freeing it from suffering and the deeprooted causes of suffering. The practice leads step-by-step to the highest spiritual goal of full liberation from all mental defilements.

Vipassana is a *pali* word meaning insight seeing things as they really are. It is not a blind faith or philosophy Vipassana means to see things as they really are, to explore the reality within. It is a practical method of mental purification through self-observation. This process of self-observation purifies the mind of the impurities of illusions and delusions. Its goal is to purify the mind, to eliminate the tensions and negativities that make us miserable.

Vipassana is taught in ten-day residential courses under the guidance of a qualified teacher. A student must stay within the course site, suspend all rites and rituals, surrender to the teacher and the technique and maintain Noble Silence. There are three steps to the training. First, he undertakes to abstain from actions which causes him harm by undertaking five moral precepts : abstention from killing, stealing, lying, sexual activity and the use of intoxicants. This allows the mind to calm down sufficiently to proceed with the next step. For three and a half days, the student practices Anapana meditation by observing the natural breath to concentrate the mind. One then proceeds to Vipassana. The choiceless, effortless, equanimous observation of body sensations leads to mental purification and the realisation of the universal truths of impermanence, suffering and egolessness. There are no charges for teaching Vipassana. The entire cost is met through the wholesome volition of gratitude and generosity, by donations of students who have benefited from completing a course.

This is practical way to examine the reality of one's own body and mind, to uncover and solve whatever problems lie hidden there, to develop unused potential, and to channel it for one's own good and the good of others. Although its purpose is never simply to cure physical diseases, as a by-product of mental purification, many psychosomatic diseases are eradicated. It is an art of living, (Hart, 2000) which eliminates the causes of all unhappiness; like craving, aversion, etc.

Vipassana is a technique that purifies the mind, deconditioning the negativities of anger, hatred, greed, selfishness etc. by self-observation and introspection. It is insight meditation. It is looking at things as they are and not through coloured glasses. It is an effort to change the deep habit pattern of the mind, which dwells in the continuous blind reactions of craving and aversion. Our minds are constantly reacting to pleasant and unpleasant happenings in the world outside. But a deep investigation of the mind through Vipassana reveals that when we react, we are actually reacting to the body sensations that result from our contact with the outside world or our own thoughts. When a thought arises, it manifests as a sensation on the body—pleasant or unpleasant—and one starts to like or dislike it. This is a law of nature. Soon those likes and dislikes begin to consolidate and develop into negativities of craving and aversion. One starts tying knots deep in the unconscious mind. We create misery for ourselves by continuously reacting to the sensations.

In this technique we train the mind to observe all the sensations with detachment and equanimity—that is without developing craving for pleasant sensations or aversion towards unpleasant or painful ones. As one proceeds on this path, one experiences that all sensations, whether pleasant or unpleasant are constantly changing. They are impermanent (anicca) and essenceless (anatta)—without any substance. This is the inherent nature of everything that exists in the universe, whether animate or inanimate. One begins to understand experientially, not merely from book knowledge.

When one begins to be non-reactively aware of the different sensations, pleasant or unpleasant, the entire mass of the mind gradually becomes conscious and aware. The barrier between the conscious and unconscious mind is broken, and one stops reacting blindly. The mental purification-cleaning, deconditioning-strikes at the root-level, that is, the unconscious mind, where our deep-rooted defilements are stored like sleeping volcanoes, which cause us so much misery when they erupt.

To attain a stage, which is free from these sleeping volcanoes, one has to walk on the Path oneself. It does not happen overnight. One needs a long and sincere practice of Vipassana with a proper understanding of the technique. As one progresses on the Path, he learns to observe more objectively his own impurities of anger, hatred, envy, pride, jealousy etc. more objectively. Vipassana is, therefore, a process of self-purification through self-observation and introspection. It is a technique of non-verbal, self-administered "psychoanalysis" in that it sets into motion the process of tension-release.

The Buddha explored reality within—the reality of the physical and mental structure and realized that every being is a composite of physical and mental processes. Every one is very much aware with the changes taking place at our physical body. Superficially one can control the movement and actions according to the conscious will. But in our inner body there is no control over functioning of internal organs. Starting from the level of superficial, apparent reality, he penetrated to the subtleast level, and he found that the entire physical structure, the entire material world, is composed of subatomic particles called *attha kalapa*. These particles are the basic building blocks of matter. Body is composed of cells and incessant biochemical reactions occur within each cell of the body. The seemingly solid body is an aggregate of sub-atomic particles and empty space. These particles are themselves constantly arising and passing away with great rapidity-trillions of times within a second. In reality there is no solidity in the material world; it is nothing but combustion and vibrations. *Sabbo pajjalito loko sabbo loko pakampito.* Modern scientists have recognized and accepted the ultimate reality of the material universe through their own investigations. An American scientist received Nobel Prize in physics for discovering the nature of subatomic particles of which the physical universe is composed. With an instrument—a bubble chamber, he found that in one second a subatomic particle arises and vanishes 10-22 times. The truth that this scientist discovered is the same as that which the Buddha found. When one experiences personally the reality of one's own impermanence, only then does one start to come out of misery. Buddha also examined the psychic process—the mind and found that in broad, overall terms it consisted of four processes : consciousness (*vinnana*), perception (*sanna*), sensation (*vedana*), and reaction (*sankhara*). The first process, consciousness, is the receiving part of the mind, the act of cognition. It simply registers the occurrence of any phenomenon, the reception of any input, physical or mental. The second mental process is perception, the act of recognition. This part of mind identifies whatever has been noted by the consciousness. The third process is sensation—pleasant or unpleasant. In the process of reaction the mind reacts with liking or disliking. Pleasant sensations are liked and unpleasant sensations are disliked. These four mental functions-consciousness, perception, sensation, reaction occur whenever any of the other senses receives an input. This is the ultimate reality of the self. If one understands it properly by direct experience, it will give clue to lead out of suffering.

Vipassana as a Psychotherapeutic Technique

Vipassana has been successfully applied as a therapeutic technique in the treatment of drug addicts. The technique of Vipassana has been used in the addiction therapy centres for drug dependents at Cyrenian House in Perth, Australia and at "Start Again" in Zurich, Switzerland. These centers are run by Vipassana meditators since 1981 and 1992 respectively. Nissanka (1995) has applied the Buddhist technique for the treatment of different mental disorders *viz.* Depression, obsession, psych-somatic Disorder, manic-depressive psychosis, conversion hysteria, etc.

Vipassana as Tool of Behaviour Change in Jail Inmates

Vipassana has been adopted as a prison reform measure in jails. The main objective of these reforms is to shift the emphasis from a custodial to a correctional approach. This historic development has initiated a more humane approach in dealing with prisoners. There is now greater emphasis on behaviour modification, treatment, rehabilitation and psychological growth of inmates. The ultimate objective is prevention of crime and re-integration into society.

Several experiments have been conducted at prisons in India. In 1975 a course was conducted for 120 jail inmates at the Central Jail in Jaipur, the first such an experiment in Indian penal history. Encouraged by the results of this first course, the Govt. of Rajasthan organised another Vipassana course in Jan. 1977 in the same jail. Subsequently in 1990 a

Vipassana course was organised in Sabarmati Jail in Gujarat followed by one more course in Baroda. Several scientific studies have been conducted on these courses reporting positive results.

The first course at Tihar Jail was held in late November 1993 in Jail No. 2 which houses the hard core of the Tihar population, ten per cent of who have been convicted of crimes. Ninety six prisoners and twenty-three Jail staff participated. Vipassana became instantly popular among prisoners and in response to their requests, four courses were conducted simultaneously in three jails on 1st Jan. 1994 in which a total of about 300 prisoners participated. After the success of the January Tihar courses, the Ministry of Home affairs called a meeting of the Inspectors General of Prisons from all over India and a proposal was adopted to introduce Vipassana as a reform measure in all the prisons in the country. On the evening of April 4, 1994, 1003 male prisoners gathered in the huge tent in Jail No. 4 to receive the opening instructions from Sri S.N. Goenkaji himself. Simultaneously, the first Vipassana course for female prisoners began in Jail No. 1. It was attended by 49 inmates and was conducted by two female assistant teachers. Thirteen male assistant teachers, each with a group of 75 to 100, helped to conduct the male course. This was the largest Vipassana course conducted in recent history. It paved the way for the opening of the first permanent centre for the practice of Vipassana inside a prison named "Dhamma Tihar". A group of clinical psychologist, psychiatrist, social worker conducted two extensive studies to investigate the psychological effects of Vipassana on Tihar Jail Inmates in 1994. The impact of Vipassana on psychiatric illness, on some positive aspects of mental health, on hostility and feelings of helplessness, on personality functioning and psychopathy were studied. Vipassana has brought a significant positive change in the behaviour and attitude of jail inmates.

REFERENCES

Hart, W. H. (2000). *The Art of Living,* VRI, Nasik.

Jones, K. (1981). *Buddhism and Social Action,* Kendy Sri Lanka : Buddhist Publication Society.

Nissanka, H.S.S. (1995). *Buddhist Psychotherapy,* New Delhi : Vikas.

Vipassana Research Institute (1995). *Psychological Effects of Vipassana in Tihar Jail Inmates Research Report.*

7

Role of Religiosity and Spirituality in Health and Illness : Issues and Research Directions

*Shikha Dixit**, *Aparna Mehrotra***, *Rajbala Singh****

Health psychology has emerged as a significant area of research in contemporary psychology. This area of research has made significant contributions to the understanding of health behaviours and has recognized and studied a large number of factors that affect or undermine health and lead to illness (Taylor, 1990). According to Matarazzo (1980), "health psychology is defined as the educational, scientific, and professional contributions of the discipline of psychology to the promotion and maintenance of health". Other than the behavioural side of health and illness, health psychology also deals with the beliefs of people regarding their health and illness. The health belief model suggests that people's behaviour regarding their health is influenced by their perceptions of illness severity.

Belief system is an integral part of human life. People attach meanings to their lives and these meanings affect their health and illness beliefs. These meanings also contain the religious and spiritual element to a very large extent, which in turn influences people's understanding of health and illness states. These religious and spiritual influences are not new in the context of health and illness. In a variety of cultures spiritual healing, sacrifice, visiting shamans, pilgrimage etc. have been common practices in order to be relieved from illness. Illness is perceived as a consequence of unethical behaviour and sin in many cultures.

Historical Perspective

Earlier the relation between spirituality/ religiosity and health (illness) was not empirically tested. Psychologists had been less interested in the study of religiosity and spirituality. Reviews

* Associate Professor in Psychology, Department of Humanities and Social Sciences, Indian Institute of Technology Kanpur, Kanpur-208016, U.P., India E-mail:shikha@iitk.ac.in.

** Research Scholar (Psychology), Department of Humanities and Social Sciences, Indian Institute of Technology Kanpur, Kanpur – 208016, U.P., India E-mainmaparna@iitk.ac.in

*** Research Scholar (Psychology), Department of Humanities and Social Sciences, Indian Institute of Technology Kanpur, Kanpur – 208016, U.P., India E-mail:rajbala@iitk.ac.in

of empirical research in psychology (Weaver, Kline, Samford, Lucas, Larson & Gorsuch, 1998) and psychiatry (Larson, Pattison, Blazer, Omran & Kaplan, 1986) have demonstrated that impact of religious beliefs on health has not been the major focus of health related research whatever little research has been conducted, has been published in specialized journals for this purpose. These journals are not familiar to researchers in the area of health (Hill & Pargament, 2003).

Further, the focus on scientific methodology and quantitative approaches might have led the researchers to consider religion and spirituality as unscientific. Their operationalization and measurement may thus be viewed as difficult. Therefore, religiosity and spirituality have not been taken as rational concepts and have been avoided by researchers.

According to Miller and Thoresen (2003), works of James (1902) and Durkheim (1897/1951) are often cited in connection to religiosity and spirituality in the domain of health but no work prior to these is generally referred. However, McCormick (2004) has noted that, "This is a pity, as Fransis Galton, the father of differential psychology, published pioneering works 30 years earlier in his book *Hereditary Genius* (Galton, 1869) and in a paper titled *"Statistical Inquiries into the Efficacy of Prayer* (Galton, 1872)."

The above evidence proves that religiosity and spirituality are not new in the area of health. However, there is a need to explicate the reasons why religiosity and spirituality should be studied extensively in health research.

Meanings of Religiosity and Spirituality

Religion has been there in human life since long. William James regarded religion as the "feelings, acts, experiences of individual men in their solitude...in relation to whatever they may consider divine" (Miller & Thoresen, 2003). Some definitions have been given by various researchers in order to distinguish between religion and spirituality. According to Thoresen (1999), religion refers to "an organized system of beliefs, practices, rituals and symbols", while spirituality refers to "one's transcendent relationship to some form of higher power" (Holt, Lukwago & Kreuter, 2003). In other words it may be said that spirituality refers to a person's orientation toward or experiences with the transcendent or existential features of life (*e.g.* meaning, direction, purpose, and connectedness). Spirituality is also known as search for sacred in life. It is also taken as going towards the divine and being one with the divine. Religion may be viewed as, "denominational, external, cognitive, behavioural, ritualistic and public" and the spiritual as, "universal, ecumenical, internal, affective, spontaneous and private" (Harris, Thoresen, McCollough & Larson, 1999). Religiosity can also be understood as the external manifestation of being spiritual. Glock (1962) has suggested five core dimensions of religiosity.

(a) The experiential dimension : Being religious can be understood as experiencing the divine and feeling one with Him. This oneness with the supreme leads to the feelings of gaiety and peace.

(b) The ritualistic dimension : Being religious can be seen as performing some rituals like, praying, going to temples, etc.

(c) The ideological dimension : This constitutes of some beliefs that people hold about religiosity and notions regarding the world according to those religious beliefs.

(*d*) The intellectual dimension : This dimension contains peoples' knowledge regarding religion and is somewhat similar to the ideological dimension.

(*e*) The consequential dimension : This dimension deals with the effect of religious beliefs, practices and knowledge on the attitudes and behaviours of people.

An interesting point to note is that though religiosity and spirituality have been differentiated, a large number of researchers have used the two concepts interchangeably (Hill & Pargament, 2003; Woods & Ironson, 1999; Stuckey, 2001; Mytko & Knight, 1999). The present paper has also used the two concepts synonymously.

Objectives

In this paper an attempt has been made to delineate the issues regarding the relationship between spirituality/ religiosity and health. The following issues have been discussed in this connection :

What is the rationale behind including religiosity/spirituality in the area of health studies and why scholars have neglected its role? Is religion an illusion or can it be conceived as realized? How religiosity/spirituality is related to adjustment and coping with illness? Whether religious beliefs always facilitate adjustment and coping with illness or sometimes it they function as therapeutic obstacle? What are the motivational, psychodynamic and cognitive perspectives of religiosity/spirituality? Can we draw parallels between the Western and Indian perspectives of religiosity/spirituality? What are the suitable approaches to understand the role of religiosity/spirituality in health related behaviours?

Existing research directions and questions pertaining to them will be discussed in the following section.

Existing Research Directions and Major Issues

Rationale for Including Religiosity and Spirituality in the Area of Health

The concepts of spirituality and religiosity have been considered as nonscientific and have been neglected by many researchers. It has been assumed that spirituality cannot and should not be studied scientifically. Scholars making these assumptions view spirituality and religiosity as non-material, beyond sensory perception and therefore not amenable to objective scientific observation.

However, Miller and Thoresen (2003) suggest that these assumptions are not valid. Thomson (1996) argues that science, by definition does not provide appropriate ways of studying spirituality. It is therefore evident that this is a matter of epistemological debate. According to Miller and Thoresen (2003), although science does not provide any appropriate methods to study spirituality/religiosity, there are incidences when science has studied phenomenon, which were not directly observable and could be inferred. Therefore, to state that religiosity/spirituality cannot be measured is inappropriate.

According to Carone and Barone (2001), "Religious beliefs are an important part of clients' culture, whether acknowledged or not". Knowing the patients' religious belief system can help the health professionals to understand the coping efforts that are guided by these beliefs. They can use these beliefs as a part of the therapeutic procedures. According to Powell, Shahabi and Thoresen (2003), religion and spirituality work twofold. Among healthy individuals they provide the basis for the disease prevention mechanism and serve the purpose of a coping device among patients. In the Indian context health is seen from a totally different perspective. It is believed that our body is a gift of God and we all are here to fulfill a purpose. In this connection Sharma (2004) has quoted Gandhi: Man came into the world in order to pay off the debt owed by him to it, that is to say, in order to serve God and (or through) His creation. Keeping this point of view in front of him, man acts as a guardian of his body. It becomes his duty to take such care of his body as to enable it to practice the ideal of service to the best of its ability.

In Indian Vedas, health is directly related with spirituality. So in order to understand the concepts of health and illness in India, spirituality and religiosity should be included as important research topics. Thus, there seems no convincing reason why spirituality and religiosity cannot or should not be studied in the context of health and illness. In order to explicate the relationship between religiosity/spirituality and health it is imperative to first understand the nature of religiosity/spirituality. There has been a controversy regarding the nature of religion. Some scholars view religion as an illusionary concept whereas some view it as a realized phenomenon.

Religion as Illusion *vs.* Religion as Realized

There is a debate regarding the nature of religion. In research literature religion is considered both as illusion and realized. Religion has been described as "unimportant", "bad science" and "not real" and such statements function as barriers and prevent researchers to accept the positive role of religion in health (Levin, 1994; as cited in Chamberlain & Hall, 2000). Sigmund Freud is one amongst those who conceive religion as an illusion. According to him, religion is nothing but, "a childish, wishful desire to explain God, the origin of life, and the mastery of death." He also conceived religion as "the universal obsessional neurosis of humanity... a system of wishful illusions together with disapproval of reality" (Chamberlain & Hall, 2000). Further, people believe in someone powerful like God to reduce their unconscious anxiety, which is the cause of all psychopathologies.

In contrast to Freudian thinking, scholars like Chamberlain and Hall (2000) have taken a practical approach where religion serves to promote people's life, both at macro and micro level. This can be possible only when the elements of religion are realized in daily life. The term realized refers to bring religion into concrete existence. And this can be achieved by practicing faith and trust (two important elements of religion) in one's life. Empirically it has been reported that realized religion brings better health, higher well-being, higher marital satisfaction, less addiction etc. When religion is realized at macro level, it leads to overall development of a society. It makes society more functional by promoting social cohesion and fosters social, cultural and religious values and norms among the members of society. In addition, when religion is realized at micro or individual level, it brings meaning, purpose and hope in individual's life.

Religious Involvement and Health

Empirical evidence report that the benefits of religious/spiritual involvement on health may exist at several levels such as, physiological, psychological, behavioural and socio-cultural. As cited in Miller and Thoresen (2003) a large numbers of studies have found that patients (especially those who practice religion regularly) like to discuss spiritual issues pertaining to their illness with their caregivers (Daaleman & Nease, 1994; Ehman, Ott, Short, Ciampa, & Hansen-Flaschen, 1999; King & Bushwick, 1994) and generally people rely on their religious beliefs in order to cope with illness and stress (Dein & Stygal, 1997).

As noted by Thoreson (1999), McEwen (1998) and Seeman and McEwen (1996) identified health problems related to "chronic distress." The body's ability to maintain physiological stability may be lost because of "long term distress" and a major consequence of this loss would be a disruptive influence on metabolism, brain functions, cardiovascular system and immunity. However, people with religious involvement manage these problems in better way. According to him, perceived loss of control, lack of social emotional support, poverty, and low social status have been suggested as examples of sources that contribute to excessive and chronic allostatic load. Conceivably those more religiously involved or spiritually active may benefit greatly in drawing upon the resources provided by others in religious organizations and/or by their own spiritually enhancing beliefs, practices and experiences. Doing so could reduce the level of allostatic load, thus enhancing overall physiological functioning.

It thus appears that religious involvement and a spiritual way of life may reduce the disease risk associated with errant physiological functioning. Several psychosocial and sociocultural mechanisms have also been identified by researchers. These mechanisms have been used to explain the connection between health and religious-spiritual factors (Pargament, 1997; Kleinman & Becker, 1998; both cited in Thoresen, 1999). In this connection health behaviours (*e.g.* cutting down on smoking and exercising regularly), cognitive processes (*e.g.* self perception of worth and social acceptance by society and/or God) and interpersonal resources (*e.g.* shared religious beliefs and group meditation) have been studied. The socio-cultural factors, such as beliefs and symbols about illness and suffering, connected to spiritual and religious factors may also help to create the kind of social context that promotes health-enhancing behaviour, cognitions and interpersonal relationships.

Cultural norms have also been found to have an important influence on health beliefs within a religious setting. Such an influence has been studied in African-American churches in the United States. The church provides an environment of protection and nurturance. This in turn leads to positive changes in health related habits and cognitions (McCrae & Carey, 1998; as cited in Thoresen, 1999), pp. 296.

Adjustment and Coping Through Religious Beliefs

Carone and Barone (2001) have discussed the role of religious beliefs in coping strategies and adjustment to health problems. Freud did not believe in the positive therapeutic role of religion. However, psychoanalysts like Jung and James and other pragmatists have recognized and appreciated the positive role of religion in health related beliefs. As noted by Carone and Barone (2001), religious beliefs can influence health positively and enhance adjustment to illness in following ways :

(a) Religion is used by people as a coping strategy and also as a justification. Illness and hardship are justified and explained by attributing them to the workings of the all powerful God who knows what is best for human beings.

(b) Attributing everything to *Karma* and belief in rebirth can also help in alleviating the stress levels associated with illness and hardships. Believing in *Karma* and a life after life may help in dealing with an impending death associated with severe illness.

(c) Religion is employed to deal with loneliness psychotic disorders Parkinson's disease, HIV and death due to murder.

(d) Religion may provide a way of enhancing health and well-being through the perception of God as a source of love, protection and care. Such perceptions enable us to perceive God as a secure attachment figure.

Research has shown that secure attachment to a caregiver can help individuals develop positive internal working models of the social world. A secure attachment has also been found to be strongly related to low level of anxiety and to high levels of self-esteem curiosity and creativity. Thus, having a caring, responsive God or other spiritual being as a substitute attachment figure could improve one's well-being.

(e) Most religions propagate forgiveness as an exalted form of reaction to distress. Forgiveness entails replacing negative feelings and emotions for the offender with positive feelings. As noted by Carone and Barone (2001) :

The main function of forgiveness is that it allows one to replace negative feelings with positive ones, such as empathy and love toward the offender. As such, therapists have recommended using forgiveness as a way for patients to deal with issues such as anger, sexual abuse, betrayals in marriage, posttraumatic stress disorder and suicide.

Alferi, Culver, Carver, Arena and Antoni (1999) have studied the effect of religious involvement on distress in early stage breast cancer patients. They found that religious/ spiritual coping patterns were quite frequently used. Believing in one's religious faith was the most common among all the religious coping strategies. Further, they have compared the coping patterns of Catholic and Evangelical women. Results demonstrated that religious involvement resulted in less distress among Evangelical women but in high distress among the Catholics. On the basis of these findings an issue emerges whether the effect of religious coping is mediated by the religious affiliation. Park, Cohen and Herb (1990) have obtained similar findings with reference to Catholics and Protestants. They discussed their findings in the light of the nature of stressor. They found that religious coping works as a buffer against distress in the case of controllable stressor for Catholics and vice-versa for Protestants. But when there an uncontrollable stressor was involved Protestants reported less distress than Catholics (as cited in Alferi *et al.*, 1999). Though these findings seem interesting but future researches are needed to examine the role of religious commitment and religious coping across various groups practicing different religions.

Alferi *et al.* (1999) have cited some studies to show that stressful situations lead people towards religiosity in order to find peace and support. These studies have demonstrated the positive effect of religious affiliation on coping with cancer, depression, other chronic illnesses and adverse conditions. Religious coping has also been found to enhance physical and psychological well-being.

Feher and Maly (1999) tried to find whether religious coping helps the elderly women diagnosed with breast cancer in reducing their distress. They found that having religious/ spiritual faith enhances the feeling of emotional and social support. Religious belief gave them a sense of security and despite being ill the patients felt protected being close to God. Another reason of feeling protected by God was patients' belief that their doctor was being guided by the Almighty. Koenig, George and Siegler (1988) found that patients have faith in

God and they believe that God is the one who gives strength to overcome any stressful situation (as cited in Feher & Maly, 1999).

Taylor, Outlaw, Bernardo and Roy (1999) reported that people, who believe in the efficacy of prayer, pray more in case of illness. Prayer is an intimate coping strategy and has been found to benefit patients suffering from various diseases, such as sickle cell disease pain. In general prayer has been found to be a successful coping mechanism. Many researchers have conceived prayer as a "psychologic or cognitive coping strategy". All studies in this paragraph are cited in Taylor *et al.* (1999).

Spirituality and Religiosity as Intervention Programmes

This section is based on the findings of Cole and Pargament (1999). They studied the role of religiosity and spirituality in intervention programmes that are run for people suffering with chronic illnesses. Spiritual resources are likely to play an important role in intervention programmes. People confronting life threatening diseases face many kinds of existential problems. Spiritually oriented people turn towards spiritual resolution for these existential concerns. Spiritual intervention has been reported to be beneficial for cancer patients. Facing cancer evokes concerns about limits of control, identity, relationship with others and meaning. Spiritual people surrender the uncontrollable into the hands of some transcendent power and thus by accepting the human limitations they generate a sense of security and peace. Spirituality also helps the person to find meaning in the event and an enhanced identity. This is because the patient connects himself to the eternity and some higher power. Finally spiritual orientation eases alienation, facilitates experience of oneness with all existence and as a result positively impact relationship with others and creates a sacred interconnectedness with others. Empirical evidence shows that religious beliefs decrease levels of pain, anxiety, hostility, social isolation, and increase life satisfaction (Jenkins & Pargament, 1995; Yates, Chalmer, St. James, Follarnsbee & McDegney, 1981; Musick, Koenig, Larson & Matthews, 1998; all the studies cited in Cole & Pargament, 1999).

Cole and Pargament (1999) developed an intervention programme that used spiritual coping and fostered a holistic healing process in coping with cancer. It was found that this healing process improves relationships with others, increases sense of identity and people start realizing that everything is not under their control. This decreases their level of depression and pain. Meditation has been found to be helpful in the enhancement of general well-being. Besides enhancement of well-being, meditation based interventions have been useful in the treatment of anxiety, addictions, pain management and also as a supplement to psychotherapy (Carrington, 1998; Kabat-Zinn, Massion, Kristeller, Peterson, Fletcher, Pbert, Lenderking & Santorelli, 1992; Rubin, 1996; studies cited in Kristeller & Hallett, 1999).

Cognitive-behavioural interventions have been used to treat clinical disorders by using spiritual and religious thinking process. It has been found that religious imagery treatment lowers the level of depression much more than non-religious imagery. Meditation based interventions have also been used to treat the patients. This is mainly an eastern concept, which is now accepted in the west also. Meditation has been a part of health intervention studies for two decades. And it has been observed that it helps in stress reduction, both physiological and psychological. Meditation enhances self-regulation and integrates the physiological, emotional, cognitive and behavioural aspects of human functioning. As a relaxation technique, meditation may decrease both emotional and physiological reactivity in such disorders as essential hypertension. Another treatment programme that has spiritual element in it is the Twelve-step fellowship programme. This programme is run for those who are addicted to alcohol and drugs. Alcoholics Anonymous is another similar kind of intervention programme for such people. Both intervention programmes have spiritual elements in them (Harris, Thoresen, McCullough, & Larson, 1999).

Some intervention programmes have been prescribed by Indian philosophy. According to ancient literature like, Vedas and scripts of famous people like, Charak, a person is believed to be having five bodies and intervention corresponding to those bodies is prescribed. First is the physical body (*annamaya kosha*) and six activities are prescribed for it : *neti dhauti, kapal bhati, tratak, nauli, vasti* and *yogasanas*. Second is etheric body (*pranamaya kosha*) and activities pertaining to it are : *pranayama*, walking, *pranvidya* and *mantra vidya*. For mental body (*manomay kosha*), meditation, concentration, recitation, and *yoga nidra*, for intellectual body (*vigyanmaya kosha*), study of Vedas, religious literature, meditation, vipasyana, and for causal body (*anandamaya kosha*) *samadhi*, liberation, peace, bliss and *sat-chit-anand* are prescribed (Sharma, 2004).

The present evidence leads the discussion towards a conclusion that religiosity/spirituality positively affects health. However, there are some incidences that focus on the role of religiosity/ spirituality as an obstacle in the therapeutic procedures. This issue has been discussed in the next section.

Religious Beliefs as Therapeutic Obstacle

Religious beliefs do not always facilitate therapeutic treatment but sometimes they work as an obstacle to treatment. Such impediments may be of different types. Some of these influences have been discussed by Carone and Barone (2001) :

(1) Rigidity due to religious beliefs may prevent patients from following the advice of the doctor. In such cases religious beliefs interfere with adopting appropriate strategy to deal efficiently with the disease. For example, a religious lady may think that it is her duty to nourish her children and serve her husband despite her poor health.

(2) Religious beliefs also interfere with the treatment when suggestions given by the doctor contradict with the religious belief a person holds. An example may be that patients' caregivers deny blood transfusion because of their religious beliefs.

(3) Religious beliefs also interfere with therapeutic interventions because both follow different approaches. Religion either follows the moral model or the enlightenment model. The moral model of religion blames persons for their problems and also expects that people should solve their problems on their own. Enlightenment model of religion also blames people for their problems but at the same time believes that people cannot solve their problem without the guidance of almighty. On the contrary, medical model given by the medical professionals mainly focuses on biological causes of the disease. It believes in giving the proper remedy or medical intervention to a patient as suggested by a health professional.

(4) Religious beliefs can interfere with the therapeutic interventions if the doctors or therapists do not properly deal with the religious beliefs a patient hold. For example

there is a greater likelihood of occurrence of a problem if a therapist challenges or refutes the religious beliefs of the patient. Problems may also occur if the suggestions given by the therapist are not consistent with notions held by the patient. As noted by Carone and Barone (2001) :

> A Buddhist client from India may come to see a counselor because she argues with her husband a lot. Because Buddhism is a religion that emphasizes self-sacrifice, this client may express a desire to defer to her husband's wishes in order to avoid any further disputes. The client's attempt at self-sacrifice is inconsistent with the modern western view that healthy marriages are based on fairness and equality. The counselor thus runs the risk of imposing his or her view on the client, which can disturb the client's value system and cultural practices as well as the therapeutic relationship. (p. 996)

Despite these obstacles there is more evidence in support of religiosity and spirituality. These beliefs work as motivating forces, which has been discussed briefly in the next section.

Religiosity and Spirituality as Motivating Forces

Religiosity and spirituality can lead people towards their real destinations in life. The spiritual strivings make people attain their goals by providing them essential support and confidence. These beliefs further direct people towards the correct path to reach their destinations. And this is not applicable in smooth times only but also in adverse situations. Hill and Pargament (2003) further state that, "...religion and spirituality can be understood, for some people, as overarching frameworks that orient them to the world and provide motivation and direction for living."

Have psychometrically measured the motivating force that is enhanced by religiosity. It has been found that well-being, satisfaction and greater purpose in life were positively associated with spiritual strivings. In addition, people who had high spiritual strivings were found to have fewer conflicts related to their goals of their life and better mental health, self-esteem, family relations, etc. Factors that were found to be negatively related to spiritual beliefs were alcohol abuse, drug abuse and sexual promiscuity. In addition to religiosity/spirituality as motivating force in life it has also been reported that they enhance the overall quality of life.

Religiosity and Spirituality as Enhancers of Quality of Life

Mytko and Knight (1999) have discussed the issue whether religiosity/spirituality should be included in Quality of Life (QOL) research or not. Literature shows that religiosity/spirituality were part of QOL theoretically but were not included in psychometric research. The existing literature has been reviewed in order to see the role of religiosity/spirituality in QOL measurement. QOL refers to a multidimensional construct that constitutes the physical, mental and social well-being of a person. Research shows that spiritual well-being has a stress reducing effect which in turn increases QOL. In general various studies have found a positive relationship between levels of religiosity/spirituality and QOL.

Health and People's Attribution to God

The studies focusing on the relationship between health status and peoples' attribution to God have been reviewed by Exline, Yali and Lobel (1999). Generally people attribute positive events to God. However, unexplained negative life events may also be attributed to God. The parents tend to attribute God in case of their child's sudden death due to sudden infant death syndrome. People often get angry with God for the pain and suffering that exist in this world. Role of forgiveness has been studied in this context. If people forgive God for the negative life events, the distress occurred by those events decreases. It has been emphasized that the effects of forgiving are on various outcomes like, family life, mental and physical health. The consequence of anger towards God has been studied which report that it can lead to poor mental health and poor coping outcomes. Exline *et al.* (1999) further found that difficulty in forgiving God can lead to anxious and depressed mood. These areas further need to be investigated as to what are the factors that lead to attribution of negative events to God and why this happens.

Indian and Western Perspectives of Health : Can We Draw Parallels?

In the present section, a comparison has been made between the Indian and the Western perspectives of health on the basis of their conceptualization, aim, and the cognitive aspect.

Conceptualization and Aim of Health

There exists a fundamental difference between the Indian and Western conceptualization of health. From the Indian perspective the concept of health has its roots in Vedic and Vedantic scriptures, Yoga school and Ayurveda. The Indian conceptualization of health emphasizes the integration of mind, body and spirit and suggests that a complete harmony among these is the basis for ideal health (Dalal, 2001).

However, according to the western perspective, there exists a dichotomy between mind and body. Rene Descartes who proposed "mind-body dualism" suggested that mind and body are two different faculties. Mind and body do not interact and work independently from each other. However, in the Indian perspective, the emphasis is on "how mind, body and spirit interact and improve the health status of an individual". On the difference between the Indian and the Western perspectives on health, Bhushan (1996) states : Yoga does not believe in a dichotomy of mental and physical health. On the contrary, it holds that human happiness depends on physical fitness, mental agility and spiritual verve. It aims at developing a balanced and integrated personality of which body, mind and spirit are integral components. Western psychology accepts the importance of the first two, but rejects the third, considering it a philosophical and mystical concept. But this is closing the eyes to reality. The three are closely interlinked. (Section on Integration of body, mind and spirit, 1)

Another difference between the two perspectives regarding health are their different aims is that Western perspective basically cures and prevents the disease, whereas the Indian perspective has an additional motive of promoting one's health. The psychodynamic model focuses on mental patients and does not leave any possibility for spiritual growth of normal individuals. The modern medical science emphasizes that the cause of many diseases is psychosomatic. This idea was already conceived by the ancient Yoga school. Further : it holds that disease germinated in the mind and later manifested in somatic symptoms. Today medical science admits that most of our diseases are psychosomatic in nature. Disease originates from mental stress causing imbalance in the neuropsychological and endocrinal systems, resulting in psychosomatic disorders. (Bhushan, 1998)

Thus, on the basis of above discussion it may be said that treatment of diseases only with the help of western psychological interventions is not sufficient. Yoga psychology claims that the proper practice of Yoga heals the disease more effectively because its approach is "psycho-somato-spiritual". The recognition of this fact has popularized the Yoga practices in different sections of modern Indian society as well as the western countries.

The next section deals with the cognitive and social cognitive perspective that underlie the conception of religiosity and spirituality in both Indian and Western perspectives.

Cognitive Aspects of Health

Carone and Barone (2001) have discussed the cognitive and social-cognitive factors that underlie religious beliefs. Psychological theories, especially cognitive theories explain the function of religious beliefs. For example, social cognitive theory explains that religious beliefs work like heuristics. Heuristics are also known as cognitive shortcuts. Cognitive shortcuts are employed by people under circumstances of multi-tasking, cognitive load and/or lack of information. Such short cuts reduce the cognitive load and facilitate decision-making. Such easy and rapid decisions may lead to biases or errors but in daily life people use them because of information overload and lack of time.

Religious beliefs also function as heuristics. Religious people make rapid judgments on the basis of the beliefs they hold rather than engaging in systematic information processing. According to Snyder and Swann (1978), "A well-documented consequence of heuristic processing is the confirmatory bias, in which selective perceiving and remembering seem to validate beliefs, hypothesis, and schemas about the world even when they do not." Confirmatory bias is a tendency to believe in those experiences that support one's views and to ignore those that do not. This leads to reduction in anxiety and stress that is caused by the overload of information. In the context of religion, an example of this bias may be that in social situations Christians try to imitate the life and behaviour of Jesus.

The use of religious beliefs as heuristics has also been mentioned by Freud, who stated that mankind's helplessness in such a chaotic and unpredictable world led to the religious notion that everything that happens in this world is an expression of the intentions of an intelligence superior to us.

Indian perspective also presents cognitive basis of health but in a very different manner. In the Yoga school the role of mind has been emphasized. In Patanjali, the primary aim of Yoga is to restrict modifications or tendencies of *chitta* or mind : "*Yogaschitta vritti nirodhah.*" This means that the mind can be disciplined by controlling *vrittis* (senses). *Vrittis* have a cognitive basis. Some parallels may therefore be drawn between the ancient Indian thinking and the Western thinking that postulates the cognitive basis of behaviour. The *vrittis* may be either painful *(klishta)* or not painful *(aklishta)*. (Bhushan, 1998). He further contends that, they originate from five cognitive sources : *pramana*, proof or valid cognition; *viparyaya*, illusion or invalid cognition; *vikalpa*, fancy or objectless verbal cognition; *nidra*, sleep or unconscious cognition; and *smriti*, memory or mental recollection of past cognition. If a person's *vrittis* are only related to materialistic pleasures then *klishta vritti* becomes dominant which leads the person to pain and extreme condition of depression. On the other hand, if a person turns his/her *vrittis* towards spirituality, it will lead a person to state of bliss, which in turn makes a person both physically and mentally healthy.

Yoga emphasizes the discipline of mind, body and spirit. In this regard, Patanjali has emphasized the eight-fold path. Following this path leads a person to function in different situations in a better way. The eight-fold path consists of : *Yama* (social code), *Niyama* (personal code), *Asana* (posture), *Pranayama* (control of prana), *Pratyahara* (sense of withdrawal), *Dharana* (concentration), *Dhyana* (meditation), and *Samadhi* (superconciousness). The idea of eight-fold path has been cited by Sudarshan (2002).

The bodily responses are the result of our thoughts and feelings. The diseases are mostly psychosomatic. This suggests that they originate from the mind. Yoga reverses the process and uses the mind as a tool to cure the disease and to enhance growth, which leads to positive and healthy life.

On the basis of above discussion it can be said that studies done in the west only provide the basis for how religious beliefs work in daily life and the processes involved in using religious beliefs. Contrary to this, the Indian perspective emphasizes certain kind of life style that entails the integration of mind, body and spirit in order to attain an ideal state of health. Any kind of disintegration or disruption may lead to illness. "Yoga provides techniques for establishing harmony between the three, resulting in physical and mental well-being and higher spiritual awareness. Thus it presents a wider spectrum than the modern view of psychology.

Bhushan (1996) has discussed the existing empirical evidence in this connection. (Ornish, 1990) as cited in Bhushan, 1998) has shown that heart disease is nothing but the result of faulty living habits. He has shown that patients of heart disease reported 91% reduction in chest pain, 21% reduction in cholesterol level, a significant improvement in blood pressure, improved well-being and reduction in anxiety and depression after following the recommended life style. This life style included vegetarian diet, some Yogic techniques like, practice of *asanas, pranayamas* and meditation (with respiration and visualization).

A number of studies have reported that a life style that includes yoga benefits patients of chronic diseases. It has been reported that hypertension, anxiety, psychoneurotic symptoms are cured by Yoga practices (Kocher, 1972; Naug, 1975; Vishal, Singh & Madhu, 1987). Akhilananda (1952) and Swami Satyananda (1983) have focused on how the mental health can be managed with yogic practices. Datey, Deshmukh, Dalvi and Vinekar (1969), Deshmukh (1971) and Goyeche (1979) have also reported similar findings in the area of stress reduction, managing psychoneurotic, psychotic and psychosomatic disorders. All the above stated studies have been cited in Bhushan (1996).

So far the present paper has discussed the studies that have attempted to explicate the relationship between religiosity/spirituality and health status. It is evident from the preceding discussion that religiosity/spirituality has an overall positive impact on health and religious/ spiritual beliefs and prayer provide successful ways of coping with distress due to illness both at physical and psychological levels. However, the relationship between health and religiosity/ spirituality is often obscured by the prevailing misinterpretations. Researchers have tested the empirical reality of these myths and misinterpretations (Levin, 1996; Thoresen, 1999).

Limitations of Current Research

Many studies have been carried out to see the beneficial effect of spirituality and religiosity on health. Studies have supported the notion that religious practices are helpful in coping and adjusting to pain, discomfort and sorrow resulting from chronic diseases. Various religious/ spiritual intervention programmes have also been designed and implemented in such cases.

However, it has been observed that there exist some drawbacks or limitations in the researches carried out in this specific area. The first limitation pertains to the nature of spirituality and religiosity. Ambiguity exists regarding whether spirituality and religiosity are same or different concepts. Many scholars have used these two concepts interchangeably in their researches (Hill & Pargament, 2003; Woods & Ironson, 1999; Stuckey, 2001; Mytko & Knight, 1999). Thus there is a need to redefine these two concepts clearly.

The second limitation is regarding the parameters of spirituality and religiosity that have been taken into consideration in various researches in this area. In most of the studies only objective indicators of spirituality and religiosity such as, attending church, praying regularly, meditating, etc. have been studied. However, only focusing on the objective manifestation of spirituality and religiosity cannot reveal the true picture of their role and importance in the area of health and illness completely.

The third limitation of current research is that there is a disregard for the constructivist nature of thought. Thus, there is a need to understand how people conceptualize the concepts of spirituality and religiosity.

The fourth limitation is related with the methodology that has been adopted in researches on the issue in question. Quantitative methodologies have been used vastly in this area. However, this reliance cannot provide an understanding of the everyday meaning and lay perception of the concepts in question. Appropriate qualitative techniques have to be employed in order to study everyday meaning of religion-health relationship.

In addition to above-mentioned limitations, there is a need to operationalize several Indian concepts related to spirituality and religiosity and to examine their empirical validity. Very few researches have been carried out in this area.

Directions for Future Research

Powell, Shahabi and Thoresen (2003) have reviewed some studies regarding religiosity/spirituality and their role in health outcomes. Studies they opted to review were methodologically sound. They categorized the studies on the basis of nine hypotheses. These hypotheses emerged from the content of the studies and were based on the relationship between religious/spiritual factors and health. This section discusses these hypotheses as they provide a basis for future research. The studies discussed in connection with these hypotheses are all cited in Powell *et al.* (2003). Their first hypothesis was that church/service attendance protects against death. Out of eleven studies nine were done on healthy people and they found that church attendance leads to decreased mortality. Studies done on patients did not show any effect of church/service attendance. Although investigation has been done by to find out the possible mechanisms in this connection, further research is needed to find out the reasons for lack of relationship found between religiosity/spirituality (church attendance) and mortality.

Second hypothesis was disease specific, and in this connection those studies were reviewed that examined the relationship between religiosity/spirituality and cardiovascular disease maintaining that religion protects against cardiovascular diseases. A reduction in various cardiovascular diseases as an effect of religious involvement was reported. The results were explained on the basis of the healthy life style that is enhanced by religious/spiritual involvement. Further research can be done in order to explore the effects of daily prayers and meditation on cardiovascular diseases.

The third hypothesis was related to the effects of religion/spirituality on cancer mortality. It was found that cancer mortality reduced under the influence of attending the church regularly. The reduction in cancer mortality was not found when the previous health conditions were adjusted. However, it is possible that people who have cancer become more religious/ spiritual. This conflict in results leaves a possibility for future research in order to find the exact directionality of the relationship between religious/spiritual factors and chronic disease.

Powell *et al.* (2003) further checked whether their hypothesis that religiosity protects against death is supported by empirical evidence or not. They found that this hypothesis was not supported by the findings. But when they took patients free from functional impairment, they did find some relationship between religiosity/spirituality and mortality. Further research is thus required in this regard.

Studies have been done to see the effect of religiosity/spirituality on disability. Powell *et al.* (2003) hypothesized that these factors protect against disability. The studies they reviewed could not find any relation between religiosity and protection against disability. A very surprising finding in this area was by Haley, Koenig and Bruchett (2001). They found that physical disability was more among those who prayed and meditated daily than those who were involved in religious activities weekly. Idler and Kasl (1997b) gave an explanation that there may actually be a reverse relationship. Higher spiritual activity may be the result of increasing physical disability. There is a dearth of research in this area, which leaves some possibilities for further research.

Another hypothesis that Powell *et al.* (2003) derived from the empirical works was that the progression of cancer slowed down as an effect of religiosity/spirituality. The review of empirical studies demonstrated little relationship between religious factors and cancer progression. Future research needs to understand these findings.

Religious coping during adverse life situations leads to longer life was the next hypothesis tested by Powell *et al.* (2003). Even in this context they found that there is a dearth of research and the causal relationship between religiosity/spirituality and long life is still not definite, which is a matter of future research. In this connection educational level may be an important factor affecting religious coping.

Powell *et al.* (2003) also examined the hypothesis that religiosity and spirituality help an individual to recover from acute illness. They reviewed works of Fitchett, Rybarczyk, Demarco and Nicholas (1999) and King, Speck and Thomas (1999) etc. These studies did not support Powell's hypothesis. In fact Fitchett *et al.* (1999) and King *et al.* (1999) found that religiosity/ spirituality slows the recovery from acute illness. There is a need for more research with more sound methodology because of contradictory results. Another interesting hypothesis was developed by Powell *et al.* (2003) that whether distant praying is helpful in recovery from acute illness or not. Little evidence shows that praying from distance affects health positively, and lowers illness severity.

Future research should be done to find out the mechanisms through which religiosity/ spirituality affects health. Some findings show that act of helping as a part of religious practice affects health positively (Langer & Rodin, 1976; as cited in Powell *et al.*, 2003). More research is needed to confirm this finding.

On the basis of literature review, it is clear that scholars are now accepting that there is positive relation between spirituality/religiosity and health. However a great number of questions are still unanswered.

There is also a need to include spiritual and religiosity dimension in the study of quality of life measures. Many scholars (Eberst, 1984; Russell, 1981, as cited in Perrin & McDermott, 1997) have also taken emotional and spiritual dimensions into account while defining health. Health is one of the important dimensions of overall quality of life. World Health Organization (WHO) (as cited in Perrin & McDermott, 1997) has defined health "as a state of complete physical, mental and social well-being and not merely the absence of disease or infirmity." WHO's definition of health does not take into account spiritual and religious aspects of health. According to Russell's model of wellness, spiritual health is an umbrella concept, which includes all other dimensions related to health. Thus, it is important to include spiritual and religious dimensions of health while judging one's overall quality of life.

As already mentioned, spirituality/religiosity are based on the human belief system. Faith and beliefs are the core of spirituality/religiosity. Thus, only taking objective indicators of spirituality/religiosity and only employing quantitative techniques will not reveal the real picture of the relationship between health and religiosity/spirituality.

To fully understand the relationship between spirituality/religiosity and health it is necessary to know how spiritual and religious beliefs are formed and in what manner they influence health. In addition, it is also important to know how cultural belief systems of meaning influence the social and subjective reality of spirituality/religiosity and its relationship to health. In this context 'social representation' approach provides a way to understand the subjective reality of any concept formed within a culture. According to social representation approach analysis of everyday knowledge is required to better understand how people understand the concepts they deal with in their daily life. Moscovici's (1988) theory emerged to understand the processes that are involved in peoples' concept formation of social representation. This theory states that people from a group or community share the ideas, thoughts, images, knowledge and these form some kind of representations in their minds. He defines social representations as, "...cognitive systems with a logic and language of their own...They do not represent simply 'opinions about', 'images of' or 'attitudes towards' but 'theories' or branches of knowledge' in their own right, for the discovery and organization of reality"(as cited in Augoustinos and Walker, 1995, pp.135-136). Spirituality/religiosity and health are among those concepts about which people form such representations.

The social representation approach mainly deals with the 'social construction' of any phenomenon (Flick, 2002). The social representation approach has already been used to understand the phenomena of health and illness (Herzlich, 1973), madness (Jodelet, 1991; as cited in Flick, 2002) and technological change in everyday life (Flick, 1995a, 1996, as cited in Flick, 2002). Thus this approach can be used to understand the conceptualization of spirituality/religiosity and its role in determining or influencing health.

Conclusions

On the basis of the literature reviewed in this paper it can be concluded that scholars have recognized the importance of spirituality and religiosity as coping mechanisms in case of illness and distress. Although Freud have termed the concepts of spirituality and religiosity as 'illusionary', scholars like Chamberlain and Hall (2000) have shown in their work how realized aspect of religion benefits both individual and society. A large number of studies have reported that people employ their religious and spiritual beliefs to cope and adjust to the pain and distress caused by chronic and life threatening illness. An important point to note at this juncture is that the religion-health relationship is intricate and involves various controversies. Based on the stated limitation of the research reviewed in this paper it may be said that the everyday conceptualization and meanings of religion, spirituality, health and illness may be different from the realist epistemological meanings.

In general, it is reported in many studies that religious involvement is associated with better health and promotes healthy behaviour practices and an environment of social interaction and support. Spiritual and religious beliefs serve as a source of attachment, security, and confidence and motivate people to strive for their life goals.

Various spiritual and religious intervention programmes have been designed and implemented for patients suffering from different chronic diseases. However, sometimes spiritual and religious beliefs do not foster but hinder the recovery process. It happens when there is a discrepancy between the beliefs held by the doctor and patient. In some cases patient's spiritual and religious beliefs are so rigid that they do not allow the patient to follow the prescription given by the doctor.

As evident from the above discussion, various unanswered questions and controversies exist as far as the exact nature of the relationship between religiosity/spirituality and coping with physical and psychological distress due to illness is concerned. However, it can be safely concluded that overall the religious and spiritual beliefs provide the basis for coping with illness.

REFERENCES

Alferi, S.M., Culver, J.L., Carver, C.S., Arena, P.L. & Antoni, M.H. (1999). Religiosity, religious coping and distress: A prospective study of catholic and evangelical hispanic women in treatment for early-stage breast cancer, *Journal of Health Psychology, 4*, 343-356.

Augoustinos, M. and Walker, I. (1995). *Social Cognition : An integral Introduction*, New Delhi, Sage Publication, 134-162.

Bhusan, L.I. (1996). Asakti-anasakti : A model of mental health, *Yoga magazine*, Retrieved April 26, 2004, from http://www.yogamag.net/archives/1996/1jan96/menhelth.shtml.

Bhusan, L.I. (1998). Yogic life style and psychological well-being, *Yoga magazine*, Retrieved April 30, 2004, from http://www.yogamag.net/archives/1998/3may98/wellbe.shtml.

Bhusan, L.I. (1998). Yoga : An Instrument of Psychological Transformation, *Yoga magazine*, Retrieved March 4, 2004, from http://www.yogamag.net/archives/1998/5sep98/tranform.shtml.

Bowling, A. (1997). *Research Methods in Health : Investigating Health and Health Services*, Open University Press, Buckingham.

Brady, M.J., Peterman, A.H., Fitchett, G., Mo, M. and Cella, D. (1999). A case for including spirituality in quality of life measurement in oncology, *Psycho-Oncology, 8*, 417-428.

Carone, D.A. Jr. & Barone, D.F. (2001). A social cognitive perspective on religious beliefs : Their functions and impact on coping and psychotherapy, *Clinical Psychological Review, 21*, 989-1003.

Chamberlain, T.J. &. Hall C.A. (2000). *Realized Religion, Research on the Relationship between Religion and Health*, Templeton Foundation, Radnor.

Cole, B. and Pargament, K. (1999). Re-creating your life : A spiritual/psychotherapeutic intervention for people diagnosed with cancer, *Psycho-Oncology, 8*, 395-407.

Dalal, A. (2001). Health psychology. In J. Pandey (Ed.). *Psychology in India Revisited : Developments in the Discipline, Vol 2 : Personality and Health Psychology (pp. 356-411).* New Delhi : Sage Publications.

Exline, J.J., Yali, A.M. and Lobel, M. (1999). When God disappoints : Difficulty forgiving God and its role in negative emotion, *Journal of Health Psychology, 4*, 365-379.

Feher, S. and Maly, R.C. (1999). Coping with breast cancer in later life : The role of religious faith, *Psycho-Oncology, 8*, 408-416.

Flick, U. (2002). *An Introduction to Qualitative Research*, London : Sage Publication.

Harris, A.H.S., Thoresen, C.E., McCullough, M.E., & Larson, D.B. (1999). Spirituality and religiously oriented health interventions, *Journal of Health Psychology, 4*, 413-433.

Herzlich, C. (1973), *Health and Illness : A Social Psychological Analysis*, London : Academic Press.

Hill, P.C. and Pargament, K.I. (2003). Advances in the conceptualization and measurement of religion and spirituality : Implications for physical and mental health research, *American Psychologist, 58*, 64-74.

Holt, C.L., Lukwago, S.N. and Kreuter, M.W. (2003). Spirituality, breast cancer beliefs and mammography utilization among urban African American women, *Journal of Health Psychology, 8*, 383-396.

Kristeller, J.L. and Hallett, C.B. (1999). An exploratory study of a meditation based intervention for binge eating disorder, *Journal of Health Psychology, 4*, 357-363.

Levin, J.S. (1996). How religion influence morbidity and health : Reflections on natural history, salutogenesis and host resistance, *Social Science and Medicine, 43*, 849-864.

Miller, W.R. and Thoresen, C.E. (2003). Spirituality, religion and health : An emerging research field, *American Psychologist, 58*, 24-35.

McCormick, D.J. (2004). Galton on spirituality, *American Psychologist, 52*.

Mytko, J.J. and Knight, S.J. (1999). Body, mind and spirit : Towards the integration of religiosity and spirituality in cancer quality of life research, *Psycho-Oncology, 8*, 439-450.

Perrin, K.M. and McDermott R. J. (1997). The spiritual dimension of health : A review, *American Journal of Health Studies, 13, 90-99.*

Powell, L.H., Shahabi, L. and Thoresen, C.E. (2003). Religion and spirituality : Linkages to physical health, *American Psychologist, 58*, 36-52.

Sharma, A.K. (2004). On the revival of magic practices in the Indian systems of medicine with special reference to Gandhi, *Gandhi Marg, 25*, 435-445.

Stuckey, J.C. (2001). Blessed Assurance : The role of religion and spirituality in Alzheimer's disease care giving and other significant life events, *Journal of Aging Studies, 15*, 69-84.

Sudarshan, J. (2002). Yoga psychology and its applications in modern life, *Yoga Magazine*, Retrieved April 26, 2004, from http://www.yogamag.net/archives/2002/6nov02/yogapsy.shtml.

Taylor, E.J., Outlaw, F.H., Bernado, T.R., and Roy, A. (1999). Spiritual conflicts associated with praying about cancer, *Psycho-Oncology, 8, 386-394.*

Taylor, S.E. (1990). Health Psychology : The science and the field, *American Psychologist, 45*, 40-50.

Thoresen, C.E. (1999). Spirituality and health : Is there a relationship? *Journal of Health Psychology, 4*, 291-300.

Woods, T.E. and Ironson, G.H. (1999). Religion and spirituality in the face of illness : How cancer, cardiac and HIV patients describe their spirituality/religiosity, *Journal of Health Psychology, 4*, 393-412.

8

Integral Yoga–Its Contribution to Positive Health : Wellness

*S.N. Sinha**, *P.S. Rathore***, *O.P. Sharma****

Most universal objects of meditation are those characterized by centrality, whether, the source may be visual, *e.g.* seen-an array of illumination, verbal-name, such as 'Om', 'Allah', or 'Lord', and even 'Sunyata', 'Kensho', or 'accoustic-Naad' or 'Dhwani', (sound). All these kinds of 'images' more or less explicitly evoke the notion of a center, around which actions flow. The Center (Kendra) as a point of balance is related to source of idea of radiation, that is prominent in many widespread objects of meditation. The objects of meditation vary in different forms and practiced in a pantheistic context, as

Table 8.1 : Forms of Meditation in Various Religions in World

	1	2	3
Form	Detached	Vriti	Expresive
Manifested in	Sunyata emptiness in Buddhists form	Nirodh (concentration, transparence, absorption) Yoga, Patanjati	(Surrender) Sufisms, Christianity, Bhagvad Gita

The alternative forms of meditation represent a pantheistic–convergence. In one form or approach the individual attempts to interiorize a given form (source of energy or light, sound, Prakash, Naad) until he absorbs the object in himself (Atmsaat). In another form the individual seeks attainment to a formless (Nirakaar) depth, out of which an imagery, or an attitude of equanimity emerges or develops. The former is absorptive and introjective. The latter, is

*Emeritus Professor, Psy. & Ex. V.C., UOR, Jaipur, India.
**Associate Professor, UOR, Jaipur, India.
***Asstt. Prof., Deptt. of Psychology, UOR, Jaipur, India.

expressive, the meditator seeks to relinquish expectation (Niskam–Nirakar, Fana, Sufi), unites with Lord–surrenders to unprogrammed–spontaneity.

Although, the forms may seem to be different, they converge upon a common end-state. All the forms and symbols that traditions of mankind offer as starting points or perspectives of meditation have originated in spontaneity. Hence, in accordance with Jung's (1963) view, the images become more "collective", and therefore similar to the universal pattern of myth, root individual's self.

Basically, in all these forms of meditation the following three states have to be strived :

(a) Stilling of mind—'*Vritti*'.

(b) Separating ego functions—'*Ahm-bhav*'.

(c) Enter a domain of experience—with '*Sambhav*' or feelings of equanimity :

This reduces, meditation as a means of elucidating the experience by mediator and reflecting upon them. As to names of God, in different religions, there are also aspects of ultimate reality. It is the experience that is expressed in theistic formulation in conformity with God's will and in alternative cognitive maps, it is also expressed as a surrender to Dharma (a Law of the Universe). Thus, meditation constitutes an exercise of attention, and it is also a practice in centeredness, a practice in being oneself and knowing oneself.

Integral Yoga

In a book entitled "Practical Guide to Integral Yoga" (1955) a publication from Sri Aurobindo Ashram, Pondichery, the optimal relevance of Integral yoga has been stated in the words of Sri Aurobindo, that "the nuclear idea of relevance of yoga to life and health by yoga, we not only seek the infinite, but we call upon the infinite to unfold itself in human life." Sri Aurobindo, while elaborating upon the ameliorative efficacy of yoga further, said that 'By Yoga we can rise from falsehood to truth, out of weakness into force, out of pain and grief into bliss ... out of darkness to light, out of confusion into purity, out of imperfection into perfection, out of self-division into unity ... ." The practical ideas as suggested by Sri Aurobindo is that 'When God in his perfection embraces everything, we must also become all embracing and absorbing."

The secularistic or pantheistic view of Puran or Integral Yoga is that the dualities have to be replaced by unity, egoism by divine consciousness, struggle and effort by self-centered divine force. All this has been called by great saint in securalistic view of Integral yoga by saying that "all this is called in the language of Christ as bringing down the kingdom of heaven on earth, or in modern language, realising and effectuating God in the world.

The concept of positive health has been visualized by Aurobindo, as a process of Transformation of a psychic nature. This transformation would take place or it can be effectuated, through the action of inner consciousness to higher states of consciousness—and produces–or transforms, or creates an image of its own. The obstacles and difficulties encountered in this process of transformation have been mentioned as it is hard to get rid of old biases, or maladaptive 'stress including responses', yet the resistance has to be overcome.

Gita Vedantic View and Integral Yoga

These forms of yoga–contain all that is essential in Gita Yoga. Sri Aurobindo's Integral

Yoga also posits complete surrender, and the truth embedded in supramental consciousness, so that it provides the power to work on life and matter. Gita, follows, the vedantic tradition. The twin notion of insight into pathologies, can be arrived at both by supreme realization and surrender.

Another practical implication of therapeutic value imparts resilience to life stressors, lies in Aurobindo's message of "consciousness as the means of the complete transformation of earthly life." In support of Gita based Yogic method Sri Aurobindo mentioned in Ashram's, publication on Integral yoga. "I suggested the Gita method for you because the opening, which is necessary for yoga, may seem to be difficult, so the way of 'GITA IS ITSELF A PART OF YOGA'. ...The Gita yoga—"as potent contributor to positive Health—lies in the conquest of desire, egoless and desireless action, an entering into cosmic consciousness and the sense of unity with all creatures."

Conze, (1956) in his book on "Buddhist Meditation", says, that in Buddhist formulation, there is no such things as self, one can only convey the experience of attainment of 'Sunyata' or 'emptiness'. The empty aspect of meditative state may be seen as a direct extension of concentrative form of mediation. Buddhist term this state as "bare attention". The culmination of this ego state of ego dissolution is achieved in 'Nirvana' and 'fana-fillilah' in Islam. Nirvana is an awakening to reality and the finding that one's identity is in the emptiness that contains all things—in themselves. Upekkha, is the goal of Buddhist meditation, which leads to peace equanimity, and compassion.

It must be noted that it is not only Buddhism that bears the epithet of compassion. In Christianity and Islam also love and compassion are the most prominent aspects of goodness. In Islam, again, the Compassionate and the Merciful are the terms used in almost each chapter of the Koran. For Tibetans, there is a condition in which equanimity has been considered as the foundation of love, peace and as source of 'selfless caring'.

The psychological process of giving oneself rests on a measure of non-attachment. Hence, the bliss of meditation state is a joy beyond hedonistic notions of pleasure and pain, a sense of attunement with the infinite body, that takes place upon surrender, as is stated in Bhagavad Gita "Feelings of heat and cold, pleasure and pain, are caused by the contact of senses with the objects. They come and go, never last long. You must accept them with equanimity and hedonistically. A serene spirit and person with positive health, accepts pleasure and pain as part of life, with an even mind and is unmoved either."

REFERENCES

Chang, C. (1959). *The Practice of ZEN*, N.Y. : Harper Brothers.

Conze, E. (1956). *Buddhist Meditation*, London : Classics of East-West.

Deikman A. (1966). Deautomatization of Mystic Experience, *Psychiatry*, *29*, 324-28.

Jung, C.T. (1963). *Essays on a Science of Mythology*, Princeton : Princeton University.

Shah, U. (1969). *The Sufis*, London.

Sri Aurobindo (1955). *A Practical Guide to Integral Yoga, Pondicherry*, Aurobindo Ashram Publication.

9

Wellness Programming in Organisations and Training in Mental Silence : Psychological Perspectives

S.S. Kaushik* & Abhilasha Singh**

"He who has health has hope, and he who has hope has everything."

As citizens of the universe, possible persons on the threshold of a rapidly evolving global network, our vision of the possible profession is to promote the holistic development of all persons for living productively and harmoniously in the technologically complex, culturally diverse, and increasingly interdependent world of tomorrow.

As we approach this topic, it may be helpful to discuss the meaning of the terms health, wellness etc.

Wellness may be defined as the level of functioning at which individuals feel comfortable and are considered healthy to be for them and for society. Wellness commonly involves a multidimensional schema that values balancing the various tasks of life such as vocation, family, recreation, and physical, emotional, social, intellectual and spiritual health. Positive health enhancing activities include eating natural foods, taking vitamins, meditating and participating in regular exercise. In past researches, there is a strong support for the idea that regular exercise can have a beneficial effect on people's physical and psychological health. During recent years, there has been an increased emphasis among psychologists on positive wellness, that is health related activities that are both preventive and remedial and have a therapeutic value for those individuals who practice them consistently (Witmer & Sweeney, 1999). For the person to be a whole, healthy, functioning organism, one must evaluate the physical, psychological, intellectual, social, emotional and environmental process (Carlson & Ardell,1998.). Signs of the holistic movement toward health and wellbeing are apparent everywhere and are spilling over in their impact globally across all ages.

*Professor & Head, Deptt. of Psychology, M.M.V., BHU, Varanasi.
**Asstt. Prof., School of Management Sciences, Varanasi.

Research backs up the basis for the wellness movement and in some ways continues to lead it. In an extensive review of literature on the effectiveness of physical fitness on measures of personality, Doan and Scherman, (1987), found strong support for the idea that regular exercise can have a beneficial effect on people's physical and psychological health. Kaushik and Pathak (1993) have explained in detail about exercise adherence. The plethora of research supports psychologists who prescribe healthy habits to accompany regular counseling practices especially in stressed organizations. Thus wellness programming or "whole person" programming incorporates integration of mind, body and spirit. Psychologists/Counselors who work in organizational settings should emphasize a wellness approach focusing on prevention and education. They should take into account the mental, physical and social spheres of life and in the process recognize how they can focus on avoiding or minimizing external or internal disruptive forces. In my opinion, building up personality in general would have positive consequences for overall growth of organizations. Personality development can occur at any age and health, well-being and development are better promoted by dwelling more on possibilities and potentialities than on difficulties, weaknesses and failures.

Wellness and illness overlap and are actually two ends of a continuum. We need an active self-regulatory psychological programme in organizations where we practice relaxation daily.

Trained psychologists can initiate the programme but learning is of little value unless it is practiced. So maintenance and follow-up are essential. Some of the psychological techniques which may be useful for reducing the stress in organizations are given below :

- The Progressive Muscles Relaxation, introduced by Jacobson in 1929, is useful for overcoming the symptoms of tension, generalized anxiety, insomnia, headaches, neck and back pain, etc. The basic assumption is that muscular tension is related to anxiety and stress, and an individual will experience a marked and comforting reduction in the felt anxiety or stress if the tense muscles can be made to be flaccid. An efficient method for achieving such a state of muscle relaxation involves the successive tensing and relaxing of voluntary muscles in an orderly sequence until all the main muscle groups of the body are relaxed.
- The second technique is Systematic Desensitization developed by Wolpe (1958). In desensitization an attempt is made to substitute relaxation for anxiety on the principle of counter conditioning, through learning procedures. (Wolpe and Lazasur, 1966)
- The third technique of relaxation is Autogenic Training developed by Schultz. He used hypnosis and stated that through "mental concentration", one can produce similar sensations such as hand warmth & limb heaviness. Autogenic training helps clients to relax, it lowers their blood pressure and serves as a useful cognitive distraction technique.
- Bio-feed Back Technique is another such useful technique. Its uses have been highlighted by Palmer (1990). It provides the person with information regarding his physiological processes as heart beat, muscle tension, blood pressure, skin conductivity and temperature when he relaxes mentally. It is effective for tension headaches, migraine, asthma and the instrument gives immediate feedback, which has the effect of positive reinforcement (reward).

- Since stress may be related to cognitive appraisals and may be based frequently on misperception or irrational beliefs cognitive behaviour therapy has been developed to help persons cope better with stress that they experience. Ellis (1970, 1993) and Meichenbaum (1993) have given different techniques based on the same idea.

Some of the major assumptions underlying Cognitive Behaviour Therapy (CBT) are :

- Individuals are active processors of information.
- Thoughts, appraisals, expectancies and beliefs can trigger mood, physiological processes, social interactions and behaviours.
- Conversely, the mood, physiological changes, environmental factors and behaviours can influence the nature and content of a person's thought processes.
- Individuals are capable of learning more adaptive ways of thinking, feeling and behaving to feel more comfortable.

Based on the above assumptions, it may be stated that the objectives of CBT include, helping clients to view their problems as being manageable rather than overwhelming and to view themselves as active, resourceful and competent to handle problems and thereby work towards changing their maladaptive patterns of behaviour. The three major processes in CBT *viz*; cognitive restructuring, coping skills acquisition and training in problem solving are of immense benefit in reducing the level of stress in organizations and thus need special reference.

- Cognitive Restructuring is used to replace stress provoking thoughts or beliefs with more constructive and realistic thinking, leading to reduction of the perception of threat or harm to self.
- Coping Skills Acquisition aims to help clients develop a repertoire of skills for managing or dealing with stress and anxiety. Although these skills include cognitive restructuring, they encompass other techniques such as relaxation, distraction, imagery and generation of positive coping self statements.
- Problem Solving Training includes a step by step approach in dealing with the problem. The seven important steps are problem identification, goal selection, generation of alternatives, consideration of alternatives, consideration of consequences, decision-making, implementation and evaluation. This approach has been found highly effective in stress and crisis management in organizations.

To conclude with, it is suggested that if one desires to keep all his dimensions in a state of wellbeing, he must think positive, feel vigilantly relaxed, learn and practice deep muscle relaxation twice daily, do exercise or brisk walking or jogging for 20 minutes at least five days a week, quit smoking and alcohol, eat low fat, low sugar, low salt diet and thus transform the life at present, as well as pave the path for healthy aging!

REFERENCES

Beck, A.T. (1975). *Cognitive Therapy & the Emotional Disorders*, New York : International University Press.

Carlson, J. & Ardell, D.B. (1998). Physical fitness as a pathway to wellness and effective counseling. In R. Hayes & R. Aubrey (Eds.), *New Directions for Counseling and Human Development*, pp. 383-396, Denvor, Co : Love.

Doan, R.E., & Scherman, A. (1987). The therapeutic effect of physical fitness on measures of personality : A literature review, *Journal of Counseling and Development*, *66*, 28-36.

Ellis, A. (1970). *The Essence of Rational Psychotherapy : A Comprehensive Approach in Treatment*, New York : Institute for Rational Living.

Ellis, A (1993). Changing rational emotive therapy (RET) to rational emotive behaviour therapy, (REBT). *The Behaviour Therapist*, *16*, 257-258.

Jacobson, E. (1929). *Progressive Relaxation*, Chicago University, Chicago Press.

Kaushik, S.S., & Pathak, A. (1993). Exercise behaviour for promoting sports excellence. In J. Mohan, N.K. Chadha & Dr. S. Akhtar (eds.), *Psychology of Sports : The Indian Perspective*, pp. 45-51, New Delhi, Friends.

Meichenbaum, D. (1993). Changing conceptions of cognitive behaviour modification; Retrospect and Prospect, *Journal of Consulting and Clinical Psychology*, *61*, 202-204.

Palmer, S. (1990). Uses of biofeedback techniques in cognitive behavioural therapy, *Bulletin of the Association of Behavioural Clinicians*, *8*, 29-34.

Witmer, J.M., & Sweeney, T.J. (1999). Toward wellness : The goal of helping. In T.J. Sweeney (Ed.), *Adlerian Counseling : A Practitioner's Approach*, Philadelphia : Taylor & Francis.

Wolpe, J. (1958). *Psychotherapy by Reciprocal Inhibition*, Stanford; Stanford University Press.

Wolpe, J., & Lazarus, A.A. (1966). *Behaviour Therapy Technique : A Guide to Treatment of Neurosis*, Oxford : Pergamon.

SECTION—II

Health in Psycho-Social Perspective

10

Pattern of Mental Health in Adolescents

Farzana Alim*

Health is a valuable asset for every individual. According to an Arabian proverb, "A man, who is healthy, has an optimistic view and who has optimistic view, has everything." In evaluating, judging and assessing the quality of a person's adjustment, generally we use terms such as good adjustment, bad adjustment and scmetimes maladjustment. Good adjustment and mental health are almost synonymous these days. An individual who has achieved good adjustment will be called mentally healthy. Mental health is more often conceptualized as a personal quality even though the person might be having difficulty in adjusting to a particular situation. However, mental health is also related to physical health. Physical health is incomplete without mental health. Mental health is related to mind's happiness, satisfaction and peace. In recent years adjustment problems have increased, specially problems of interpersonal relationship. In modern age everybody is under stress and tension. Under such circumstances the individual cannot adjust himself to his environment. If a person's mental health is good the coordination between himself and the environment also remains good.

To a large extent mental health seems to be a function of emotional security, and the roots of this security are embedded within the home and family. In the present situation one must understand the tremendous role played by home and family in shaping the individual's personality and, consequently, in laying the foundations for a mentally healthy person. Home is the matrix of an individual's personal traits. How his parents, brothers, sisters, other relatives and grandparents treated him like a child, may serve to account for his present shyness, boldness, nervousness, depression and ill health. That is why family background is important as it shapes beliefs, attitudes and ideas of a growing child. A home atmosphere, where there is mutual trust adds to one's feelings of security and aids mental hygiene. The child who feels unwanted or rejected by one or both parents is likely to become the victim of feelings of inferiority. Building up a sense of security in a child is thus a major parental responsibility. There are certain self-evident precautions to be observed in the way of not

*Reader in Home Science, Women's College, Aligarh Muslim University, Aligarh.

playing favourites by being more generous with one child than with another because there are so many psychological dangers of playing favourites.

The concept of mental health has different meaning in different cultures, however, it can be viewed as self-esteem, happiness, tolerance, adjustment in a typical situation, feeling of security and confidence in general. Adequate self-knowledge, adequate life goal, environmental mastery, growth and learning from experiences in life and integration and consistency of personality are also the other aspects of mental health.

Jahoda (1958) identified the different aspects of positive mental health as an attitude of an individual toward his own self, the accessibility of the self to consciousness, the correctness of the self-concept, its relation to the sense of identity and the acceptance by individual of his own-self, growth and development or self-actualization, integration, autonomy, perception of reality and environmental mastery.

So, mental health is an integral component of health through which a person realizes his or her own cognitive, affective and relational abilities. With a balanced mental disposition, one is more effective in coping with the stresses of life, can work productively and fruitfully and is better able to make a positive contribution to his or her community (WHO, 2001). For Clausen *et al.* (1966) a mentally healthy individual maintains good adjustment with social situation, and is engaged in some or the other project intended to benefit society.

Verma, Nehra and Puri (1998) proposed a dual theory of mental health. This theory regards mental health as an absence of mental illness and a presence of certain factors of positive mental health. The positive mental health factors include a sense of well being, satisfaction, hope, adjustment, ego-strength, superego, creativity, ability to enjoy, happiness, honour, quality of life, self-realization, and social support.

Some negative aspects of mental health such as tension, anxiety; worry depression, frustration instability, lack of confidence, drug addiction and antisocial behaviour have been identified. It may also include insomnia, hypertension, short temper and attention deficit disorder. Mental health is concerned with the prevention of inadequate adjustment or with those processes or methods that help the maladjusted individual to readjust himself with the society. The aim of mental health is to enable every individual in society to make good adjustment with the environment. Some of the individuals are born with a strong constitution but some are not. So the individuals, with strong constitution, are able to strive hard. The study of personality gives us some insight into the aspects of mental health. The behaviour and personality of child is determines his interaction with other people and this is directly related to mental health. Thus, the status of mental health is one of the most important core issues of human existence.

Larry (1998) explained mental health as absence of mental illness, appropriate social behaviour, freedom from worry and guilt, personal competence and control, self acceptance and actualization, unification and organization of personality, open mindedness and flexibility.

Thus, the family, one's personality characteristics and other socio-cultural factors, economic condition, discrimination, patterns of relationship as emotional security and ability to give and receive affection and love influence mental health of an individual.

The present study has been taken up with the objective to study the pattern of mental health in male and female adolescents (14-17 years).

METHOD

Sample

A sample of 100 children (50 males and 50 females) in the age range of 14-17 years was randomly selected from population of secondary school students of Aligarh.

Tool

A self-structured questionnaire developed by the investigator was used to measure mental health pattern of children in the age range of 14-17 years.

Procedure

The data was collected from the children in the age range of 14-17 years irrespective of caste, class, religion and to socioeconomic status. The investigator informed the subjects that their information would be kept confidential. Subjects, generally, took 20-25 minutes to complete the questionnaire.

RESULTS AND DISCUSSION

The mental health scores of the male and female respondents were computed separately on eight dimensions. These have been shown in Table 10.1.

Table 10.1 : Mental Health Scores on Eight Dimensions and the Significance of Difference Between Male and Females

S. No.	*Dimension/Aspects of Mental Health*	*Males (n=50)*		*Females (n=50)*		*t*
		Mean	*S.D.*	*Mean*	*S.D.*	
1.	Integration of personality	13.24	1.40	11.50	0.92	9.88**
2.	Depression, insomnia, worries, anxiety and headache	21.22	4.47	21.84	4.85	0.129
3.	Examination stress, home work, tuition and coaching	30.30	11.22 9	29.44	11.10 7	0.385
4.	Time pressure, traffic, noise, pollution, hectic schedule	38.00	5.85	41.40	6.05	7.34**
5.	Parental pressure, expectation and household work	36.62	4.54	41.94	3.95	6.57**
6.	Self realization/actualization	6.00	0.63	6.34	1.02	1.61
7.	Adjustment to home environment	8.41	1.89	10.16	1.39	7.29**
8.	Freedom to play; recreation and creativity	16.76	7.87	11.46	6.15	4.90**

$p<.01$.

Data presented in Table 10.1 shows the mean scores on various dimensions of mental health for males and females separately. The mean of integration of personality was more for males (13.24) as compared to females (11.50). Statistically, the difference between males and females was found to be significant ($t = 9.88$, $p<0.01$).

The mean scores for the second aspect of mental health related to depression, insomnia, worries, anxiety and headache was more in females (21.84) as compared to males (21.22). But this difference was statistically insignificant ($t = 0.129$, $p > 0.05$). The mean of examination stress, homework, tuition or coaching was more (30.30) in males as compared to females (29.44). This difference was also was found to be insignificant ($t = 0.385$, $p>0.05$).

The mean of time pressure, traffic noise, hectic schedule was higher in females group (41.40) as compared to male group (38). Significant difference was found between males and females ($t = 7.34$, $p<0.01$).

The mean of parental pressure expectation and household work was higher (41.94) in females as compared to males (36.62). Statistically, this difference was found to be significant ($t = 6.57$, $p<0.01$).

The mean of adjustment to home environment was higher in the females group (10.16) as compared to group of males (8.41). Statistically, the difference was found to be significant between males and females in this mental health aspect ($t = 7.29$, $P<0.01$).

The mean of freedom to play, recreation, and creativity was more (16.76) in males as compared to females (11.46), the difference between the two means was found to be significant at .01 level. ($t = 4.90$, $P<0.01$).

The results of the present study revealed that males and female differed significantly from each other in terms of integration of personality, time pressure, traffic noise, hectic schedule, parental pressure and expectation, adjustment to home environment, freedom to play and recreation/creativity.

Thus the present study indicated a difference in the pattern of mental health of females and males. These results can be discussed in terms of the impact of the stress which has gained widespread attention in recent years. More and more children are being exposed to severely stressful life situations due to rise in competition, hectic schedule, traffic jams, noise pollution, peer pressure etc. Parents' focus has shifted to success, career and social aspects, which also contributes to the same problem. In this situation, children's emotional needs, individual attention, physical and mental health are oftenly ignored.

All children irrespective of their gender exhibited problems related to time pressure, lack of sleep, stress, headache etc. These behavioural and emotional problems, lead to major life stresses. Kataria, Swanson and Trevathan (1987) have also reported that the sleep disturbances common in early childhood tend to persist in the later school years and the same trend has been found by the present investigator. The persistence of sleep disturbances may be indicative of the presence of stress in the child's environment.

It can be concluded that expecting the anxiety stress related and self realization/ actualization aspects of mental health male and female adolescents differed significantly. The, female adolescents scored higher than male adolescents on time pressure, parental pressure and adjustment to home environment dimension of mental health. Further, the home environment has been found to be an important determinant of stress and mental health of children.

Parents should be made aware of the importance of physical and mental health, which depends upon healthy eating habits, exercise, games and healthy environment. School adjustment is related to academic achievement. So those children who do well academically tend to be socially adequate while those who have academic problems tend to have more problems like disturbed personality and mental ill health. In some representative studies, 20 to 42 percent of the children have been found to be moderately maladjusted, and 1 to 12 percent have been identified as seriously maladjusted. Boys are much more likely to be considered maladjusted than girls.

Use of consultation services, continuing evaluation of pupils, sophistication of both teachers and pupils and a greater emphasis on teacher parent cooperation are some of the effective mental health programmes which have been advocated. Child development workers and counselling workers must try to arrange camps, workshops, programmes and seminars relating to the promotion of mental health of children.

REFERENCES

Arkoff, A.B.E. (1968). *Adjustment and Mental Health,* Sydney : McGraw Hill.

Clausen *et al.* (1966). *Contemporary Social Problems,* New York : Harcourt Brace.

Jahoda, M. (1958). *Current Concepts of Positive Mental Health,* New York : Basic Books.

Kataria, S., Swanson, M. S., & Trevathan, G.E. (1987). Persistence of sleep disturbances in preschool, *Journal of Pediatrics, 110,* 642-646.

Larry, V.W. (1998). The relationship between religion and mental health, *Journal of Social Issues, 51,* 33-48.

Verma, S.K., Nehra, A. & Puri, A. (1998). Quality and quantity of mental health, *Journal of the Indian Academy of Applied Psychology, 24,* 59-62.

World Health Organization Brochure (2001).

11

Social Commitment and Well-Being

Geeta Rani Magoo*

Health has been conceptualized as a concept much broader than illness. It is generally considered to be a state a complete physical, social and mental well being which includes absence of disability and freedom from symptoms. Stress, personality factors, life style factors can have both positive and negative health consequences. The individual social circumstances are also of particular importance in determining the way in which patients cope and in the degree of success that coping strategies can have in regulating their health and well-being. Epidemologic studies have shown that simple measures of social network are significant predicators of longevity. These include marital status, number of close friends and membership to religious groups and institutes.

Berkman and Breslow (1983) reported that men with weak social networks were 2.5 time as likely to die within a definite period than those with extensive networks. However, the benefit was more pronounced in women. Reduced emotional stress resulting from automobile accident injuries and higher self esteem and life satisfaction in burn patients who have support from family and friends have also been observed (Davidson, Bowden and Tholea, 1979; Porrit, 1979). Hintikka, Koskela, Kontula Koskela and Viinamaeki (2001) studied the association between the number of close friends and mental well being and found that mental distress was increased in men with no friends and among those who had 1 or 2-4 friends as compared with those who had more friends. Social relations were related to increase in satisfaction with life and reduction in loneliness. Further, assertiveness and perceived social support from family and friends correlated negatively with depressive symptomatology (Rolon, 2001). Having a good social support system is a significant predictor of good health maintenance, by contrasts being alone and lonely predicts multiple illnesses and death from multiple causes (Hafen, Karren, Frandsen & Smith, 1996). Lynch (1977) in a book entitled 'The Broken Heart', argues convincingly that the relatively high incidence of heart disease in industrialized communities stems in part from the absence of positive human relationships. Psychiatrist Spiegel (1991) reported that a group of seriously ill breast cancer patients who had been assigned to group

*Lecturer in Psychology, Hindu Girls College, Sonepat.

therapy survived on average twice as long as a comparable group of women given only standard medical treatment due to the development of strong, mutually supportive ties.

Thus, it appears that received support helps in coping with stress. However, the mechanism by which close relationships protect against illness is not well understood, Cohen and Syme (1985) identified two rival explanations for this relationship. The stress buffering model assumes that social relationships buffer the impact of stress, while the main effect model assumes that social relations influence, health outcomes independently of stress, in a variety of ways such as through modelling reinforcement of healthy behaviours, encouragement, peer influences etc.

Beckmann (2001) has studied the demands of care giving and care-giver health and well-being. Results revealed that care-givers who reported receiving more instrumental and affective support from others also reported greater satisfaction with the support they received or the support they perceived as available to them; a higher sense of care-giving self-efficacy; and lower depression, better physical and emotional health and higher sense of positive well-being. Earlier, studies have shown that mere expression of stressful events by healthy respondents *i.e.* writing about real or imagined stressful experiences, lead to a reduction in visits to hospital for minor ailments (Pennebaker, Kiecolt-Glaser and Glaser, 1988). Thus, giving support, leads to strengthening and expansion of ones own social support system. It might also benefit the individual directly as it helps in developing positive coping strategies and may enhance well being *via* the empathetic behaviour.

The focus of research with regard to the effect of social support has been on the receiver. The present investigator felt that it might be fruitful to study the influence of social commitment on well being. It was hypothesized that social commitment would enhance well being.

METHOD

Design

In the present investigation a two group design was used to study the differences in well being, of a socially committed group (consisting of respondents who were actively associated with an NGO) and a socially non committed group, who were not members of any socially active group.

Sample

A purposive sample of 100 subjects (Socially Committed group 50, Non Social-Commitment group : 50), whose age ranged between 35-50 years who voluntarily agreed to participate in the study was taken. All the respondents were at least graduates and belonged to the middle socio economic status.

Tool

A Well-Being Scale (WBS) by Sindhu consisting of 50 statements, divided equally in 10 statements for 5 different aspects of well-being was used. The 5-point Likert rating scale (Very Much, Rather So Much, Average, To Some Extent and Not So Much) was used to indicate the how strongly one agreed with each of the statement. The scale has 29 positive items and 21 negative items.

Procedure

Well-Being scale was administered individually to each subject. Subjects were approached at their residence by the investigator and they were instructed and requested to answer each item using the numerical ranking (1-5) indicating how strongly they agreed with each of the statement. The instructions were clearly specified on the top of the scale. It was also ensured that subjects responded to each of the items of the scale. They were also briefed about the Well-Being scale and it's purpose. Finally the responses of the subjects were scored and the data was statistically analysed.

RESULTS AND DISCUSSION

The mean well being scores of the two group of subjects on the Physical, Mental, Social, Emotional and Spiritual dimensions were computed. Further, the Total well being score of both the groups were also calculated. The difference between the mean scores of the two groups was statistically analysed by applying t test.

Table 11.1 Significance of Difference Between Mean Well Being Scores

	Social Commitment Group	*Non-Social Commitment Group*	*t value*
Total Well-Being Score	197.45	182.80*	3.43 p<.01
Physical	41.45	36.80*	3.73 p<.01
Mental	37.55	36.80	n-s
Social	39.65	37.60	n-s
Emotional	38.55	37.55	n-s
Spiritual	42.15	34.05*	3.96 p<.01

From Table 11.1 it is evident that the socially committed group was significantly higher on the total well being score ($t = 3.43$, $p < .01$). Thus the results show that involvement in social activities did enhance the well being of the respondents.

Further comparisons on the individual dimensions show that the mean scores of the socially committed group was higher on all the 5 dimensions. However a significant difference was observed only in case of the physical and spiritual dimensions ($t = 3.73$ and 3.96, respectively). These results are in line with those of Beckmann (2001) who also reported higher sense of well being in the care giver group.

Serving others or commitment for society enhances the well-being and positivity of a person and it is evident that helping others compensates the negative aspect of a person, enhances the feeling of self-worth, self-efficacy, coping strategies, contentment, social communication skill, promotes group culture, makes the person strong, develops internal happiness, peace of mind, spiritual growth and understanding about life in general and specific which further lowers depression and reduces stress. The effect of received social support has already been established, however service-givers also benefit in the process of serving others.

The present results are in line with the main effect model of stress. Involvement in social activity encourages healthy behaviours as it makes the individual more aware of the potential hazards and may be leading to development of positive coping strategies. Further, the active involvement results in a more active lifestyle, whereby physical well being is increased. The spiritual well being is also enhanced as the individual is involved in the process of giving and the empathy experienced by the individual might lead to spiritual upliftment.

The results also in congruence with those of Berkman and Breslow (1983), who also found that extensive social networks had a beneficial effect on health.

Thus it appears that perceived social support, has a positive effect on the well being of an individual, where not only the receiver but the giver also benefits. Active social involvement reduces social isolation, increases perceived social support and may help in development of positive coping strategies.

REFERENCES

Beekman, N.R. (2001). *Famiy Caregiving, Dementia, and Social Support. (Caregiving, Alzheimer's disease)*, U. Michigan, US.

Berkman, L.F. & Breslow, L. (1983). *Health and Ways of Living : Findings from the Alameda Country Study,* New York : Oxford University Press.

Davidson, T.N., Bowden, L. & Tholen, D. (1979). Social support as a moderator of burn rehabilitation, *Archives of Physical Medicine and Rehabilitation, 60,* 556.

Hafen, B.Q., Karren, K.J., Frandsen, K.J., & Smith, N.I., (1996). *Mimd/Body Health : The Effects of Attitudes, Emotions and Relationships,* Needham Heights, MA : Allyn & Bacon.

Hintikka, J., Koskela, T., Kontula, O., Koskela, K., Viinamaeki H. (2001). *Men, Women and Friends : Are there Differences in Relation to Mental Well-being?* Kuopio University Hospital, Dept. of Psychiatry, Kuopio, Finland.

Lynch, J.J. (1977). *The Broken Heart,* New York : Basic Books.

McAuley, E., Blissmer, B., Marquez, D.X., Jerome, G.J., Kramer, - A. F., Katula, J. (2001). *Social Relation, Physical Activity and Well being in Older Adults.* U Illinions, Dept. of Kinesiology, Urbana, IL, US.

Pennebaker, J.W., Kiecolt-Glaser, J.K. and Glaser, R. (1988). Disclosure of trauma and immune function : Health implications for psychotherapy, *Journal of Consulting and Clinical Psychology, 56,* 239-245.

Porrit, D. (1970). Social support in crises : Quality or Quantity, *Social Science and Medicine, 13A,* 715-721.

Rolon, R. (2001). *An Exploration of the Impact of Social Support and Assertiveness on the Psychological Well being of Puerto Rican Women in New York City.* City U New York, US.

Spiegel, D. (1991). A psychological intervention and survival time of patients with metastatic breast cancer, *Advances, 7,* 10-19.

12

An Exploration of Self-Actualization and Personality Correlates Among Professionals

*Nishat Afroz** & *Ranjana Mitra***

Maslow's main premise was 'what makes some people live up to their full potential' or 'what makes some people self-actualize'. Maslow's concept of self-actualization has been based on hierarchy of needs. His argument is that if social and physical environments can fulfill basic physical and psychological needs, an individual has the chance to go ahead for satisfying his meta needs, *i.e.*, the desire for justice, unity, beauty and order. The basic needs lead to his physical growth and meta needs lead to his psychological growth and self-actualization. Self-actualization is dedicated to wholeness of human life—and it is his main contribution to humanistic psychology. The essential meaning of the concept, self-actualization is found in the discovery of the real self and its expression and development. Self-actualizing people are seen as seeking meaning and accomplishment in their work and life. Their other needs become well satisfied. As a result these people tend to be primarily self motivated, capable of being mature on the job, and willing to integrate their own goals with those goals of their profession or the organization in which they work.

Interest in Maslow's (1962, 1970) theoretical conception of self-actualization or optimal personality functioning has increased rapidly within recent years. One of the major factors in upsurge of interest is the humanistically based realization that the growth and development of inherent human potentialities is not only important for mental health and well being of the individual but also for the community, the organization and the world at large. Maslow's meta psychological model of the self-actualizing being has been extensively investigated by different researchers (Wilkinson, 1979; Frick, 1982; Woolpert, 1982; Baaumeister, 1987; Coan, 1991).

Many investigators (McAlindon, 1981; Cangemi, 1987; Wacks, 1987; Schostac, 1989) have put forward the view that education is a creative source which will help in attaining self-

*Lecturer, Psychology Section, MMV, B.H.U., Varanasi.
**Reader, Psychology Section, MMV, B.H.U., Varanasi.

actualization. The purpose and aim of education, for example, the development of skills and potentialities, achievement, psychological nourishment, creativity is if inculcated in the individual, should lead to self-realization and help the individual self-actualize or be able to reach one's self-appointed goals. It has been suggested (McAlindon, 1981) that education in its broadest sense is the real hope for improving the quality of future generations. Learning to become a fully-functioning person can improve organizations, neighbourhood, families and societies. Cangemi (1984) suggested that institutions of higher education should critically evaluate their objectives to determine where they stand regarding the process of self-actualization. The views of the eastern philosophers are compared to the views of Maslow (Ghaskadei, 1981) and the authors feel that both focus attention on individual behaviour, self-fulfillment and self-awareness, and the goal and activities of education must be based on Maslow's hierarchy of needs and should be attainable to sustain interest in learning.

Self-actualization provides a means by which each educator whether he be parents, teachers, friends, or community can view each individual as an unique personality, full of special abilities and potentialities which should be nurtured, leading not only to individual gains by having a fully integrated and healthy personality but one who is equally important for the benefit and growth of a rich and vibrant society (Farmer, 1984).

A crucial element of Maslow's (1954) theory is that self-actualization, the highest need is the weakest biologically. This characteristic, in addition to many examples of failure to achieve self-actualization after satisfying the more basic needs suggests that self-actualization requires some auxiliary source of strength and support (Frick, 1982). Frick argued that strong conceptual support provided by growth enhancing concept is an essential variable for achieving self-actualization. Keeping all this in mind the present study proposes to explore the personality correlates of the self-actualization amongst professionals.

In the light of the above argument put forward by Frick (1982) the present investigation proposes that high education and learning, skill training and highly placed professional careers will provide many growth enhancing conditions for the subject of this study to be able to self-actualize. Further, the present study proposes that certain distinctive personality traits should emerge for professionals who have been able to self-actualize and to determine whether self-actualization as measured by a western tool is an adequate measure to understand how highly educated individuals of an entirely diverse culture like India view and understand the concept.

METHOD

Sample

The sample of the study consisted of 300 professionals. Professionals have been characterized as those individuals who are able to see practical results and impact of their high education and training for the benefit and development of the society. In the study 200 professionals were selected from the Institute of Medical Sciences, Institute of Technology, Faculty of Management Sciences, Faculty of Arts, Faculty of Social Sciences, Faculty of Science and Faculty of Commerce of Banaras Hindu University and 100 professionals were taken from the city of Varanasi as practicing doctors, engineers and lawyers.

Tools

Biographical data sheet to provide necessary demographic details about the selected samples.

Personal Orientation Inventory (POI), developed by E.L. Shostrom (1963) was used to select respondents who were self-actualized and those who were not self-actualized. It is a 150 two-choice item self-report questionnaire which reflects the values and behaviour of major importance in the development of self-actualizing person. The items are scored twice, first for two basic scales of personal orientation, inner-directed support (127 items) and time competent (27 items) and second for ten subscales each of which measures a conceptually important element of self-actualizing (1) Self-actualizing Value (SAV), (2) Existentiality (Ex), (3) Feeling Reactivity (Fr), (4) Spontaneity (S), (5) Self-regard (Sr), (6) Self Acceptance (Sa), (7) Nature of Man (Nc), (8) Synergy (Sy), (9) Acceptance of Aggression (A), (10) Capacity for Intimate Contact (C).

16 P.F. Questionnaire: The personality assessment tool was originally designed by Cattell (1964). The Hindi version by Kapoor (1970) was employed to carry out the study. The norms used were the original ones.

Procedure

The selected subjects were contacted individually. After aprising them of the aim of the study they were assured of confidentiality of their responses. After a complete rapport, now they were given the tools mentioned above and were requested to fill them up. The scoring was done as per the manuals. The Ss were divided into low & high self-actualized Ss and their scores on personality questionnaire were tabulated separately. Now the scores were put to analyses. t-test and correlation were used for statistical analyses.

RESULTS AND DISCUSSION

Overall finding was that out of 300 subjects 18 subjects were found to be self-actualized while the remaining subjects were not able to reach the required level for self-actualization. Though self-actualized and non self-actualized professionals have more or less same personality profile except on one factor of emotional stability on which self-actualized were found emotionally stable as compared to non self-actualized who were emotional. Although they (NSAZ) also have the supportive personality traits that makes them develop into individuals who are healthy, creative, intelligent and have the ability to express their creative potentialities in diverse and original ways while facing the challenges of their professional demands of work and dealing effectively with them, yet they were not able to reach the required level of time competency and inner-directedness to be able to self-actualize.

Table 12.1 : Mean, SD and Comparison of Differences Between Self Actualized (N = 18) and Non Self-actualized (N = 282) Professionals on the POI Scales

		Self-actualized		*Non-self-actualized*		
S.No.	*POI Scales*	*Mean*	*SD*	*Mean*	*SD*	*T*
1	2	3	4	5	6	7
1.	Time Competence (Tc)	18.55	.511	14.09	2.45	7.67**
2.	Inner-Directed (I)	90.11	4.71	75.66	7.89	7.66**
3.	Self Actualizing Value (SAV)	19.50	1.88	18.16	2.98	1.87
4.	Existentiality (Ex)	18.72	5.23	15.65	3.73	3.28*
5.	Feeling Reactivity (Fr)	14.44	3.03	13.03	2.71	2.12*
6.	Spontaneity (S)	11.88	2.37	10.60	2.14	2.44**

(Contd.)

Contd.

1	2	3	4	5	6	7
7.	Self-regard (Sr)	12.55	1.42	11.89	1.96	1.39
8.	Self-Acceptance (Sa)	16.77	3.42	13.59	2.81	4.58**
9.	Nature of Man (Nc)	11.72	1.36	11.58	1.78	.311
10.	Synergy (Sy)	7.00	1.57	6.29	1.39	2.06*
11.	Acceptance of Aggression (A)	15.16	3.01	14.19	2.68	1.48
12.	Capacity for Intimate Contact (C)	18.88	4.01	15.24	3.34	4.42**

*p<.05, **p<.01.

Table 12.1 gives the Mean, SD and Significance of difference between self-actualized and non-self-actualized professionals as identified by POI norms. Self actualized and non self-actualized professionals significantly differed on the scale of Time Competence (7.67, < .01), Inner-directedness (7.66, < .01), Existentiality (3.28, <.01), Feeling Reactivity (2.12, <.05), Spontaneity (2.44, <.01), Self Acceptance (4.58, < .01), Synergy (2.06, < 05), and Capacity for Intimate Contact (4.42, < .01). They did not differ on the scales of Self-actualizing Value, Self-regard, Nature of Man and Acceptance of Aggression.

The mean indicates that self-actualized professionals are time competent, inner-directed, flexible in application of values, sensitive to own needs and feelings, able to freely express feelings behaviourally, accept their self inspite of weaknesses, see opposites of life as

Table 12.2 : Mean, SD and Comparison of Differences between Self-actualized (N = 18) and Non Self-actualized (N = 282) Professionals on the 16 PF

		Self-actualized		*Non-self-actualized*		
S.No.	*POI Scales*	*Mean*	*SD*	*Mean*	*SD*	*T*
1.	Reserved vs Outgoing (A)	4.22	1.43	4.52	1.36	-.898
2.	Less Intelligent vs. More Intelligent (B)	7.22	1.39	7.28	1.54	-.164
3.	Emotional vs. Emotionally Stable(C)	6.55	1.46	5.40	1.88	2.53**
4.	Humble vs. Assertive (E)	5.44	1.38	5.44	1.32	.004
5.	Sober vs. Happy-g-lucky (F)	4.33	2.02	3.86	1.89	1.02
6.	Expedient vs. Conscientious (G)	6.66	1.74	6.01	1.71	1.56
7.	Shy vs. Bold (H)	5.55	2.25	5.56	1.70	-.011
8.	Tough-minded vs. Tender-minded (I)	5.16	1.58	5.20	151	-.096
9.	Trusting vs. Suspicious (L)	6.22	1.51	6.58	2.33	-.644
10.	Practical vs. Imaginative (M)	5.22	2.07	5.40	1.77	-.425
11.	Forth-right vs. Shrewd (N)	5.55	1.68	5.90	1.97	-.733
12.	Placid vs. Apprehensive (O)	5.61	1.24	5.38	1.54	.604
13.	Conservative vs. Experimenting (Q1)	5.94	1.69	5.56	1.62	.970
14.	Group Oriented vs. Self sufficient (Q2)	6.16	1.79	6.31	1.50	-.392
15.	Undisciplined vs. Controlled (Q3)	5.83	1.04	5.58	1.52	.678
16.	Relaxed vs. Tense (Q4)	4.16	1.72	4.81	1.93	-.138

*p <.05, **p<.01.

meaningfully related and have warm interpersonal relationships as compared to non-self-actualized. Both self-actualized and non-self-actualized reject the self-actualizing values, have marginally low self-worth, see men as essentially evil and deny feeling of anger and aggression.

Table 12.2 gives the mean, SD and significance of difference between self-actualized and non-self-actualized professionals on the 16 PF. As results indicate, self-actualized and non self-actualized significantly differed on only one factor of emotional stability. Self-actualized professionals were found to be more emotionally stable as compared to non self-actualized who were found to be more emotional (2.53 < .01). On the remaining factors both groups showed the similar traits of being reserved, intellectual, humble, sober, conscientious, bold, tough-minded, suspicious, practical, shrewd, placid, experimenting. self-sufficient, controlled and relaxed.

Table 12.3 : Correlation of POI Scales Against 16 PF of Self-actualized Professionals

POI Scales	*r*
1. Inner Directed & Assertive	–.532*
2. Existentiality & Imaginative	.472*
3. Existentiality & Shrewd	.518*
4. Self-Acceptance & Controlled	.533*
5. Nature of Man & Bold	–.559*
6. Nature of Man & Imaginative	–.480*
7. Capacity for Intimate Contact & Emotionally Stable	.642**
8. Capacity for Intimate Contact & Sober	–.510*
9. Capacity for Intimate Contact & Apprehensive	.479*

*p<.05, **p<.01.

Table 12.3 presents the correlation of POI scales against the 16 PF for self-actualized professionals. Significant and positive correlation was found between Existentiality and Imaginative (.472, < .05), Existentiality and shrewdness (.518, <.05), Self-acceptance and Controlled (.533, < .05), Capacity for Intimate Contact and Emotionally Stable (.642, <.01) and Capacity for Intimate contact and Apprehensive (.479, <.05). A significant but negative correlation was found between the Inner Directedness and Assertive (–.532, <.05), Nature of Man and Boldness (–.559, <.05), Nature of Man and Imaginative (–.480, <.05), and Capacity for Intimate Contact and Sober (–.510, <.05).

Existentiality is positively and significantly correlated with the imaginative and shrewd indicating that self-actualized subjects are flexible in application of values, are found to be self-motivated, imaginatively creative and concerned with essentials. They tend to be polished, experienced and often hardheaded and analytical, have intellectual and unsentimental approach to the situation. The self-actualized professionals are able to accept themselves in spite of their weaknesses. They are controlled, socially precise and have regard for social reputation and a proper self image.

The scale of capacity for intimate contact were positively and significantly correlated with the factor of emotionally stable and apprehensive indicating that these self-actualized professionals have warm interpersonal relationship and they tend to be emotionally mature, stable, realistic about life and better able to maintain solid group morale. They were also found to be moody, and worriers having anxiety in difficulties. But the fact is that the mean was near the average value.

Inner directedness was negatively correlated with the humbleness, indicating that self-actualized professionals are independent, self-supportive, but to some extent, as the mean indicates, that they have the tendency to give way to others. They are docile, often dependent, confessing and have anxious personality traits. A negative but significant correlation between the nature of man and boldness indicates that self-actualized professionals are sociable, bold, ready to try new things, spontaneous and abundant in emotional response. On the other hand they see men as essentially evil or bad and are not synergistic.

Nature of men is negatively correlated with imaginative indicating that self-actualized subjects do not see men as essentially good. They cannot resolve the goodness-evil, masculine-feminine, selfishness-unselfishness, and spirituality-sensuality dichotomies in the nature of man. They tend to be unconventional, unconcerned over everyday matter, self-motivated, imaginatively creative, concerned with essentials. Their inner directed interests sometimes lead to unrealistic situations accompanied by expressive outbursts. Their individuality tends to cause them to be rejected in group activities.

The scale of capacity for intimate contact is also negatively correlated with the sober, this indicates that they have the ability to develop meaningful, contactful relationships with other human beings, but they tend to be serious, introspective, and sometimes dour, pessimistic, unduly deliberate and primarily correct by observers.

Table 12.4 : Correlation of POI Scales Against 16 PF for Non-Self-actualized Professionals

POI Scales	*r*
1. Time Competence & Controlled	.153*
2. Inner Directed & More Intelligent	.139*
3. Inner Directed & Controlled	.168*
4. Self-actualizing Value & Outgoing	.119
5. Existentiality & Conscientious	-.129*
6. Feeling Reactivity & Self-Sufficient	.142*
7. Spontaneity & Apprehensive	.121*
8. Spontaneity & Tense	.138*
9. Self-Acceptance & Conscientious	-.119*
10. Self-Acceptance & Shrewd	.157*
11. Nature of Man & Reserved	.126*
12. Nature of Man & More Intelligent	.147*
13. Synergy & Tense	-.121*
14. Acceptance of Aggression & Emotionally Stable	-.128*
15. Acceptance of Aggression & Tense	.156**
16. Capacity for Intimate Contact & Conscientious	-.135*

*$p<.05$, **$p<.01$.

Table 12.4 presents the correlation of POI scales against the 16 PF for non self-actualized professionals. A positive and significant correlation was found between Time Competence and Controlled (.153, <.05), Inner Directedness and Intelligence (.139, <.05), Inner directed and Controlled (.168, <.05), Self-actualizing value and Reserved (.119, <.05), Feeling Reactivity and Self-sufficient (.142 <.05), Spontaneity and Apprehensive (.121, <.05), Spontaneity and Reserved (.138, <.05), Acceptance of self and Shrewd (.157, <.01), Nature of Man and Reserved (.126, <.05), Nature of Man and Intelligence (.147, <.05) and Acceptance of Aggression and Reserved (.156, <.01). A significant but negative correlation was found between the scales of Existentiality and Conscientiousness (–121, <.05), Self-Acceptance and Conscientiousness - (.119, <.05), Synergy and Relaxed (–.121, <.05), Acceptance of Aggression and Emotional Stability (–.128, < .05) and Capacity for Intimate Contact and Conscientious (–.135, <.05).

Time competence is significantly correlated with undisciplined indicating that non self-actualizing subjects are comparatively time competent. This marked time incompetence suggests that the non-self-actualizing subjects do not discriminate well between past and future. They are excessively concerned with past and future relative to present. A person who is past oriented may be characterized by guilt, regret, blaming and resentments. They regard for social demands. They are not overly considerate, careful or painstaking.

A positive and significant correlation was found between the scale of inner directed with intelligence and undisciplined. This indicates that other directed subjects appear to have been motivated to develop a radar system to receive signals from a far wider circle than simply the parents. There is a danger that the other directed persons may become oversensitive to others' opinion in matters of external conformity. Approval by others becomes the highest goal. They tend to be slow to learn and grasp, dull, given to concrete and literal interpretation and they were also found to be undisciplined, having self conflict.

The scale of self-actualizing value was significantly and positively correlated with the reserved indicating that the non-self-actualized subjects reject the values of self actualizing people, tend to be stiff, cool, skeptical and aloof. They like things rather than people, working alone and avoiding compromises of viewpoints.

The scale of feeling reactivity was also positively correlated with group oriented. This indicates that they are insensitive to own needs and feelings, and prefer to work and make decisions with other people, like and depend on social approval and admiration. The sub scale of spontaneity is significantly correlated with placid and relaxed factors. This shows that non self-actualized subjects are fearful of expressing feelings behaviourally while they tend to be placid, with unshakable nerve and they are also found to be relaxed, composed and satisfied. In some situations over satisfaction can lead to laziness and low performance.

A significant correlation was found for the scale of acceptance of self and forth-right, indicating that these professionals are unable to accept self with weaknesses. They are also unsophisticated, sentimental and simple. A positive significant correlation of the nature of man with the factor of reserved and intelligence, indicates that they see man as essentially evil or bad and they tend to be reserved, critical and detached, slow to learn and grasp, following concrete and literal interpretation. A significant correlation found between the acceptance of aggression and relaxed indicates that these subjects deny feelings of anger or aggression, they are relaxed and unfrustrated.

A negative but significant correlation was found for the scale of existentiality and conscientiousness, indicating that professionals who are not able to self-actualize hold values so rigidly that they may become compulsive and dogmatic. They tend to be exacting in character, dominated by sense of duty, persevering and usually conscientious and moralistic.

Conscientious was further negatively correlated with the two sub scales of POI, acceptance of self and capacity for intimate contact, indicating that non self-actualizing professionals are dominated by sense of duty. They are responsible, planful and prefer hard working people to witty companions but they are unable to accept own weaknesses or deficiencies and have face difficulty with warm inter personal relationship.

The scale of synergy was negatively correlated with relaxed, clearly indicating that they have the ability to see opposites of life as meaningfully related. When one is synergistic one sees that work and play are not different but they tend to be relaxed and satisfied, that disrupts their work performance and their over satisfaction can lead to laziness and low performance. Acceptance of aggression was negatively correlated with emotional stability. This indicated that they deny feelings of anger and aggression, are mature, stable, possessing ego strength and better able to maintain solid group morale.

The above findings indicate that most of the professionals in spite of high education and stimulating careers have not been able to self-actualize. They have the required traits that could lead them in the right direction if they could manage a balance between their need to grow to their full potential and demands of their work situations and career. Pertinent literature indicates that the teachers (Hankins & Clarks, 1989), professors (Hampton & Kerasotes, 1978), managers (Mathur & Yadava, 1987), have all turned out to be less self-actualizing than were hypothesized. These results are congruent with earlier Indian & non-Indian studies in this area.

Thus it was observed in this study that in spite of high education, skill training and highly placed career, growth enhancing and stimulating environment, very few faculty members have been able to attain the level of self-actualization. This can be viewed in terms of two arguments. One is that, the work organization, the society and the community is not able to provide the support and growth enhancing conditions to its members. There is a need to critically study, evaluate and identify areas and conditions of work that are acting as deterrents to fully functioning individuals. It is important to identify and implement all those practices that will be conducive for its members to develop into rich, vibrant and dynamic human resources of not only the organization but the community, the nation and the world.

The second argument in support of the inability of large members of highly educated, trained and skilled members to self actualize could be seen in terms of their cultural, religious and social values which are built in the personality from an early age and as the individual matures, barring few 'biological elite' as Maslow terms them only few people are able to rise above the pressure and compulsions of their particular culture and traditions to be energized by the need for self actualization. The Indian culture, religion and social values are based on love, tolerance, sacrifice, the need to put the other persons interest before one's own, maintenance and respect for familial and other relationships, consideration and conformity to traditional demands. This seems to be the reason why their stimulating careers are still not functioning effectively in their development towards truly self-actualizing persons.

One important argument may be that POI measures self actualization dimension routed in the western culture where the attainment of materialistic and individualistic goals of self actualization are emphasized, where as Indian notion of self actualization is based on the realization of spirituality within oneself.

As already mentioned, out of 300 only 18 subjects were able to self-actualize though the impulse to realize one's potential is natural and necessary, only a few ever do so. Maslow (1970) himself estimated that less than one percent of the population fulfills the need for self-actualization. Maslow advances three reasons for this first, people are invariably blind to their own potentialities, and second, the social environment often stifles development towards self fulfillment. A final obstacle is the strong negative influence exercised by the safety needs. The growth process demands a contrast willingness to take risks, to make mistakes and to break old habits. This requires courage. It logically follows that any thing that increases the individual's fear and anxiety also increases his tendency to regress towards safety and security.

To conclude, the study indicates towards very less number of professionals who could self actualise. However, the number in this small sample was quite high *i.e.* 6% of the sample taken as compared to 1% as indicated by Maslow. It is suggested to find out the causes for lack of self actualisation and implement the policies at individual and social level.

REFERENCES

Baaumeister, R.F. (1987). How the self becomes a problem : A psychological review of historical research, *Journal of Personality and Social Psychology, 52,* 163-176.

Cangemi, J.P. (1984). The real purpose of higher education : Developing self-actualizing personalities, *Education, 105* , 151-154.

Cangemi, J.P. (1987). Education and self-actualization, *Journal of Instructional Psychology, 14*, 164-175.

Cattell, R.B. (1964). *Handbook of 16 PF*, Institute of Personality and Ability Testing Illinois : Champaign.

Coan, R.W. (1991). Self-actualization and the quest for the ideal human, *Journal of Social Behaviour and Personality, 6,* 127-136.

Farmer, R. (1984). Humanistic education and self-actualizing theory, *Education, 105,* 162-172.

Frick, W.B. (1982). Conceptual foundations of self-actualization : A contribution to motivation theory, *Journal of Humanistic Psychology, 22,* 33-52.

Ghaskadei, V.Y. (1981). Self-actualization and east-west synthesis, *Indian Psychological Review, 20,* 40-41.

Hampton, J.D., & Kerasotes, D.L. (1978). Faculty level of SAZ in relation to student rating instructors, *Educational and Psychological Measurement, 39,* 971-975.

Hankins, N.E., & Clark, H. (1989). Self-actualization : Do teachers need it? *Journal of Human Behaviour and Learning, 6,* 7-13.

Maslow, A.H. (1954). *Motivation and Personality,* New York : Harper.

Maslow, A.H. (1962). *Toward a Psychology of Being,* New York : Van Nostrand Reinhold.

Maslow, A.H. (1970). *Religious Values and Peak Experiences,* New York : The Viking.

Mathur, P., & Yadava, S.R. (1987). Managerial effectiveness, leadership styles and SAZ, orientation of middle level managers in public sectors organizations in India, *Social Science International, 3,* 1-12.

McAlindon, H.R. (1981). Education for SAZ, *Training and Development Journal, 35,* 85-91.

Schostac, J. (1989). The play of education, Special issue : New directions for educational theory : II. Conceptualizing the problems of educational change, *Cambridge Journal of Education, 19,* 207-223.

Shostrom, E.L. (1963). Edits manual for POI, *Educational Industrial Testing Services,* San Diego, California.

Wacks, V.Q. (1987). A case for self-transcendent as a purpose of adult education, *Adult Education Quarterly, 38,* 46-55.

Wilkinson, K.P. (1979). Social well being and community, *Journal of the Community Development, 10,* 5-16.

Woolpert, S. (1982). A comparison of rational choice and self-actulization theories of politics, *Journal of Humanistic Psychology, 22,* 55-67.

13

Self-concept and Cognitive Style of Physically Disabled Adolescent Girls

*Nishi Tripathi**

The physical aspect of physical disability in itself may not be as challenging as its social consequence, especially in those cases where the handicap is visible. It is only recently that the 'Disability' has been replaced by 'Challenge'. The bias against disability is revealed in the terminologies locally used for referring to these individuals, which are often derogatory and limiting. Such individuals grow up with a very negative self-image resulting in low motivation and aspiration. They grow up with the belief that they 'cannot do' where as when the disability is offered as a 'challenge' their outlook towards life changes. But the modern attitude and outlook is still not prevalent and thus these individuals still have a tough challenge to face.

The past decades has seen a greater emphasis on the study of self-concept for understanding and predicting the many facets of human behaviour. Self-concept is one of the most dominating factors influencing an individual's behaviour; on the other hand life experiences also affect the self-concept. Thus physical disability which is a dominent life event also affects the self-concept. Successes and other pleasurable events in life lead to the enhancement of self-concept while failure, frustration and other denigrating experiences tend to lower the concept of one's self. Self-concept is considered to be the most significant factor in human life as everyone is continuously striving toward self-actualization, self-realization and self-enhancement, and is constantly wishing to avoid self-condemnation and self-lowering experience. The foundations of the self-concept are laid during the early months when the infant begins to delineate himself form the environment through exploration and experience. As he goes out of the home, he learns about the worlds around him and later hears stories from books, radio and television of what children like him are doing. Any, if not all, of these experiences are less accessable to the handicapped child and it is almost, always found that a handicapped child's development is slower, to a greater or lesser extent, then that of a normal child, even though the handicapped child is of normal intelligence. Being given a name and being addressed by it is a basic part of the development of a concept of oneself.

* Coordinator of the Counselling Centre, Department of Psychology, University of Allahabad, Allahabad.

For Harre (1998), self-concept relates to the individual's strength and weaknesses, and hence is concerned with abilities. Self-concept can include attitudes and beliefs and may extend to temperamental matters. Self concept is highly dependent on the kind of situation a person perceives him or herself to be acting in, "Knowing myself, then involves, not only knowing my dispositions and abilities but the situations and conditions in which I may be able (or liable) to have them". According to social constructionists, 'self' is a learned construct. They forward the claim that gender is learned in the same way as learning about the other objects of the world, that is, a human attribute, through inductive process of categorization and classification, serves the function of acquiring social knowledge (Bigler & Liben, 1992; Das & Ghadially, 1988; Gupta, 1994; Heller, 1993; Liben & Signorella, 1980; Slaby & Frey, 1975). Miller (1990) also writes that even though in infancy both girls and boys are matched in a complex and 'interacting' sense of self, 'Girls are encouraged to augment their abilities to "feel as the others feel", and to practice "learned about" the other(s)'. Self-concept is the some total of an individual's belief about his or her own personal attributes.

Thus, self-concept is the set of ideas that a person has about himself. These ideas run through all his emotional experiences, habits, memories, trades and values. It refers to an attitudinal structure, which tends to be self-sustaining. An individual's evaluation of self-concept as dominant or submissive, emotional or calm, social or seclusive will be dependent to some extent upon the group with which consciously or unconsciously he/she compares himself/herself. No one is born with a fully framed self-concept. It develops as we experience approval and criticism, success and failure. It goes with our family, our friends, our place in society, and our perception of the world around us, it is modified as our bodies mature and we evaluate our physical, social and emotional characteristics.

Psychologists have paid attention to the different aspects of development of self-concept in physically handicapped persons. Hopkins (1973) studied the self-perception of disabled persons and reported that handicapped children attribute their disability to themselves. Physical appearance serves as a critical variable in the process of personality development for the physically handicapped children. Dreikurs (1948) reported that nearly half of a sample of 40 severely crippled children deliberately used their abilities to appear inferior and more helpless than they really were. All of them showed poor self-concept, their self-image was distorted and they blamed themselves. They experienced more fears and feelings of guilt than able-bodied children. All these exhibit their poor self-concepts. Shakespeare (1975) surveyed those studies of handicapped people where better-adjusted and poorly adjusted people were compared. He found that better adjusted people had positive self-concept, more self esteem and more readily saw themselves as making a worthwhile contribution to society. His findings also showed that better adjusted people are less anxious and have less need of social approval.

Everything we do is shaped and defined by our unique life style; it determines which aspects of our total environment we will attend to or ignore and what attitudes we will hold. To understand how the style of life develops we must return to the concept of inferiority feelings and compensation, for they form the basis of our life style. The life style so formed becomes the guiding framework for later behaviour. The nature of lifestyle will depend on the nature of the relationship between parent and child as the child works to find a way to compensate for his or her sense of inferiority. For example; a girl who has been neglected may feel inferior in coping with the demands of life (negative self). Adler (1927) expressed that the individual creates the 'self'. The person "does not relate himself to the outside world in a predetermined manner. He always relates himself according to his own interpretation of himself." This is the basis for the construction of attitude of the disabled person towards life.

Another important concept which has been used to account for the attitude of the disabled persons is relational attitude. According to Berry's (1980) theory of acculturation, when people from two different cultures are in contact, they can establish a relation in a number of different ways. Two factors that will determine the mode of relationship are, how much they value the maintenance of cultural identity and how much weightage they bestow on maintaining relationships with other groups. These are : assimilation, integration, separation and marginalization. These concepts are well known in the literature of disability. It is suggested that we can assess attitudes towards people with disability in the same way as acculturation attitudes are assessed (Berry, Kim, Power, Young & Bujaki, 1989; Berry & Dalal, 1994). In this sense, assimilation implies that persons with disability should be treated exactly like other people, integration implies that persons with disability, while acknowledging their special needs should be integrated into the larger group, separation implies that persons with disability are different and should be treated accordingly, while marginalization implies that persons with disability have no special needs and have no role in the community life. Thus, these four options or modes of adjustment reveal different kinds of attitudes which people have.

Cognitive Style

Psychological differentiation a broader construct of field dependence-field independence cognitive style can be studied with the help of Embedded Figure Test (FET). Witkin, Dyk, Faterson, Goodenough and Karp, (1974) first introduced the concept of psychological differentiation in the course of studies of individual differences in cognitive style. "Differentiation" refers to the complexity of structure of a psychological system (Witkin, 1978). In another study of a similar kind Berry (1966) compared the Temne and the Eskimo groups and found that the Temne children who were severely disciplined and physically punished were more field dependent than Eskimo children who were given much freedom, were rarely punished and were encouraged to assume responsibility early in life. A number of studies have given similar results. Studies have shown that family experiences and socialization (Dyk, 1969; Dyk & Witkin, 1965; Witkin, 1965; and Witkin *et al.*,1974) are important determinants of psychological differentiation. Therefore, there are reasons to believe that children in these two types of families will differ in the extent of psychological differentiation. Families with greater parental involvement were likely to have field independent children (Busse, 1969; Dawson, 1967; and Dreyer, 1975) and extended family structure was associated with field dependence while a nuclear family structure was associated with field independence (Witkin *et al.*,1974; Holtzman, Diaz Guerrero & Swartz, 1975). The modes of adaptation (Berry & Kim, 1988) and support systems available to individuals (Caplan & Killilea, 1976; Cohen & Wills, 1985) have been implicated as important factors in the experience of stress associated with changes in life style. It is evident that individuals, who adopt integration, coexistence and assimilation strategies, experience less stress while those who adopt separation or marginalization strategies experience greater stress (Berry, 1990; Berry & Kim, 1988; Mishra, Sinha & Berry, 1996). With regard to social support mechanisms, it was found that social isolation of individuals heightens the levels of stress (Cohen & Wills, 1985; Fondacora & Moos, 1987). Individuals own psychological make up is also an important variable in the experience of stress. For example, field-independent individuals, who happen to be cognitively controlled, experience stress to a lesser extent than field-dependent individuals, who seem to be less cognitively controlled (Berry & Annis, 1974; Mishra *et at.*, 1996).

In view of the importance of self concept in determining the aspiration and behaviours of an individual, and the role of cognitive style in experience and dealing with stress, this study was conducted to study self-concept and cognitive style of physically disabled girls.

METHOD

Sample

The sample comprised of 54 physically disabled and 30 non-adolescent girls studying in different Girls Intercolleges of Allahabad city from 8th to 12th standard.

Tools

Demographic Information : This section of the questionnaire focused on eliciting the following demographic information :

Age : The age of the respondents were recorded in years by rounding off months. For example if she reported that she was 16 years and 6 months old, then she was recorded as 17 years of age and if she reported that she was 16 years and 5 months old then she was recorded as being 16 years of age.

Education : The education of the disabled girls was noted down. On the basis of the obtained educational information, a coding scheme was developed. Thus class VIII to X = 1, class XI to XII = 2.

Socio-economic Status : For recording the socio-economic status as perceived by the respondent, four categories were given in the questionnaire : Higher SES, High middle SES, Low middle SES, Lower SES coded as 1, 2, 3, 4 respectively.

Family Structure : Family structure was recorded as joint or extended family = 1 and nuclear family = 2.

Self-concept Measure : Self-concept measure (how you describe yourself?) was used to assess the self-concept of the physically disabled adolescent girls. This scale was adopted from Disability, Attitude, Belief, and Behaviour (DABB) Project (Dalal, Pandey, Dhawan, and Punetha, 2000). This scale consists of eight items (bi-polar adjectives), which are answered on five-point scale ranging from negative attitude (1) to positive attitude (5). There were some negatively framed items (1, 3, 7, 8) indicated by R, which required reverse scoring order. In the context of the present study, this scale was again tested. The coefficient correlation of this scale was found to be 81.

Relational Attitude Measure : Relational attitude was used to assess the attitude of the physically disabled adolescent girls towards their disability. This scale was also taken from Disability, Attitude, Belief, and Behaviour (DABB) Project (Dalal, Pandey, Dhawan, and Punetha, 2000). The original scale had 20 items, 4 categories and 5 items in each category using a five-point scale. In the present study two items from each category were dropped, as their inter-item correlation was very low. The final version of the scale had total 12 items with 3 items in each category, [*a*] marginalisation (item no. 10, 13, 14, r =.83); [*b*] separation (item no. 7, 9, 11, r = .66); [*c*] assimilation (item no. 5, 6, 12, r = .65); and [*d*] integration (item no. 2, 18, 20, r = .47). The total correlation coefficient of this scale was found to be 64.

Cognitive Style Measures : Cognitive Style was measured using Embedded Figures Test. A short form of Witkin's (1984) EFT was used. The short form included the following patterns (following Witkin's numbering system) : C1 D1 E1 A2 C2 G1 A3 H1 E3 C3 D2 and E5. In the present study EFT was used for physically disabled girls and on their counter-parts normal girls to measure their cognitive style of field-dependent vs. independent.

Procedure

Initially a pilot study with 5 physically disabled girls was conducted. It was observed that these girls found no difficulty in understanding the questionnaire, indicating that there was no ambiguity in framing of the questions.

For the main study each respondent was visited in her school and the questionnairn were administered. Disabled girls were told about the objectives of the study. A good rapport was established. Then, they were assured that their responses would be used only for research purposes. In order to ascertain the differences in the cognitive styles of disabled/non-disabled individuals, the cognitive style measure was administered to 30 normal girls in addition to the disabled group.

RESULTS AND DISCUSSION

The demographic information of the disabled sample was compiled in term of percentages.

Table 13.1 : Demographic Profile of the Respondent

Demographic Information	*Disabled Girls N = 54*
Age	14-19 yrs. M = 16.5
Education	37.4% 8th-10th standard 62.96% 11th-12th standard
Family structure	68.5% joint family 31.5% nuclear family
Perceived social status	74.1% high middle class 22.2% low middle class 3.7 lower class
Total Family Income	1200-30000 /- Month M = 5507.41

From the table it can be seen that the average age of the physically disabled girls was around 17 years. Among them 37.04% girls had 8th -10th grade education and 62.96% girls had 11th-12th grade education. 68.5% girls were from joint family and 31.5% girls were from nuclear family. 74.1% girls perceived themselves as belonging to higher middle class and 22.2% girls perceived themselves as belonging to lower middle class, only 3.7% girls perceived themselves as lower class. Their average family income per-month was 5507.41.

Table 13.2 : Correlations Between Demographic Variables, Self-concept, EFT and Relational Attitude

Psychological Variables	*Age*	*Education*	*Family Income*	*Social Status*
Self-concept	–.24	–.31*	.15	–.15
EFT (mean score time)	.31*	–.09	.23	.22
RAS-Assimilation	.02	.07	.16	–.07
RAS-Integration	–.07	.06	–.11	.05
RAS-Marginalization	.31*	.23	.06	.04
RAS-Separation	.22	.08	–.22	.20

* $p<.05$.

The scores of the respondents were obtained on self concept, relational attitude and EFT (Mean Time Score) and correlation were computed with the demographic variables. Table 13.2 suggests that disabled girls with increasing age were more field dependent as they had taken more time on embedded figure test than younger disabled girls. The results also show that higher the age of the disabled girls more marginalized they were. The findings further reveal that more educated disabled girls had more negative self-concept.

Table 13.3 : Correlations Between Self-concept and Relational Attitude

Self-concept and	*Relational Attitude Measure*			
Measures	*Assimilation*	*Integration*	*Segregation*	*Marginalization*
Self-concept	.73***	.12	–.76***	–.63**
RAS-Assimilation		.26	–.62***	–.63***
RAS-Integration			–.05	–.13
RAS-Segregation				.75***
RAS-Marginalization				

*p<.05,**p<.01,***p<.001.

In order to study the relationship between self concept and relational attitude, correlations were computed between the scores of the respondents on the two measures. Table 13.3 shows that disabled girls who had a positive self-concept towards themselves were more assimilated and less marginalized and less separated. The results further show that disabled girls who were more assimilated were less separated and marginalized. More marginalized disabled girls were also more separated. (This also indicates the direction of the scale).

Table 13.4 : Mean Scores (time) on Embedded Figures Test

EFT	*No. of Cases*	*Time taken (Mean)*	*S.D.*	*t-value*	*2 tail-significant*
Disabled girls	54	72.40	18.38	2.74**	.008
Non-disabled girls	30	64.85	6.32		

**p<.01.

The EFT had been administered to both disabled and non disabled girls. The difference between the means of the two groups was analysed by applying t-test. Table 13.4 shows that t-value 2.74 (P<. 008) was significant. This indicates that there is significant difference between the disabled and non-disabled group on EFT, where mean value of disabled group was higher than non-disabled. It indicates that disabled girls were more field-dependent than non-disabled girls.

Table 13.5 : Correlations of Self-concept & Relational Attitude Measure with Embedded Figures Test

Self-concept & Relational Attitude Measure	*Embedded Figures Test*
Self-concept	–.44**
RAS-Assimilation	–.27
RAS-Integration	–.27
RAS-Segregation	.47***
RAS-Marginalization	.46**

* p<.05, **p<.01, ***p<.001.

Lastly, correlations were computed between the scores on EFT and self-concept/relational attitude. Table 13.5 shows that disabled girls who perceived themselves positively took less time on EFT and were more independent. Similarly in the relational attitude scale, separation and marginalization had positive significant correlation with EFT. This suggests that more field dependence disabled girls were more separated and marginalized.

Considered together these results indicate that the disabled girls despite their disability attended schools with other non-disabled girls. This suggests that these disabled girls were in frequent interaction with those who were different from them. There were only few girls in the colleges sampled who were physically disabled hence they were visible, easily identifiable and in a minority.

On scanning the relationship between demographic and psychological variables, the finding suggests that older girls had negative self-concept that nothing could be done for their disability. It was also evident that older girls were more field dependent, since from their childhood, and due to longer experience of disability they felt more frustration and experiences greater insecurity. Further older girls felt more marginalized. This suggests that those disabled girls who felt more marginalized were withdrawn from social interactions with others non-disabled as well as disabled people and experienced anxiety, alienation and tension (Berry & Kim, 1988). The findings further suggest that more marginalized disabled girls had more negative self-concept.

The findings also suggest that the more educated girls had more negative attitude towards themselves and were less hopeful about their future improvement. It appears that with increasing age and educational experiences these disabled girls had become realistically aware about their own capacities and abilities hence were not hopeful about their future improvement and perceived their disability as being more severe.

However, disabled girls having positive self-concept felt more assimilated and less marginalized and separated. It seems that the self-concept provides an extension of self, which is reflected in positive perception of others (assimilation and integration) and leads to adjustment (Rogers, 1961; Maslow, 1954; Jung, 1955; Allport, 1961). Similarly the findings further reveal that those disabled girls who felt more assimilated were less segregated and marginalized and who felt more segregated were more marginalized. These findings support those of Berry & Dalal (1994). In another similar study according to Berry & Kim (1998), assimilation is merging with the mainstream culture. It seems that the disabled girls who had positive self-concept could extend 'selves' to others without any defense; they were willing to perceive themselves similar to the non-disabled people. They did not isolate themselves from the mainstream society and thus were well adjusted. The findings further suggest that those disabled girls who had a positive self-concept were not segregated and marginalized. It seems that those girls who were withdrawn, did not intend to associate with the non-disabled people. They kept themselves isolated because they perceive themselves different from non-disabled people. These girls from their childhood were facing difficulties in adjustment, could not perceive themselves positively and therefore they were unable to perceive others positively. This further created difficulty in adjustment with others. They could not perceive themselves positively, therefore they felt insecure and they developed a basic sense of mistrust from childhood (Erickson, 1968). Such a state of affair makes individuals maladjusted to a great extent (Berry & Kim, 1988). The intergroup relations theory which assumes that the minority group who do not interact with majority group suffer from conflict, stress and tension appears to hold true here.

The findings further suggest that those girls who have positive self-concepts were more oriented towards field independence. This means that person dependent on the external field can easily differentiate between self, others and environments. The result further shows that the marginalization and segregation was positively correlated with embedded figure test. It indicates that disabled girls who were more marginalized and more segregated were more field dependent and had more undifferentiated perceptual style. This indicates that socialization experience was the determining factor in shaping, cognitive style. It is important to note that self is an important determinant of behaviour, that is, how one perceives one self and others determines the mode of adjustment also. The results of a number of studies have documented a positive relationship between self-esteem and adjustment to disability (Heinemen & Shontz, 1982; Linkowski & Drunn, 1974; Wissel, 1981). In a review of studies on self-concept and adjustment to disability, Linkowski (1988) found a positive relationship between self-concept and adjustment to disability, regardless of age, disability or other characteristics. Adler (1927) found that individuals with defective organs typically try to compensate for their weaknesses by intensive training. It is further clear from the present results that those disabled girls who felt themselves assimilated perceived their disability as less severe and hence needed less help in their daily routine activities. Similarly those disabled girls who were segregated, felt that they needed more help in their daily routine activities. On the same pattern more marginalized disabled girls felt that their disability problem was more severe and correspondingly they needed more help in their daily routine activities. Result shows a different trend that marginalized disabled girls were not hopeful about future improvement. This shows that they felt more insecure. The findings further suggests that disabled girls who have more control beliefs were more hopeful about future improvement, perceived their disability problem less severe and correspondingly they needed less help in their daily routine activities. Those who depended on God's will and law of Karma were more satisfied with the help they received and those disabled girls who attributed internal causes responsible for their disability reported that they needed less help in their daily routine activities.

It was also found that older girls were more field dependent, more separated, more marginalized as compared to younger girls. This suggests that longer duration of stress places more negative impact on self-concept. The finding also suggests that education is also one of the most determining factors of self-concept. It further suggests that formal education must be imparted to disabled girls to make them self-dependent and enhance their self-concept.

It is clear that in traditional Indian society belief in God and in the law of Karma is part of the Dharma (religion). These enduring, culturally prescribed beliefs may be the reason why the disabled girls belonging to joint families reported that they received more help from various sources/places. However, in the interpersonal sphere these girls were less assimilated and more marginalized in comparison to disabled girls of nuclear families. It is reasonable to state that the economic status of the family provided resources, which could meet the additional needs of the disabled child.

The findings of Embedded Figures Test showed that the disabled girls who by necessity were dependent on others for their daily routine activities, showed a similar trend. This test also measures the socialization aspect of dependency. When Embedded Figure Test scores of disabled girls were compared with the scores of non-disabled (normal) group, it was found that there was significant differences indicating that the disabled girls were more field dependent. It appears that in due course of time physical dependency inculcates a need for dependency and sense of dependency on others. This finding also suggests that the disabled girls become dependent due to their disability, therefore, they should be given support and help in order to achieve autonomy in functioning which would eventually enhanced their well being.

Thus disabled girls, who are dependent by nature and necessity, must be given help to the extent that they can be independent and develop a healthy self-concept. As age increases the perceived severity of disability also increases, so older disabled girls require additional support. Education is also one of the positive factors, which enhance self-concept of the disabled girls and fosters independence.

REFERENCES

Adler, A. (1927). *Understanding Human Nature*, New York : Greenberg.

Allport, G. (1961). *Pattern and Growth in Personality*, New York, Rinehart and Winston.

Berry, J.W. (1966). "Temne and Eskimo Perceptual Skills". *International Journal of Psychology, 1*, 207-229.

Berry, J.W. (1980). Psychology of acculturation : Understanding individuals moving between cultures. In R. Brislin (Ed.), *Applied Cross-cultural Psychology*, 232-253, Thousand Oaks : Sage.

Berry, J.W. (1990). Psychology of acculturation : Understanding individuals moving between cultures. In R. Brislin (Ed.), *Applied Cross-Cultural Psychology*, 232-253. Thousand Oaks : Sage.

Berry, J.W., & Annis, R.C. (1974). Acculturative stress : The role of ecology, culture and differentiation, *Journal of Cross-Cultural Psychology, 5*, 382-406.

Berry, & Dalal, A.K. (1994). *Attitudes, Beliefs and Behaviours in Relations to CBR Programmes : A Cross-Cultural Perspectives*. Paper presented at the Asian Regional Symposium on Research and Evaluation in CBR, Bangalore, December 5-7.

Berry, J.W., & Kim, U.(1988). Acculturation and mental health. In P.R. Dasen, J.W. Berry, and N. Sortorius (Eds.) *Health and Cross-Cultural Psychology, Toward Applications,* 207-236, Beverly Hills : Sage.

Berry, J.W., Kim, U., Power, S., Young, M. & Bujaki, M. (1989). Acculturation attitudes in plural societies, *Applied Psychology, 38*,185-206.

Bigler, R.S. & Liben, L.S. (1992). Cognitive mechanisms in children's gender stereotyping, Theoretical and educational implications of a cognitive based intervention, *Child Development, 63*, 1351-1363.

Busse, T.V. (1969). "Child-rearing Antecedents of Flexible Thinking", *Developmental Psychology, 1*, 585-591.

Caplan, G., & Killilea, M. (1976). *Social Support Systems and Mutual Help : Multidisciplinary Explorations*, New York : Grune Stratton.

Cohen, S., & Wills, T. A. (1985). Stress, social support, and the buffering hypothesis, *Psychological Bulletin*, 98, 310-357.

Dalal, A.K., Pandey, N., Dhawan, N., Dwijendra, D., & Berry, J.W. (2000). *The Mind Matters : Community Based Rehabilitation,* Indian : Allahabad, University of Allahabad.

Das, S. & Ghadially, R. (1988). Parental; sex role orientation and sex stereotypes of children. In R. Ghadially (Ed.), *Women in Indian Society : A Reader*, New Delhi : Sage.

Dawson, J.L.M. (1967). " Cultural and Physiological Influences upon Spatial Perceptual Processes in West Africa"- Part II, *International Journal of Psychology, 2*, 171-185.

Dreikurs, R. (1948). The Social-psychological dynamics of Physical Disability : A review of the Adlerian Concept, *Journal of Social Issues, 4*, 39-54.

Dreyer, A.S. (1975). " Family Interaction and Cognitive Style : Situation and Cross-sex Effects". In H.B. Biller (Chair). *Beyond Father Absence : Conceptualization of Father Effects*, Symposium presented at the meeting of the Society for research in Child Development, Denver.

Dyk, R.B. (1969). "An Exploratory Study of Mother-Child Interaction in infancy as related to the Development of Differentiation in Children," *Journal of the American Academy of Child Psychiatry, 8*, 657-691.

Dyk, R.B. & Witkin, H.A. (1965). "Family Experiences Related to the Development of Differentiation in Children," *Child Development*, 30, 21-55.

Erickson, E. (1968). *Identity, Youth and Crises,* New York : Basic Books.

Fondacora, M.R., & Moos, R.H. (1987). Social support and coping : A longitudinal analysis, *American Journal of Community Psychology, 15*, 653-673.

Gupta, J. (1994). *Gender Differences in the Development of Moral Orientations in 10-15-year-old Children*. M.Phil. Dissertation (Child Development), Dept. of Human Development and Family Studied, Faculty of Home Science, Maharaja Sayagirao University of Baroda, Vadodara, Gujarat.

Harre, R. (1998). *The Singular Self*, New Delhi, Sage Publication.

Heller, W. (1993). Gender differences in depression. Perspectives from neuropsychology, *Journal of Affective Disorders, 29*, 129-143.

Heinemann, A.W., & Shontz, F.C. (1982). Acceptance of disability, self-esteem, sex role identity, and reading aptitude in deaf adolescents, *Rehabilitation Counseling Bulletin, 25*, 197-203.

Holtzman, W.H., R. Diaz-Guerrero, & J.D. Swartz (1975). *Personality Development in Two Cultures : A Cross-Cultural Longitudinal Study of School Children in Mexico and the United States*, Austin, Texas: University of Texas Press.

Hopkins, M.T. (1973). Patterns of Self-destruction among the orthopedically disabled, *Psychological Abstract, 50*, 6,11509.

Jung, C.G. (1955). *The Interpretation of Nature and Psyche*, New York : Pantheon Books.

Liben, L.S. & Signorella, M.L. (1980). Gender-related schemata and constructive memory in children, *Child Development, 51*, 11-18.

Linkowski, D.C. (1988). *The Acceptance of Disability Scale : An Update*, 1969-1983. Unpublished manuscript, George Washington University, Washington, D.C.

Linkowski, D.C., & Dunn, M.A. (1974). Self-concept and acceptance of disability, *Rehabilitation Counseling Bulletin, 17*, 28-32.

Maslow, A.H. (1954). *Motivation and Personality*, New York : Harper & Row Publishers.

Miller, J.B. (1990). The development of women's sense of self. In C. Zanardi (Ed.), *Essential Papers in the Psychology of Women*, New York : New York University Press.

Mishra, R.C. Sinha, D., & Berry, J.W. (1996). *Ecology, Acculturation and Psychological Adaptation : A Study of Adivasis in Bihar*, New Delhi : Sage.

Rogers, C.R. (1961). *On Becoming a Person*, Boston : Honghton Muffin Company.

Shakespeare (1975). *The Psychology of Handicap*, London : Methuen and Company Limited.

Slaby, R.G. & Frey, K.S. (1975). Development of gender constancy and selective attention of same-sex models, *Child Development, 46*, 849-856.

Witkin, H.A. (1965). "Psychological Differentiation and Forms of Pathology," *Journal of Abnormal Psychology, 70*, 317-336.

Witkin, H.A. (1978). *Cognitive Styles in Personal and Cultural Adaptation, 11*, 1977, Hoinz Werner Lecture Series, Clark University Press.

Wissel, E.A. (1981). *Analysis of Self-concept and Acceptance of Disability with the Traumatic Spinal Cord Injury : A Doctor Dissertation*, The Catholic University of America, Washington, D.C.

Witkin, H.A., R.B. Dyk, H.F. Faterson, Goodenough, D.R., and Karp, S.A. (1974). *Psychological Differentiation*, Potimac, Md. Erlbaum (Originally published, Wiley, 1962).

14

Noise Sensitivity, Traffic Noise and Health

*Prabha Bhatia** & *Sonika Chhabra***

The problem of noise pollution in recent years has become a serious threat to human health. Noise pollution is the unwanted sound dumped into the environment without regard to its adverse effects, it may have on the person exposed to it. Bhatia, Muhar, Malhotra and Mahajan (1995) reported that environmental noises can play havoc with human extra auditory physiological functioning and can make the person liable to various cardiovascular disorders. It has been reported in a study by Environmental Management Centre (1997) that noise pollution alters the heart beats and respiration rate and can cause hypertension and diabetes.

Sound is called noise when it becomes loud or disagreeable and particularly when it results in physiological or psychological harm. The menace of noise pollution is growing throughout the world day by day due to population explosion, rapid industrialization and urbanization. Stansfeld, Sharp, Gallacher and Babisch (1998) said that the major possible sources of noise pollution fall into the major categories of transportation or traffic noise, industrial, household and loudspeakers. The noise from vehicles, construction, air traffic, home appliances and surface transportation are of greater concern than other type of noises.

It has been reported by (Misra, 1999), a Professor of Medicine at AIMS, Delhi, that the tremendous noise can cause a condition called Insulin Resistance Syndrome (IRS). That is single most important factor for heart attacks. IRS is a condition in which there is resistance to insulin secreted by the pancreas and the body begins to secrete more amounts of the hormones to affect this. The extra insulin has adverse effects on the heart, blood-pressure, and cholesterol. IRS is the harbinger of several disorders such as diabetes, high blood pressure, blood cholesterol and coronary artery disease (CAD).

In western countries one rarely blows automobile horns on the roads. The horns fitted to the automobiles are very mild and are governed by law. Whenever, one blows horn in west, it immediately attracts the attention of the general masses that something has gone wrong.

*Reader, Department of Psychology, M.D. University, Rohtak.
**Ex-Student, Department of Psychology, M.D. University, Rohtak.

But the position in our country is at the other extreme. In 2002 All India Institute of Medical Sciences, New Delhi, reported that average environmental traffic noise is more than twice the internationally acceptable limit. In metropolitan cities, the traffic noise levels, even during night, never fall below 60 decibels. Sometimes at the busy interactions, loudspeakers are used to control traffic and pedestrian movements. One can fit as many high pitched horns to the vehicles as one wishes. Pressure horns are popular with young generation. Pressure horns are though banned in metropolitan cities but the vehicles coming from the other states have this type of horns, so they create noise pollution.

It has been reported repeatedly that exposure to persistent noise, even if low, causes hearing problem. Human ear can take sound upto 60 to 80 dB without damage to ears or hearing loss. Any sound above 80 db is potentially dangerous. Noise causes hearing loss, interferes with our sleep, and is an annoyance in our everyday life. According to Dr. Ogale (2005), Head of the ENT department at KEM Hospital, Mumbai, continuous traffic noise interferes with our conversation, concentration, relaxation, leisure and work. It can also provide persistent favourable background for the development of nervous and mental disorders of many kinds.

Thus in view of the immense importance of noise research, the present investigator decided to work in this area. The present study was undertaken to study the effect of traffic noise on physiological health. It was hypothesised that both the high noise sensitivity group and low noise sensitivity group would be spending greater physiological energy under the noisy condition as compared to quiet condition. In order to measure the effect of noise on health, the physiological energy expenditure which was inferred from systolic/diastolic blood pressure and pulse rate was taken into account.

METHOD

Design

In multigroup design with four groups, of low and high noise sensitivity groups, Ss worked exactly under similar conditions for 36 minutes except in experimental conditions, where prerecorded traffic noise was switched on additionally. The Ss were required to do a numerical task, when they were exposed to traffic noise.

Sample

A sample of 120 Ss—60 belonging to high noise sensitivity group and 60 belonging to low noise sensitivity group—was selected from the population of 600 Ss after administering a noise sensitivity scale on them.

Instrumentation

Tools

Indian adaptation of Weinstein's Noise Sensitivity Scale by Bhatia, Malhotra and Muhar (1989).

Multiplication charts, Philips Stereo Cassette Deck F6121 to record and play the traffic noise; Taped traffic noise recorded from one of the busiest area *i.e.* I.T.O. bridge, New Delhi and Compact Digital Wrist Blood Pressure Monitor (Model R4) with fyrrylogic.

Procedure

After administering noise sensitivity scale, on 600 Ss belonging to high noise sensitivity group and 60 Ss belonging to low noise sensitivity group were selected on the basis of their scores on noise sensitivity scale. Digital wrist blood pressure monitor was tied up at the left wrist of each subject. When the blood pressure and pulse readings, got somewhat stabilized, and subject was totally relaxed his basal readings were noted down. Then changes in the systolic and diastolic blood pressure and pulse rate were noted down after every five minutes. This procedure was exactly identical for low and high noise sensitivity groups, when they worked under quiet and noisy conditions. In quiet condition, no noise was played, whereas in noisy condition, the pre-recorded traffic noise was played at 100 decibels. Each subject's readings of systolic and diastolic blood pressure and pulse rate were noted down for 36 minutes at the interval of five minutes.

The obtained readings were calculated in terms of increase (difference) in terms of percentage from the basal readings. Then those percentages were converted into arc sin transformation scores before applying statistical analysis.

RESULTS AND DISCUSSION

The obtained statistical data of low and high noise sensitivity groups, after applying critical ratio are being presented in the various tables.

The data related to systolic blood pressure is presented in Table 14.1.

Table 14.1 : Showing Significance of Differences on t-test Between the Mean Percentage Increase in the Systolic Blood Pressure of Low Noise Sensitivity and High Noise Sensitivity Groups Under Quiet and Noisy Conditions

Low Noise Sensitivity Group			
Condition	*Mean*	*Difference*	*t-value*
Quiet	15.23	9.59	5.95**
Noise	24.82		
High Noise Sensitivity Group			
Quiet	20.71	6.54	3.87**
Noise	27.25		

** $p > 0.01$.

The results presented in the above table show that in low noise sensitivity group mean increase in systolic blood pressure is 15.23 in quiet condition and 24.82 in noisy condition. There was a mean difference of 9.59 between the quiet and noisy conditions of low noise sensitivity group. In order to know the significance of difference between the two conditions of low noise sensitivity group, 't' test was applied.

The obtained t-value is 5.95 which indicates that this value is significant at .01 level. Thus the difference between the means of two conditions is highly significant, showing that this group had spent greater physiological energy under noisy condition.

In case of high noise sensitivity group mean increase in systolic blood pressure is 20.71 in quiet condition and 27.25 in noisy condition. There was a difference of 6.54 in the means of quiet and noisy conditions of high noise sensitivity group and t-value relating to the significance of difference between the two means is 3.87 which is significant at .01 level. The results based on t-tests clearly show that there is significant difference in the physiological energy spent by both the high as well as low noise sensitivity groups under quiet and noisy conditions.

These results clearly indicate that in both the groups *i.e.* low noise sensitivity and high noise sensitivity, physiological energy expenditure was more in noisy condition as compared to quiet condition. Increase in systolic blood pressure is indicative of increase in physiological energy expenditure. Thus, it is quite evident from the obtained results that noise had significant deteriorating effects on systolic blood pressure which was taken as one of the physiological parameters for energy consumption under different conditions—quiet and noisy.

Now the data relating to the effect of noise on diastolic blood pressure is being examined (Table 14.2).

Table 14.2 : Showing Significance of Differences on t-test Between the Mean Percentage Increase in the Diastolic Blood Pressure of Low Noise Sensitivity and High Noise Sensitivity Groups Under Quiet and Noisy Conditions

Condition	*Mean*	*Difference*	*t-value*
Low Noise Sensitivity Group			
Quiet	18.46	4.02	2.61**
Noise	22.48		
High Noise Sensitivity Group			
Quiet	18.18	8.33	4.78**
Noise	26.51		

** p>0.01.

The results presented in Table 14.2 show that mean increase in diastolic blood pressure is 18.46 in quiet and 22.48 in noisy condition. There was a mean difference of 4.02 in quiet and noisy conditions of low noise sensitivity group and the 't' value relating to the significance of difference is 2.61 which is significant at .01 level. Thus in noisy condition physiological energy expenditure, which is inferred from mean percentage increase in diastolic blood pressure is more than the quiet condition.

In high noise sensitivity group mean increase in diastolic blood pressure is 18.18 in quiet and 26.51 in noisy condition. The difference between the means of two conditions is 8.33. The obtained t-value is 4.78 and is significant at .01 level. It is clearly evident from the results that both the groups *i.e.* low noise sensitivity and high noise sensitivity group consumed more physiological energy under noisy condition compared to quiet condition. It can be concluded that noise had significant role to play in bringing changes (increase) in the blood pressure.

Now the pulse based data is being analysed as it was used as one of the physiological indices for the measurement of energy expenditure.

Table 14.3 : Showing Significance of Differences on t-test Between the Mean Percentage Increase in the Pulse Rate of Low Noise Sensitivity and High Noise Sensitivity Groups Under Quiet and Noisy Conditions

Condition	*Mean*	*Difference*	*t-value*
Low Noise Sensitivity Group			
Quiet	14.32	7.13	4.85**
Noise	21.45		
High Noise Sensitivity Group			
Quiet	16.99	6.11	4.42**
Noise	23.10		

** p>0.01.

The results presented in the above table show that mean increase in pulse rate is 14.32 in quiet and 21.45 in noisy condition. There is a difference of 7.13 in the mean increase of pulse rate between quiet and noisy condition of low noise sensitivity group. t-value relating to the significance of differences between two means is 4.85 and is significant at .01 level.

In case of high noise sensitivity group mean increase in pulse rate is 16.99 in quiet and 23.10 in noisy condition. There is a mean difference of 6.11 between the two conditions and the t-value relating to the significance of difference is 4.42 and is significant at .01 level. This clearly indicate that noise affected the energy expenditure of both the groups under noisy condition.

The results presented in tables show that noise significantly affected the pulse rate. There was increase in pulse rate with the introduction of noise. In case of both low noise sensitivity and high noise sensitivity groups magnitude of energy expenditure inferred from pulse increased under noisy condition.

Statistics presented in table 14.1, 14.2 and 14.3 are enough to prove that in both low noise sensitivity and high noise sensitivity groups, physiological energy expenditure was more in noisy condition than in quiet condition. Noise remained costlier in terms of energy expenditure. Since higher systolic/diastolic blood pressure and pulse rate imply that subjects had to spend higher physiological energy under noisy conditions.

The hypothesis which had predicted that both high noise sensitivity and low noise sensitivity groups would be spending greater physiological energy under the noisy condition as compared to the quiet condition has been supported. Both the systolic/diastolic blood pressure and pulse rate were significantly affected by noise. From the present findings it can be inferred that traffic noise. environmental noise play an adverse role with human physiological functioning that may result in various cardiovascular disorders, hypertension and even diabetes about which common people may not be aware of. Today the kind of society we are living in, it becomes necessary to have public awareness campaigns about traffic noise pollution which is first and far most way to control traffic noise. The education about the harmful effects of traffic noise pollution should be spread among common people through the mass media like television, radio and newspapers.

To create a civic sense about traffic noise pollution some elementary chapters at school level should be added to existing syllabus. There should be also proper encouragement from the voluntary organizations which are campaigning to teach people about the harmful effects of traffic noise pollution.

There should be proper enforcement of existing laws regarding traffic noise like prohibition of use of pressure horns and placement of audio/visual and radio in motor vehicles. The offenders should be strictly punished according to the law when they use pressure horns. There should be proper encouragement of initiatives on noise less technology in production of motor vehicles. Some developed noiseless technology in the motor vehicles should be adopted at manufacturing stage as is done in west. It is, though, impossible to have a total elimination of annoying sounds, but it can certainly be minimized by taking into account such factors as reduction of noise at source and duration of noise exposure. Noise has become so much a part of our life that its long term, unseen, unnoticed harmful effects on our body and mind are often overlooked, though funding agencies like the University Grants Commission, Indian Council of Social Sciences Research and Indian Council of Medical Research are encouraging the research in this area. In this context, Ministry of Information and broadcasting, government of India (2005) issued a notice in public interest that loud noises cause permanent hearing loss, insomnia, headaches and hypertension. It has been recommended that 'Experience the joy of sounds but don't silence your ears for ever."

REFERENCES

Bhatia, P., Muhar, I.S., Malhotra, S. and Mahajan, K.K. (1995). Extra Auditory Physiological Effects of Noise on Work Efficiency, *Indian Psychological Review*, *44*, 15-20.

Bhatia, P., Malhotra, S. & Muhar, I.S. (1989). *Manual for Shor Sanvedi Mapak*, Hindi Adaptation of Weinstein's Noise Sensitivity Scale (WNSS), Agra, National Psychological Corporation.

Mishra, A. (1999). Time to shut down the noise. *The Tribune*, July, 12th, pp. 3.

Ministry of Information and Broadcasting (2005). Experience the joy of sounds, but don't silence your ears forever, *The Hindustan Times*, 29th Sep., pp. 3.

Ogale, C. (2005). All that noise can knock you out, *The Hindustan Times*, pp. 5.

Stansfeld, S.A., Sharp, D., Gallacher, J. and Babisch, W. (1998). Road Traffic Noise, Noise Sensitivity and Psychological Disorder, *Psych-Medicine*, *23*, 977-85.

15

Attributional Style in Relation to Sense of Well-Being

Samreen Hasan Khan* & Musaddiq Jahan**

People have different kinds of feelings ranging from negative mental states (anxiety, depression, dissatisfaction, unhappiness, etc.) to positive states (good health, satisfaction, happiness, etc.). Literature review indicates that unhappiness, ill-being and other negative aspects of human behaviour have been explored in-depth whereas happiness, well-being and other positive aspects of health are neglected. So many terms such as happiness, satisfaction, morale, hope, optimism, quality of life, positive affect and positive mental health etc. have been used in literature synonymously and often interchangeably. Psychologists have recently focused their attention on the concept of well-being which includes affective, cognitive and motivational aspects of life experiences with subjective feeling of satisfaction, achievement, belongingness, support and worth etc.

Schwanrz and Clore (1983) formulated a cognitive model based on attributions to explain the tendency of human beings to acquire happiness. The model suggests that good events bring most happiness if they are attributed to internal and stable factors. However, there may be some events that can lead to happiness, regardless of the attributions made, because of the positive subjective perception the individual made about the event.

Attribution is a complex process that refers to our efforts or attempts to understand the cause behind other's behaviour and occasionally, the cause behind our behaviour too. Thus attribution is the individual's perception of causation and his perspective and framework through which he views life. The term attributional styles emerged out of the theory of learned helplessness (Maier and Seligman, 1976; Seligman, 1975). The theory states that after experiencing uncontrollable events a variety of organisms show cognitive, motivational and emotional deficits. Ickes and Layden (1976) describe attributional style as consistent way of ascribing the causes of positive or negative events.

---

*Research Scholar, Department of Psychology, Aligarh Muslim University, Aligarh.
**Senior Lecturer, Women's College, Aligarh Muslim University, Aligarh.

A study conducted by Tiggemann, Winefield, and Goldney (1991) demonstrated that attributional style was relatively stable and was correlated with measures of psychological well-being. They used ASQ, measures of depressive affect (DAF) and hopelessness (HPL) in their study. Subjects who scored highest on DAF and HPL attributed good outcomes more externally and less stable and bad outcomes to relatively stable and global causes.

Moreover, attributional styles have relevance to various important matters related to health and illness (Peterson, 1988, 1995), depression (Seligmann, Abramson, Sameel and von Baeyer, 1979; Sweeney, Anderson and Barley, 1986; Dua, 1994), success and failure (Zeleski, 1988), interpersonal relationships, achievement etc. which are undoubtedly related to the well-being of an individual.

There are various evidences regarding the relationship between attribution style and health or illness. Individuals who believed that stable plus global factors caused bad events, experienced more days of illness in a month and visited physicians more frequently in a year (Peterson, 1988). Optimist individuals who explain bad events with external, unstable and specific causes experience better health than the pessimist, who explain bad events with internal, stable and global causes (Peterson, 1995).

In the present study the investigator has tried to probe three attributional style dimensions—*(i)* Internal Vs External, *(ii)* Stable Vs Unstable, & *(iii)* Specific Vs Global, as given by Abramson, Seligman and Teasdale, (1978); Abramson, Garber & Seligman (1980).

The aim of the present study is to explore the relationship between the attributional style and the psychological well-being of individuals. The major research question is—Do the persons having high sense of well-being differ in attributional style from those who have low sense of well-being?

METHOD

Design

Two groups design was used for conducting the study.

Sample

The sample consisted of 50 Ss (age ranging from 14 to 50 years) selected through non-random procedures. Their participation was purely on voluntary basis.

Tools

(i) Psychological well-being scale (PWS)—In the present study psychological well-being scale, developed by Bhogle and Prakash (1995) was used to assess over all well-being of the subjects. It consists of 24 items that measure perceived satisfaction in different life settings, such as peer relationship, marriage, health, social support and satisfaction with social support.

(ii) Attributional style questionnaire (ASQ)– ASQ was originally developed by Peterson, Semmel, von Baeyer, Abramson, Metalsky and Seligman (1982) and revised by Peterson and Seligman (1984). It presents 12 hypothetical events, 6 good and 6 bad. Additionally half of the events are interpersonal/affiliative while half are achievement related. The test-taker is asked to write down one major cause of each event and then to rate the cause along a 7-point continuum for each of the three causal dimensions.

Procedure

First of all, the Ss were presented with psychological well-being scale (PWS). On the basis of scores on this scale, Ss were divided into two extreme groups, cut-off points being Q_1 & Q_3. Subjects scoring below Q_1 were taken as low well-being (LWB) group and those above Q_3 comprised high well-being (HWB) group. 15 Ss fell in each group and then the ASQ was administered. After collecting the required data from all the 30 Ss both the groups were compared on 8 dimensions of attributional style, with the help of t-test.

RESULTS AND DISCUSSION

Table 15.1 : Comparison of Attribution Scores of Subjects Experiencing H.W.B. (High Well Being) and L.W.B.(Low Well Being), for Different Attributional Style Dimensions

Group	*Attributional Style Dimension*	*N*	*Mean*	*SD*	*t*
H.W.B.	Composite positive	15	16.63	2.19	2.66*
L.W.B.	Composite positive	15	14.67	1.99	
H.W.B.	Internal-External positive	15	5.70	1.19	3.06**
L.W.B.	Internal-External positive	15	4.36	1.28	
H.W.B.	Stable-Unstable positive	15	5.46	0.92	0.10
L.W.B.	Stable-Unstable positive	15	5.43	0.72	
H.W.B.	Specific-Global positive	15	5.13	1.36	0.40
L.W.B.	Specific-Global positive	15	4.97	0.84	
H.W.B.	Composite negative	15	11.67	1.54	1.83
L.W.B.	Composite negative	15	13.36	3.39	
H.W.B.	Internal-External negative	15	4.18	0.89	1.01
L.W.B.	Internal-External negative	15	3.81	1.19	
H.W.B.	Stable-Unstable negative	15	3.67	0.56	3.93**
L.W.B.	Stable-Unstable negative	15	5.14	1.39	
H.W.B.	Specific-Global negative	15	3.51	1.36	2.39*
L.W. B.	Specific-Global negative	15	4.67	1.39	

* P<.05, ** P<.01.

From Table 15.1, it is observed that subjects having high sense of well-being and low sense of well-being differ significantly on 4 out of 8 dimensions of attributional style, namely, Composite positive, Internal-External positive, Stable-Unstable negative and Specific-Global negative dimensions. The subjects having high sense of well-being are more internal on positive dimensions of attributional style, while subjects having low sense of well-being are more stable and global on negative dimensions of attributional style.

The obtained results reveal that there is a relationship between the experience of well-being and attributional style, and this difference holds good for both positive and negative events.

Persons having high sense of well-being emerged more internal on their attributions about positive events and unstable and specific for the negative events. On the other hand, the attributions of the persons having low sense of well-being are found to be more external for positive events and specific and global for the negative events. This attributional style is somewhat similar to that of person experiencing depression, which Seligman, Abramson, Semmel and Baeyer (1979) had brought out. The attributional style-depression linkage suggested by them, suggests that depressed persons make internal, stable and global attributions for negative events. Sweeney, Anderson and Barley (1986) also supported this conclusion. They reported that for negative events, attributions to internal, stable and global causes had reliable and significant association with depression. The obtained results are indicative to some degree of this trend.

The attributional style of H.W.B. Ss shows that they themselves take credit for all the pleasant events while they attribute negative events to environmental factors, for example, the score on Internal-External dimension of positive events shows that the subjects themselves take responsibility for the positive events, that is, they perceive the positive outcomes as a result of their own doings (for example, their skills, abilities, efforts, etc.) and the negative outcomes as a result of environmental factors (for example luck, task difficulty, situational constraints etc.). They are of the view that problems in their life may not last long and with the time they will fade away. They feel helplessness only in a situation *per se* and do not generalise it.

On the other hand, L.W.B. Ss have the typical attributional style associated with depression. For negative events their attribution is more stable and global. This suggests that they find the cause of negative events to be more persistent and general. Under similar negative conditions or situational cues they always experience helplessness which may not last over a period of time. In addition to this, their attributions about negative events affect expectancy and hence their performance in many situations. These findings are clearly endorsed by the results of the study conducted by Peterson and Vaidya (2001) who have reported that generalised expectations resulting from the stability and globality of explanatory styles lead to depression.

On the basis of the findings the answer to the research question is that persons experiencing H.W.B. differ from those experiencing L.W.B. on their attributional style. The Ss with high well being show significantly higher composite positive & internal-external positive attributional styles than the LW.B subject. On the other hand the L.W.B. subjects exhibit significantly higher levels of stable-unstable negative and specific global negative attribution styles to interpret various situations and behaviours in their daily routine.

REFERENCES

Abramson, L.Y., Garber, J., & Seligman, M.E.P., (1980). Learned helplessness in humans : An attributional analysis. In Garber and Seligman (Eds.), *Human Helplessness,* New York : Academic.

Abramson, L.Y., Seligman, M.E.P., & Teasdale, J. (1978). Learned helplessness in humans : Critique and reformulation, *Journal of Abnormal Psychology, 87,* 49-74.

Bhogle, S. & Prakash, I.J. (1995). Development of the Psychological Wellbeing (PWB) Questionnaire, *Journal of Personality and Clinical Studies, 11,* 5–9.

Dua, J.K. (1994). Comparative predictive value of attributional style, negative affect and positive affect in predicting self reported physical health and psychological health, *Journal of Psychosomatic Research, 38,* 669-680.

Ickes, W. & Layden, M.A. (1976). Attributional Styles. In J. Harvey (Ed.), *New Directions in Attribution Research (pp. 119 –152),* Hillsdale, NJ : Earlbaum.

Maier, S.F. & Seligman, M.E.P. (1976). Learned helplessness : Theory and evidence, *Journal of Experimental Psychology : General, 105*, 3-46.

Peterson, C. (1988). Explanatory style as a risk factor for illness, *Cognitive Therapy and Research, 12,* 119-132.

Peterson, C. (1995). Explanatory style and health. *In* Buchaman, G. McClelland and Seligman, M.E.P. (Eds.), Explanatory style, pp. 8058-92, Lawrence, Erlbaum.

Peterson, C. & Seligman, M.E.P. (1984). Causal explanations as a risk factor for depression : Theory and Evidence, *Psychological Review, 91,* 347-374.

Peterson, C., Semmel, A., von Baeyer, C. Abramson, L.Y., Metalsky, G.I. & Seligman, M.E.P. (1982). The Attributional Style Questionnaire, *Cognitive Therapy and Research, 6,* 287-299.

Peterson, C. & Vaidya, R.S. (2001). Explanatory style, expectations, and depressive symptoms, *Personality and Individual Differences, 31,* 1217-1223.

Schwanrz, N. & Clore, G.L. (1983). Mood, Misattribution and judgements of well-being, Informative and directive functions of affective states, *Journal of Personality and Social Psychology, 45,* 513-532.

Seligman, M.E.P. (1975). *Helplessness : on Depression, Development and Death,* San Francisco : Freeman.

Seligman, M.E.P., Abramson, L.Y., Semmel, A. & von Baeyer, C. (1979). Depressive attributional style, *Journal of Abnormal Psychology, 88,* 242-247.

Sweeney, P.D., Anderson, K., & Barley, S. (1986). Attributional style in depression : A meta analytic review, *Journal of Personality and Social Psychology, 50,* 974-991.

Tiggemann, M., Winefield, A.H., Winefield H.R., & Goldney, R. (1991). The stability of attributional style and its relation to psychological distress, *British Journal of Clinical Psychology, 30,* 247-255.

Zeleski, Z. (1988). Attribution and emotion related to future goal attainment, *Journal of Educational Psychology, 80,* 563-568.

16

Self-efficacy Beliefs and Causal Attributions

***Vandana Sharma*[*] & *Bhavneet Kaur Gill*[**]**

Individuals possess a self-system that enables them to exercise a measure of control over their thoughts, feelings and action. It includes the ability to symbolize one's own behaviour and engage in self-reflection. Bandura (1982) labeled this self-system as "Self-Efficacy" which is instrumental in defining individual's choices, emotional reactions and also provides and avenue through which he interprets his surroundings. Attributional theory (Weiner, 1986) describes how people explain their experiences and what type of information they use in making those causal inferences. Bandura proposed that self-efficacy provides information from which causal attributions are made which in turn influence the subsequent formation of self-efficacy. Self-efficacy plays an important role in dealing effectively with negative feedback and failure. Self-efficacy helps to account for such diverse phenomena as changes in coping behaviour produced by different modes of influence, level of physiological stress reactions, self-regulation of refractory behaviour, resignation and despondence to failure experience, achievement striving, growth of intrinsic interest and career pursuits. Self-efficacy beliefs are not simply reflective imprints of past performance rather the impact of past performance in self-efficacy depends on the cognitive appraisal of perceived performance (Bandura, 1977). Fosterling (1985) suggested that the causal attributions made by individuals are important to maintain their self efficacy beliefs. Low self-efficacy individuals perceive the things to be tougher than they really are and as a result suffer from stress, depression and narrow vision. Whereas, individuals with high self-efficacy beliefs approach difficult task as a challenge to be mastered rather than as threat to be avoided. High self-efficacy beliefs enhances performance through cognitive, affective or motivational intervening processes and are also associated with better physical and psychological well being (Bandura, 1978).

Self-efficacy refers to beliefs about one's capabilities to learn or perform behaviour at designated levels. Efficacy beliefs influence how people feel, think, behave and motivate

[*]Professor & Head, Dept. of Psychology, Punjabi University, Patiala.
[**]Researcher Scholar, Dept. of Psychology, Punjabi University, Patiala.

themselves. It is defined as individual's conviction about his/her abilities to mobilize cognitive, motivational and behavioural faculties needed to successfully execute a specific task within a given context (Stajkovic & Luthans, 1998). It is grounded in social cognitive theory, which postulates that human achievement depends on interactions between one's behaviours, personal factors (*e.g.* thoughts, beliefs) and environmental conditions (Schunk, 1984, a, b, c). Self-efficacy beliefs influence the choices people make and the courses of action they pursue. Individuals tend to engage in tasks about which they feel competent and confident and avoid those in which they do not.

Self-efficacy is a social cognitive theory of personality which postulates a triadic reciprocal interaction between an individual's personal factors, environmental events and behaviour. Introduced by Bandura, perceived self-efficacy has been defined as "a generative capability in which cognitive, social, emotional, and behavioural subskills must be organized and effectively orchestrated to serve innumerable purposes". It mediates between an individual's ability and his purposive action. Perceived self-efficacy influences the course of action adopted, effort invested, endurance and resilence in the face of obstacles and failures, coping, and the level of accomplishments. Bandura states that people with high self-efficacy is enhanced. In its role as a mediator between task capability and action, self-efficacy is dependent on one's belief in control capability. "Perceived self-efficacy is concerned with people's belief in their capabilities to perform in ways that give them some control over events that affects their lives" (Bandura, 1997).

However, it can be assumed that attribution and self-efficacy have a bi-directional causal relationship (Schunk & Pagares, 2002) Attributions affect appraisal of self-efficacy and perceived self-efficacy biases causal attributions. Bandura concludes that when intelligence is viewed as an incremental skill, effort, perseverance in the face of obstacles and task-orientation are the pattern of behaviour in attaining a goal. Similarly Anderson (1999) contends that self-efficacy is determined as one developed by : *(a)* self-efficacy of one's ability vs effort at a task, and *(b)* attribution of success/failure to ability or effort. Attribution is the process of perceiving the dispositional properties of objects including other persons in the environment. It is the process by which people use information to make inference about the causes of behaviour or events. The events which serve as objects of perception might consist of the actions of social others, one's own actions, and or environmentally produced effects. Attribution theory is a social psychological theory that relates to the way in which people explain their own behaviour and that of others. The concept of attribution was introduced by Heider (1958) who viewed that an individual cannot be described as a lone subject in an impersonal environment but must be viewed as a part of the total situation. Heider's attribution theory explains that persons action or behaviour has significant effect upon others. When we observe a change in a person's actions, we may attribute it to internal or personal causes, to external or environmental cause.

Recently, relationship between gender and self-efficacy has become a focus of research (Hackett, 1995). In general, researchers report that boys tend to be more confident than girls in academic areas related to mathematics, science, and technology (Pajares and Miller, 1994; Wigfield, Eccles, and Pintrich, 1996), whereas in areas related to language and arts, male and female students exhibit similar confidence despite the fact that the achievement of girls typically is higher. Pajares (1995) asked the elementary and middle school students to provide self-efficacy judgement and to make comparative judgments regarding their writing ability. Results revealed that girls judged themselves to be better writers than the boys. With this background the present study was designed to investigate as to what extent high self-efficacy individuals (girls and boys) and low self-efficacy individuals differ in terms of their attributional styles relating to different academic outcomes (success and failure), with the following objectives :

(1) To study the effect of levels of self-efficacy (high and low) on attributional styles.

(2) To study the effect of academic outcome (success/failure on an academic task) on attributional styles.

(3) To study the effect of gender on attribution.

It was hypothesized that :

(1) The high self efficacy (HSE) individuals as compared to low self efficacy (LSE) individuals would attribute academic success to internal causes.

(2) HSE individuals as compared to LSE individuals would attribute academic failure to external causes.

(3) Males, would attribute success to internal factors and failure to external factors in comparison to females.

METHOD

Design

The present study was conducted by following a 2 × 2 × 2 factorial design with two levels of self-efficacy (high/low), outcome on academic performance (success/failure) and gender (male and female). Participants were randomly assigned to each cell.

Participants

A total of 80 participants (40 boys and 40 girls) in the age group of 16-17 were randomly selected from a school with their prior consent for participation.

Material used

Two sets of anagrams (solvable and unsolvable). Attribution scale (Anderson, 1999)

Children's Perceived Academic Self-Efficacy Scale (Jerry & Morgan, 1999) : The scale was used to identify self-efficacy beliefs of individuals regarding academic achievement. This scale is applicable to students of age group of 14-17 year having 30 statements including four sub-scales-talent, effort, task difficulty and context. The overall reliability coefficient of the inventory is 82. Each participant was contacted individually and the test was administered, in the experimental room.

Procedure

Experimental task : The experimental task consisted of 2 sets of anagrams. One set contained solvable anagrams (very easy to solve) and the other set contained unsolvable anagrams. Anagrams were in jumbled form and the S was required to put the letters of the words in their correct order so as to make a meaningful word. In solvable task, all the 14 anagrams were solvable but in unsolvable task out of a list of 14 anagrams only 5 were solvable.

The task was similar to the task used by Baumeister and Tice (1985) for manipulation of success and failure feedback. Subjects were given 8 minutes to work on anagrams.

Manipulation of Experimental Situation : Overall two conditions were manipulated, success condition (in which solvable task was given) and failure condition (in which unsolvable task was given). Ss in success condition were made to believe that they have got success over the task they had performed, whereas, Ss in failure condition were made to believe that they have failed over he task they had performed.

Each S participated in the experiment one by one and was made to sit comfortably as he/she entered the experimental room. Each of them received a set of general instructions as follows :

"You are going to participate in an experiment and as the requirement of the experiment you have to perform on a task that consists of 14 anagrams. I am going to show you a sample anagram and the necessary steps for solving it. See, here is a word 'EOSN'. If we change the position of the letters E and N, it makes a meaningful word, *i.e.*, "NOSE". Due to time limit of 8 minutes, please don't waste time. Start when I say 'Ready' and stop when I say 'Stop'."

When S finished the task, the E pretend to 'score' the S's performance. When the E ostensibly finished scoring, the outcome feedback, was presented. Further, a set of specific feedback was given to the Ss in the success and failure conditions.

Failure Conditions : In success condition in which Ss were given the solvable task so as to achieve success, they were told : "You have done well and have scored in the 89th percentile. It was one of the best score I have seen since I have been administering the test." Thus, they were made to believe that they have got success over the task they had performed.

In failure condition in which Ss were given unsolvable task, they were told, "You have done quite badly and have scored in 21st percentile. I'm surprised, this is one of the lowest score I have seen since I have been administering the test". Thus, they were made to believe that they have failed over the task they had performed.

After the outcome manipulation a five point rating scale was used to determine the subjects' attributional styles in relation to different academic outcomes (success and failure). Finally, participants were carefully debriefed and thanked for their participation.

RESULTS AND DISCUSSION

The scores of the participation on the attribution rating scale were analysed by applying three way ANOVA.

Table 16.1 : Summary of Anova

Sources of Variation	*S.S.*	*Df*	*Ms*	*F*
Self Efficacy A	195.31	1	195.31	20.30*
Academic Outcome B	2.11	1	2.11	0.21
Gender C	5.51	1	5.51	0.57
SS AB	15.51	1	15.51	1.61
SS AC	12.01	1	12.01	01.24
SS BC	25.31	1	25.31	2.63
SS ABC	436.31	1	436.61	45.38*
SS Within	692.28	72	72	9.62

* P < .01.

The mean attribution score of the HSE group was found to be higher (27.075) than of the LSE group (23.95). Analysis also showed that main effect of self efficacy ($F = 20.30, P < 0.01$) was significant. However the main effects for academic achievement success : 25.675; Failure : 24.4 $F = 0.21$) and Gender (Males : 25.25; Females : 25.77; $F = 0.57$) were not found to be significant. However, interaction between self-efficacy, academic outcome and Gender ($F = 45.38$) was found to be significant.

As the means show, HSE individuals were found to be more internals ($M = 29.60$) than their LSE counterparts. ($M = 21.75$). SHE individuals attributed their success to internal causes and failure to external causes. On the other hand LSE individuals attributed their failure to internal causes and success to external causes. These finding can be explained in terms of self-consistency theory Swann, 1990 which holds that people strive to acquire information that confirms their self-conceptions because self-confirmatory information seems especially trustworthy, diagnostic and accurate. High self-efficacy individuals perceive themselves favourably, confident (Baumeister, Smart & Boden 1996), more competent of greater worth (Baumgardner, 1990). On the other hand, Low self efficacy individuals evaluate themselves less favourably (Baumgardner, 1990), and view themselves to be less competent (Brown & Dutton, 1995) and inadequate (Brown & Mankowski, 1993). Both of the SE groups as such strive for those situations where these attributes are confirmed. As people develop attitudes and behave in ways that maintain their level of self-esteem. Brockner (1988) suggested that HSE individuals, in particular, have strong positive beliefs concerning their qualities, as such, they are not easily affected by external cues, rather they make more internal attributions. In contrast, LSE individuals have strong negative beliefs concerning their self and as such have greater susceptibility to be influenced by external attributions. The attribution style of both SE groups is result of these cognitive basis which help to sustain self-perceptions. Findings of the experiment prove that HSE and LSE are self-maintaining. This could be reason as to why HSE individuals are internal in their attributions, whereas, LSE individuals are external in their attributions.

Findings can also be explained in terms of model of self-certainty (Campbell, 1990; Baumgardner, 1990). This term refers to the degree to which people are clear about who they are. Individuals with LSE are less sure of who they are than are HSE individuals (Campbell & Faireym, 1991). They are generally more uncertain as to where do they stand on any given attribute than are HSE individuals as their self concept is characterized by uncertainty. Uncertainty increases the doubts of LSE individuals concerning their ability (Tang & Reynolds, 1993) which as such decreases their confidence. The extent to which people possess their attributional styles is also influenced by the extent to which they are certain of their selves.

The difference in the attributional styles of both SE groups can also be explained in terms of associative network model of Brown and Mankowski (1993). Individuals with LSE in general have richer association with external causes *i.e.* luck etc. (Brockner, 1988). On the other hand, HSE individuals have richer association with internal factors *i.e.* ability etc. (Tang & Reynolds, 1993). LSE individual possess stronger external, unfavourable and negative self-associations (Isen, 1984), whereas, HSE individuals possess stronger internal, positive and favourable self-associations (Jussim, Coleman & Nassam, 1987). This could explain why LSE individuals were found to possess external attribution and HSE possessed internal attribution.

According to self enhancement motive (Brown & Dutton, 1995), people have a desire to maximize feelings of self-worth to the extent to which they can view themselves positively. HSE people are especially apt at satisfying this need (Brown and Mankowski, 1993). People are more apt to reject or otherwise dismiss the negative implications of failure. They consistently respond to events in a way to restore or maintain feelings of self-worth and as a result perform better by increasing their efforts (Tang & Reynolds, 1993). Researchers have demonstrated that through positive feedback, academic achievement and desirable self attributions (*e.g.* I succeeded on the mathematics task because I have the ability to do well in mathematics) can be increased. Self enhancement contribute to assisting children with LSE to regard themselves as worthwhile and feel good about themselves and their abilities, which can help them to live better and healthy living.

REFERENCES

Anderson, C.A. (1999). Attributional style, depression, and loneliness : A cross-cultural comparison of American and Chinese students society for *Personality and Social Psychology*, Inc., *25*, 482-499.

Bandura, A. (1977). Self-efficacy : Toward a unifying theory of behaviour change, *Psychological Review*, *84*, 191-215.

Bandura, A. (1978). The Self-efficacy in reciprocal determinism, *American Psychologist*, *3*, 334-358.

Bandura, A. (1982). Self-efficacy mechanism in human agency, *American Psychologist*, *37*, 122-147.

Baumeister, R.F., Smart, L., & Boden, J.M. (1996). Relation of threatened Egotism to Violence and Aggression : The dark side of the high self-esteem, *Psychological Review*, *103*, 5-33.

Baumgardner, A.H. (1990). To know oneself is to like oneself : Self-certainty and self-affect, *Journal of Personality and Social Psychology*, *58*, 1062-1072.

Brockner, J. (1988). Low self-esteem and behavioural plasticity : Some implications for personality and social psychology. In L. Wheeler (Ed.), *Review of Personality and Social Psychology*, Vol. 4, (pp. 237-271), Beverly Hills, CA : Sage.

Brown, J.D., & Dutton, K.A. (1995). The thrill of victory, the complexity of defeat : Self-esteem and people's emotional reaction to success and failure, *Journal of Personality and Social Psychology*, *68*, 712-722.

Brown, J.D., & Mankowski, T.A. (1993). Self-esteem, mood, and self-evaluation, Changes in mood and the way you see you, *Journal of Personality and Social Psychology*, *64*, 421-430.

Campbell, J.D. (1990). Self-esteem and clarity of the self-concept, *Journal of Personality and Social Psychology*, *59*, 538-549.

Campbell, J.D. & Fairey, P.J. (1991). Effects of self-esteem, hypothetical explanations, and verbalization of expectancies on future performance, *Journal of Personality and Social Psychology*, *48*, 1097-1110.

Forsterling, F. (1985). Attributional retraining : A Review, *Psychological Bulletin*, *98*, 495-512.

Heider, F. (1958). The Psychology of interpersonal relations, *New York*, Willey.

Hackett, G. (1995). The role of mathematics in self-efficacy in the choice of math related majors of college women and men : A path-analysis, *Journal of Counseling Psychology*, *32*, 47-56.

Isen, A.M. (1984). Toward understanding the role of affect in cognition. In R.S. Wyer, Jr., & T.S. Srull (Eds.), *Handbook of Social Cognition*, Vol. 3, (pp. 179-236). Hillsdale, NJ : Erlbaum.

Junks, J., Morgan, v. Jerry, Vicky Morgan (1999). *Children's Perceived Academic,* Self-Efficacy : An Inventory Scale.

Jussim, L., Coleman, L., & Nassau, S. (1987). The influence of self-esteem on perceptions of performance and feedback, *Social Psychology Quarterly*, *50*, 95-99.

Pajares, F. & Miller, M.D. (1994). Mathematics self-efficacy and mathematics outcomes, The need for specificity of assessment, *Journal of Counseling Psychology*, *42*, 190-198.

Pajares, F. (1995). Self-efficacy beliefs in achievements setting, *Review of Educational Research*, *66*, 543-578.

Pajares, F. & Schunk, D.H. (2001). Self-beliefs and schools success : Self-efficacy, self-concept, and school achievement. In R. Riding & S. Rayner (Eds.), (2001), *Self-perception* (239-266), London : Ablex Publishing.

Pajares, F. (2002). Overview of Social Cognitive theory and of self efficacy. http://www.emory edu/ EDUCATION/ mfp/efftalk.html.

Pajares, F. (in press). Self-efficacy beliefs, motivation, and achievement in writing : A Review of the Literature, Reading and Writing Quarterly.

Stajkovic. A.D. & Buthans, F. (1998). Self-efficacy and work-related performances : A meta-analysis, *Psychological Bulletin*, *124*, 240-261.

Stajkovic, A.D., & Sommer, S.M. (2000). Self-efficacy and Casual Attributions : Direct an Reciprocal Links, *Journal of Applied Social Psychology*, *30*, 707-737.

Schunk, D.H. (1991). Self-efficacy and academic motivation, *Educational Psychologist*, *26*, 207-231.

Schunk, D.H. (1984a). Self-efficacy perspective on achievement behaviour, *Educational Psychologist*, *19*, 48-58.

Schunk, D.H. (1984b). Sequential attributional feedback and children's achievement behaviours, *Journal of Educational Psychology 76*, 1159-1169.

Schunk, D.H. (1984c). Enhancing self-efficacy and achievement through rewards and goals, Motivational and informational effects, *Journal of Educational Research*, *78*, 29-34.

Schunk, D.H. & Pajares, F. (2002). The development of academic self-efficacy. In A. Wigifeld & J. Eccles (Eds.), Development of achievement motivation (pp. 16-31). *San Diego : Academic Press.*

Shaw, Marvin, E. & Costanzo, Phillip R. (1985). *Theories of Social Psychology*. (2nd printing), McGraw, Hill. Inc.

Swann, W.B. (1990). To be adored or to be known : The interplay of self-enhancement and self-verification. In R.M. Sorrentino & E.T. Higgins (Eds.), *Motivation and Cognition*, *2*, 408-448, New York : Gulford Press.

Swann, W.B., Jr., Griffin, J.J., Jr., Predmore, S.C., & Grainer, B. (1987). The cognitive-affective crossfire : When self-consistency confronts self-enhancement, *Journal of Personality and Social Psychology*, *52*, 881-889.

Tang, T.L.P., & Reynolds, D.B. (1993). Effects of self-esteem and perceived goal difficulty on goal setting certainty, task performance, and attributions, *Human Resource Development Quarterly*, *4*, 153-170.

Wigfield, A., Eccles, J.S. & Pintrich, P.R. (1996). Development between the ages of 11 and 25. In D.C. Berliner & R.C. Calfee (Eds.), *Handbook of Educational Psychology* (pp. 148-185), New York : Simon & Schuster Macmillan.

Wiener, B. (1979). A theory of motivation for some classroom experiences, *Journal of Educational Psychology*, *71*, 3-25.

Wiener, B. (1986). An attribution theory of motivation and emotion, New York : Springer-Verlag.

Zimmerman, B.J., Bandura, A. & Matrinez-Pons, M. (1992). Self-motivation for academic attainment : the role of self-efficacy beliefs and personal goal-setting, *American Education Research Journal*, *29*, 663-676.

17

Childhood Rearing and Mental Well-Being

Vidhu Mohan*

Happiness is a state of mind, which every one aspires to attain; yet very few know how to do it. Mental well-being and a state of tranquility, satisfaction, happiness, are handmaidens of each other. The type of attitudes and values ingrained in the individual by the parents or surrogates usually lay down the foundations of how one is going to behave as an adult. The earlier socialization of the child is an important landmark in his/her development of personality. Parental attitude, values, behaviour, has a great impact on shaping the personality of the child. The mother, in the Indian set up, is known to be the first "Guru" or teacher of the child. Hence a mentally healthy mother lays down the foundations of a healthy personality.

In the Indian trilogy, the concept of 'Sat', 'Chit' and 'Anand' reside in the perception of 'Satyam Shivam, and Sundaram'. Truth is the handmaiden of ultimate peace and tranquility. What is beautiful, leads to joy in our heart. Maslow's Self-Actualization came very near to our Self-realization, or knowing of the true self, which is truth beauty and eternal joy. This is supposed to give one the highest sense of attainment and happiness. But how to get is and what is its ambit we do not understand to the full extent.

In Bhagvad Gita the chapter 14 & 17 gives a full description of the Triguna personality. The Sattavic Guna is 'purity, causing illumination and health..... by attachment to happiness and knowledge'. The Rajasic Guna is 'passion, nature of attraction springing from craving and attachment which binds one to action'. The Tamasic Guna, is characterized by inertia, slothfulness, and heedless indifference'. It is quite obvious from this that when Sattavic Guna will prevail upon the other two Gunas the individual will be in a state of bliss; but when Rajasic Guna will prevail in one's life, one would be always running after the mirage, and delusions of life; when Tamasic Guna will prevail, one would be lazy, slack, and negligent. Hence 'Rajas' and 'Tamas', would only generate misery, dejectedness, and discontent in life.

* Prof. Vidhu Mohan, Formerly Professor and Chair Person, Psychology Dept. Punjab University and Hony Secretary, Indian Council for Child Welfare, Chandigarh : Present address : 587-D, Section 21, Panchkula (Haryana).

E-mail mohanvidhu@hotmail.com

In early childhood, the parents should see to it that action & habits related to Sattavic Guna should be inculcated in the child. In a recent work the author (Mohan & Kataria, 1998) found that delinquency prone adolescents were more maladjusted in terms of 'home', 'health', 'social', and 'emotional' spheres in comparison to the non delinquent adolescents. In terms of the Triguna, the non-delinquents scored higher on Sattavic Guna, and the delinquents scored higher on Rajasic and Tamasic Guna. Inculcating spiritual values of "Sattavic Guna' in the formative years of the child is a must for positive mental health and well being of the child. These days we see so much of violence like rape, murder, road rage, fights and what not. Apart from physical violence there is a log of psychological violence—such as hurting the feelings of others by either commission or omission.

The Author (Mohan, 1999) developed a module for 'Self Growth Skills'. This module comes very near to the concept of developing EQ. This in turn comes very close to Maslow's self-actualization and Sattavic Guna. Some of the aspects of 'Self Growth Skills' include—interpersonal skills, sensitivity, communication skills including listening, self knowing, resolving intra-personal conflicts, motivating self, developing positive and innovative thinking, coping with the stress of life. In order to inculcate these, the initiation must take place in the early part of life for which parental training for proper child rearing practices is a must. These skills are elaborated below :

1. Interpersonal Skills

These include the ways in which we relate to others, and interact with them. Most of us don't have the tact to tell people what we feel. We become either very defensive or offensive or withdraw from the relation. (Mohan, 1999). This is integral part of developing Emotional Quotient as suggested by Golman (1995).

2. Developing Sensitivity

This is the skill to empathize with others, understand their feelings and relate to their hurts and pain. These feelings of hurt pain often dictate ones behaviour. If through empathetic understanding one goes into the shoes of the other person, then one can control the behaviour and modify, it, if necessary. (Mohan, 1999)

3. Communication Skills

Interaction with others essentially depends on our skills to communicate our thoughts to others. Effective communication imply adequate understanding of the communicate; understanding of the message to be communicated, and self knowledge of one's own capacity to relate the message. For effective communication, one must be clear about what one wishes to communicate, must have commitment to the cause one is espousing, adequate language and style to talk, good observation skills to perceive both verbal and non-verbal message, and listening skills. (Mohan, 1999) Language and Good communication is learnt first of all at home. We often lack interpersonal skills and feel diffident to interact with others. Most of us are a little uncomfortable meeting new people. Many of us are lonely but still we do not reach out. Or if we do reach out, we do what Bach and Deutsch (1970) call "rejection insurance?" We avoid getting emotionally involved with someone or we are careful to "keep pace" with our new partner and not get more involved with him or her, so that we don't get hurt! But is it necessary to protect ourselves?

4. Knowing Oneself

This part of self-development can further be subdivided into three areas :

(i) Understanding one's self with the help of Johari Window.

This window makes us perceive ourselves with the eyes of others and our own. Our understanding of self comes from our interactions with others and their feedback about how we behave. The more openly we relate to others, the more acceptable we become. The Johari Window is shown below and explained in the context of the self-perception and the perception of others.

JOHARI WINDOW SELF

Other	*I*	*II*
Known	**Public self**	**Blind arena**
	Open arena	**Bad breath**
	Free interactions	Social hindrances
	Flow of psychic energy	Not acceptable to others.
	Healthy encounters with others	
Unknown	*III*	*IV*
	Private self	**Dark arena**
	Hidden arena	**Unknown to both**
	Negative emotions	Talents as well as
	Conflicts	Liabilities
	Complex	

The Open/Public Self : This part of self represents those things that we share with others. The Open-self is directly related to the degree of closeness and openness we feel toward others. The larger the open self the more effective and dynamic we can become. It releases considerable psychic energy, which we can use freely to have better interactions with others, be more at peace within yourself.

The Blind Self : It represents those things in ourselves about which we are not aware. These may include behaviour patterns, which may prove to be irksome to others. This area can also have some good qualities about which we may not be aware. This quadrant can only be reduced if others give us a feedback about our behaviour.

The Hidden/Private Self : This quadrant contains things that an individual would like to hide from others. These could include various conflicts, complexes, negative emotions which we may not like to share with others, like jealousy, hatred, guilt feelings, anger, fears and apprehensions, or some attitudes and opinions which we may not like to share with others, due to negative consequences or we wish to avoid confrontation. The only way to reduce this quadrant is to be able to do self-disclosure and sharing with others. But every thing cannot be shared with others, one has to use discernment, caution, and the appropriateness of the person with whom we are going to share.

The Dark Arena : This part of self, which is the truly unknown, may contain some unknown talents, abilities, which the individual is totally unaware. Many of us may suffer from 'Hanuman Complex', like this legendary figure did not know his own strength and underestimated himself till a 'Jamwant' came to awaken him to his true strengths. This area may also have some liabilities about which a person may be unaware like the 'heel of Achilles' or the 'Thigh of Duryodhan'. The only way to reduce this arena is to take recourse to scientific probing through various Psychological tests. The author has successfully used various tests of ability and personality to help people explore their real self. (Mohan, 1999)

The effort of training lies in increasing quadrant I by reducing quadrants II, III, and IV. probing'. The changed Johari – Window may appear like something shown in the figure given below :

MODIFIED JOHARI WINDOW SELF

Other	*Known*	*Unknown*
Known	**I** **Increased Open Arena Free Energy** Improved inter-personal relations. More self-acceptance. Greater understanding of self and others. Release of psychic energy for productive work. Happier state of mind.	**I** **Reduced Blind Arena** by receiving Feedback from others and accepting it for changing self.
Unknown	**III** **Reduced Hidden Area** by Self-disclosure of things which need no hiding.	**IV** **Reduced Dark Arena** by scientific probing through Psychological tests.

With the help of Johari Window, the author has been able to improve the behaviour of more than five hundred commonwealth youth trainers and more than five hundred trainee counselors.

(ii) Known one's Negative Emotions and Coping with them.

In Johari Window quadrant III, a mention was made about the negative emotions. Usually these are one's major liabilities and we do not know how to deal with them. Learning skills to deal with these emotions can bring about an immense improvement in ourselves. For example if we understand what causes our anger then we can deal with it. The author while working with anger experienced by different groups of participants, deduced two main causes of anger : first is one's own expectations and demands out of others. When these are not fulfilled one feels a lot of anger and frustration. Second is the lack of interpersonal skills and ability to deal with a situation, often causes a great deal of irritation and anger, sometimes even mixed with a little apprehension. (Mohan, 1999)

(iii) Knowing one' Intra-personal Conflicts and resolving them.

As stated by Mohan (1997) "This type of conflict resides within the individual. It implies that there is a collision of motives, goals, values, interests, needs etc., of approximately equal strength, making it difficult for the individual to choose a course of action." According to Kurt Lewin (1935) there are three types of these conflicts, which an individual faces quite often in life :

Approach-Approach Conflict—in this situation a person is confronted by two equally desirable alternatives and finds it difficult to decide which to choose and which to leave.

Approach-Avoidance Conflict—here the individual is faced with a situation wherein there is both a negative and a positive aspect of the choice you make. If you choose the positive goal now then later the negative outcome is to be suffered. If you accept the negative aspect now then you suffer from feelings of despair, irritation, and apprehensions.

Avoidance-Avoidance Conflict—in this situation one is faced with two equally unpleasant or noxious choices. It is like being between the devil and the deep sea. Both alternatives have negative valences, which the individual would like to avoid, but cannot; he/she is forced to choose from one of the two unattractive alternatives.

All the three types of conflicts occur everyday in our life. But when the intensity or the extensity increases one feels disturbed. A conflict neglected has a tendency to snowball. The right thing to do is neither escape from the situation, nor loose one's calm and become aggressive, but to confront the situation adequately and deal with it, (Mohan, 1999)/Children can be taught in the early years to face the conflict rather than live in make believe, day dreams or tell lies. Some children learn to thrown a temper tantrum instead of facing their problem. Parents play a major role in reducing such behaviour.

5. Motivating Self

In order to lead a meaningful life one has to know one's aspirations in life. In order to fulfill them one must be committed to execute them, and accomplish one's goals of life. Identification of one's life goals and needs then the way to satisfy these can be identified. Awareness of one's own needs, hence becomes the first step in motivating oneself to accomplish them. These needs can be identified through exercises based on Maslow's Need Hierarchy. The author has been successfully using this model to improve upon the self-motivation of groups like medical practitioners, industrial middle level executives, police officers, bureaucrats, co-operative functionaries, youth trainers, social workers, and students. (Mohan, 1999). For children too this model can be used successfully. Instead of reinforcing children only with chocolates and the like, reinforcement of desired behaviour can be done through building self-esteem and then making the child develop internal locus of control.

6. Developing Innovative Thinking

This ability is to allow oneself to experiment with new ideas, explore new things, and take the liberty to try out new horizons. Usually in life we get tied down with set ideas, normative thinking, routine jobs and habitual acts. This makes life very regimented and routine and with lots of monotony. In order to live a full and fulfilling life one must be able to create, innovate new situations for oneself. Creative or Divergent thinking can be generated through exercises and practice. (Mohan, 1999). The author has used methods like brainstorming, developing 'fluency', 'flexibility', original ideas, problem solving, and such like enrichment programmes, (Mohan, 1999). Children have a natural curiosity to learn more. But often parents or teachers snub them when they ask questions or when they say 'why can't this be like this'.

They are put in a straight jacket of 'Convergent Thinking'. Parents & teachers should encourage 'Divergent Thinking' in children.

7. Developing Positive Attitude

We often tend to look at the dark side of the picture. Some people tend to live in an unrealistic euphoria, where their feet are rarely on the ground. These persons through their foolhardiness get hurt badly and then start blaming others. The other type are the ones who are perpetually pessimistic, fault findings, suspicious, and blaming others or situations. For a healthy and wholesome life one has to develop a realistic optimism and positive attitude in life. Authors like Dale Carnegie have written volumes on how to develop a healthy positive attitude in life. One has to learn to appreciate the assets of others and one's own. Also one should learn to cope with one's limitations, liabilities and contain them or convert them into assets. Parents and teachers can do a lot in making a healthy orientation in the thinking of children. Instead of blaming others or criticizing others or situations all the time, parents should make children appreciate things, look at the positive things happening in their life.

8. Coping with One's Stress

We live in an era of cold wars, nuclear weapons, violence—both domestic and community, scarcity, breaking down of social support systems, excessive emphasize on materialism. Children also start experiencing stress right in the early years of their life. Entry to school itself is a stressful situation. In school too there are peer group pressures and academic pressures. Parents create some of these by making very small child push into heightened competitiveness. Even the polluted ecology can cause stress for an individual so that coping strategies can be devised. In her presidential address, *Mohan* (1989) had suggested that stress can be coped through **physical means**—with the help of physical exercises, yoga, nutrition which should be balanced and health generating as described in 17th chapter of Bhagvad Gita for sattavic food and relaxation; which includes both mind and body relaxation; **Psychological means**—Bringing about a change in one's attitude develop positive thinking, learn techniques of time management, try to cope with one's conflicts by facing them and not procrastination, learn better interpersonal skills, and learn to relax and try out new alternatives; Making use of Social Support Systems like taking the help of family members—they are your allies, Seeking the help of sincere friends, in job situation by seeking the help of honest and sincere colleagues, and even religion can help in reducing stress; **Getting formal Help**—Going to a trained counselor for help, joining formal groups where training is imparted for coping strategies and joining the courses imparting self-development skills.

Positive Parenting

Parental attitude is very vital in giving a child a happy & healthy orientation in life. Parents are supposed to give the child unconditional love, but do they know its meaning? I would like to quote Swami Vivekananda's words on Love "I would like to share something on the 'nature of love' I once had a friend who grew to be very close to me. Once when we were sitting at the edge of a swimming pool, she filled the palm of her hand with a little water and held it before me, and said this, "You see this water carefully contained on my hand? It symbolizes Love." As long as you keep your hand caringly open and allow it to remain there, it will always be there. However, if you attempt to close your fingers around it and try to possess it, it will spill through the first cracks it finds. This is the greatest mistake that people do when they meet love...they try to possess it, they demand, they expect... and just like the water spilling out of your hand, Love will retrieve from you. For love is meant to be free, you cannot change its nature. If there are people you love, allow them to be free beings." Mother happens to be the first "Guru" and she can dispense love in a most healthy manner. (Mohan, 1994).

The author has developed a scale to measure how parents reflect their love for the child. (Mohan & Kaur, 1989; Mohan & Grewal, 1990; Mohan & Nalwa, 1996). Most of the socialization takes place through love. But often we don't know how to express it. The author on the basis of her research identified ten areas in which parental involvement is a must for a well-adjusted development of the child. These are also behavioural ways of demonstrating to the child that you love him/her). These areas are discussed in details below :

- **Academic or mental growth :** Taking interest in the academic affairs of the child; seeing that he/she has the necessary things for the school work; concentrating not only on school work but also giving a bigger vision of knowledge.
- **Social relations :** Taking care of the child's social relations and friends; promoting Sattavic Guna through pro-social behaviour such as helpfulness, sharing, mutual give and take, showing care and concern for friends. Parents should know the friends of their children and interact with them so that they know what type of psychosocial milieu their child is living in.
- **Recreation :** The parents should know and take interest in what the child does in his/her free time. It is the duty of the parents to plan healthy recreational activities including outdoor activities.
- **Economic self-sufficiency :** The parents should try to build the self-regard in the child by knowing his/her financial needs and give a regular pocket money by negotiating and educating the child to be frugal.
- **Nutrition :** Adequate and healthy nutritious and sattavic food should be given to the child. Now a days parents just let the children indulge in junk food intake, or lop sided nutrition for example allowing child to eat only high protein diet of non-vegetarian diet, not giving it a balance with vegetables and fruits.
- **Clothes :** Parents should provide suitable clothes. This does not mean parents should go in for very expensive branded clothes and make the child over possessive about goods. The child should be neat and clean and dressed in clothes tailor made for him/her.
- **Puberty development :** This is a highly neglected area of child rearing. Parents shy away in educating their child about the body development and the sexual growth. Teaching about the body in a scientific manner, and giving right attitude about sexuality is the duty of the parents (Mohan, 2003). Neglect in this area results in many cases of sexual experimentation, reading pornographic material, surfing such material, even contracting sexually transmitted diseases like AIDs; sometimes children become a prey to sexual abuse like rape and sodomy through sheer ignorance.
- **Demonstration of love :** "Skin hunger" or the need for experiencing love through

touch has been recognized right from the time of the famous experiment done by Harlow with chimpanzee babies. They preferred to go to the cuddly cloth mother rather than the wire mother, which gave them milk. Parents should demonstrate their affection physically also to the child.

- **Personality development :** Proper socialization leads to the development of a healthy wholesome personality. The parents can do this by trusting the child, giving autonomy, appreciate industry, respect their identity and develop their self-esteem.
- **Health :** This can be done through proper medical check up, taking the child for proper medication when sick, and alertness to any of their deficiency.

Through proper looking after and care in the said areas, the parents can inculcate the right attitude towards life with more pre-dispositions towards the supremacy of the Sattavic Guna in the child.

What Parents can do

Parents can achieve the aforesaid goals by indulging in some activities in the various areas of development. The author has conducted many workshops in this area through which she has been able to evolve these activities. These workshops were conducted on nearly five hundred people who were educated and belonged too professional class. These activities are presented below :

ACTIVITIES FOR CHILDREN

	Area	*Activity*
1.	Physical	Muscular Co-ordination, Skills; *e.g.* jumping, running, back-step walking, rope skipping, group exercises and games.
2.	Mental	Reasoning and Creative thinking; *e.g.* story telling, word building, poem recitation, singing rhymes, story building, doing small puzzles, computer, games of thinking, quizzes etc.
3.	Social	Teaching pro-social & Co-operation, Altruistic behaviour *e.g.* make children play group games, tell stories which have messages of helpful behaviour, like 'Panchtantra', 'Jatak tales', 'Story of Vikramaditya' and the like. Make children indulge in some social work, take them to places needing their help like homes for destitute etc.
4.	Emotional	Cope with Anger, fear, jealousy, sorrow *e.g.* this could be done by teaching opposite and pleasant emotions like love, joy, contentment, & happiness. Dramatization techniques can be of help.
5.	Moral	Internal values. Stories with morals are the best way to do this such as our ancient folklores like Panchtantra, Jatak tales etc.; plus dramatization, & role-playing.

A happy and healthy childhood is the right of each child. But is that what is happening? We find children suffering from psychosomatic disorders since they are under constant stress. We—the educationists and the psychologists—have a duty towards the society to educate our future parents in proper child rearing practices so that our progeny does not suffer in the hands of well meaning but ignorant parents. It is easier to give birth to the child—a matter of nine months only, but the proper rearing of the child can take years of input. An attempt has been made in this paper to help parents to improve their rearing practices.

REFERENCES

Goleman, D. (1995). *Emotional Intelligence,* Bantam Books, N. York.

Khandwala, Pradip (1984). The Fourth Eye.

Mohan, V. (1994). *Women, Education, and Child Rearing. In The Indian Girls.* Ed. V.K. Dhoundiyal, N.C. Dhoundiyal & A. Shukla, Shri Almora Book Depot, Almora.

Mohan, V. (1994). Women, Education, and Child Rearing. In 'The Indian Girls' Ed. V.K. Dhoundhiyal, N.C. Dhoundhiyal, & A. Shukla, Shri Almora Book Depot, Almora.

Mohan, V. (2003). Developing Skills : Self Awareness, Decision-making, Interpersonal value analysis & clarification. In Adolescence & Life Skills. Ed. Bhagwan Prakash, CYP, Tata McGraw Hill, N. Delhi, 190-209.

Mohan, V. (2004). Application of Psychology for the welfare of society in human behaviour & organizational excellence. Ed. M. Bhargava & S. Arora, 2004, 10-35, Sunrise, Agra.

Mohan, V. & Kaur, J. (1989). Perception of child rearing practices by children of working and non-working mothers, *Indian Journal of Community Guidance Service,* Vol. 6(1), Pp. 1-12.

Mohan, V. & Grewal, R. (1990). Perception of child rearing practices of mothers with high premenstrual tension syndrome, *J. Indian Academy of Applied Psychology,* Vol. 16(2), Pp. 23-29.

SECTION—III

Health in Socio-demographic Perspective

18

Mental Hygiene of T.B. Patients of Saurashtra Region of Gujarat State in Relation to Socio-personal Variables

D. J. Bhatt[*]

Mental health has long been recognized as an integral component of overall health of an individual. Unfortunately, even after fifty years since WHO (1946) defined it as "a state of complete physical, mental and social well being and not merely the absence of disease or infirmity," mental health has been neglected by most of the countries. Good health depends on the state of both mind and body. Each exerts a direct influence on the other but owing to the power of mind over matter good mental health is of supreme importance. Mental health is the full and harmonious functioning of the whole personality.

According to Schultz and Schultz (2004) stress-related diseases are wide spread among employees in the United States. A national survey conducted by a Life Insurance company found that nearly half of all employed adults considered their job to be extremely stressful and one of every three Americans has seriously considered quitting their jobs because of stress. As many as half of all visits to physicians are precipitated by stress. Further, a major share of physical complaints may be psychosomatic—that is actual physical disorders caused by or related to emotional factors such as stress on the job. Physical problems associated with stress include high blood pressure (hypertension), ulcers, colitis, heart disease, arthritics, skin diseases, allergies, headaches, neck and lower back pain, cancer and other diseases. The problem of mental health, stress and the patients' different kinds of physical diseases has led to a new filed of study—Medical Health Psychology. This concern for mental health and the patient's well-being can be traced back to the early years of medical psychology practice. Medical Health Psychology is the study of problems dealing with the health effects of diseases oriented stress and other aspects of patient well being. Initially some sporadic efforts were made for providing community mental health care. In 1950's measures were taken by Dr.

[*]Professor and Head, Department of Psychology, Saurashtra University, Rajkot (Gujarat).

Vidyasagar at Amritsar to involve concerned families of patients in their treatment in the hospital setting (Vidyasagar, 1971). The first rural mental health center was started in 1964 at Patna (Sharma & Palit, 1991).

Mishra & Somani (1993) suggested that the coefficient of correlation between scores obtained on mental health and occupational stress of the supervisors turned to be negative. Verma & Asthana (1993) revealed that there was significant mean difference between the cancer patients and the normal patients and their mental health aspects, *viz.* Ego-centrism, alienation, emotional stability and social non-conformity while expression was insignificant. Nakum (1995) suggested that there was significant mean difference between the cancer patients', sex, age and area and their overall mental hygiene scores.

Jagdish and Yadav (1999) indicated that home deprivation was negatively associated with positive self-evaluation, perception of reality, integration of personality, autonomy, group oriented attitude, environmental mastery and overall mental health.

Kothari (2000) expressed that there was significant mean difference between the T.B. patients' sex age, marital status and education and their overall mental hygiene whereas area, income and type of T.B. patients were non-significant.

Ojha (2002) found that social anxiety was significantly higher in orthopaedically handicapped group. Orthopaedically handicapped females, were found to be more socially anxious as compared to orthopaedically handicapped males. However, few dimensions of mental health, *viz.* group oriented attitude, integration of personality, and positive self evaluation were found to be significant on physically handicapped in general. Latha (2002) revealed that higher Trait Anger scores (< 22) and high Hostility score (< 9.29) significantly increases the risk for the coronary heart disease (CHD).

Khan (2003) said that without mentally healthy teachers we cannot aspire and expect a good society. Besides it, the teachers should be aware of and well informed about mental health care programmes and practices so that they may guide and direct the student's guardian/ parent properly and accordingly, whenever it is needed.

Akhani, Rathi & Nath (2003) showed that hostelers had more religious personal values than day scholars, and day scholars are significantly high on health personal values. There was no significant difference between mental health of the two groups.

Thus it is apparent that mental health is related with physical health. Researches specifically on T.B. patients have identified four kinds of factors which are associated with the disease. These are agent factors (Physical, chemical, food, biological and mechanical), host factors (Age, sex, marital-status, heredity, vocation, SES, habits), environmental factors (radiation, air pollution, daily underwear (cloth), medicine & social environment) and psychological factors (type of personality, perception, individual differences, attitude toward T.B. etc.)

The present study aimed at comparing the mental hygiene level of the different type of T.B. patients and to find the difference in mental health of subjects' as a function of socio-personal variables in hospital set-up.

It was hypothesized that there would be no significant difference in the overall and different factors of mental hygiene scores of subjects of different gender, age, area and type of disease (T.B.).

METHOD

Sample

The sample of the present study consisted of 160 male and female, T.B. patients who were selected through incidental-cum-purposive sampling technique from the T.B. Hospitals located in Saurashtra region. They were suffering from either lung or brain T.B. All the subjects were between 19-70 years of age. The sample mean age was 24.55 yrs with SD = 3.79 yrs. Their education level was from illiterate to graduate. The average number of the patients generally belonged to middle socio-economic status.

Tool

The Mental Hygiene Inventory (MHI) developed and standardized by Bhatt and Gida (1992) was employed to assess the mental health of the T.B. patients. This Inventory consists of 40 items with two alternative responses, namely Agree and Disagree. The Inventory measures five dimensions, *i.e.*, perception of reality integration of personality, positive self-evaluation, group-oriented attitude and environmental mastery. The test-retest reliability of the MHI was 0.87 and the split half reliability corrected by Spearman—Brown formula was 0.90 with an index of reliability of 0.94 (overall). The test-retest reliability of five factors of mental hygiene was 0.96, 0.91, 0.80, 0.97 and 0.87 respectively. The content and concurrent validity were sufficient for the Inventory.

Procedure

The above-mentioned Inventory was administered to the T.B. Patients in groups by fixing the time and day for collecting the data with authorities of the hospitals.

RESULTS AND DISCUSSION

The scoring was done with the help of manual after collecting the data. Thus, a total score indicating overall mental hygiene was obtained for each patient. The entire data was arranged in tabular form for statistical analysis.

Table 18.1 : Statistical Analysis of Mental Hygiene Inventory Scores (for Six Factors) of Male and Female T.B. Patients (N = 160)

Factors of Mental Hygiene	*Male T.B. Patients*			*Female T.B. Patients*			*t-Value*
	N	*M*	*SD*	*N*	*M*	*SD*	
1. Perception of reality	80	5.20	1.42	80	3.98	1.37	5.55**
2. Integration of personality	80	4.80	1.38	80	4.10	1.20	3.50**
3. Positive self-evaluation	80	4.80	1.50	80	3.96	1.40	3.65**
4. Group oriented attitudes	80	5.10	1.41	80	4.32	1.30	3.71**
5. Environmental mastery	80	4.40	1.21	80	4.10	1.10	1.66
6. Overall MH scores	80	24.96	3.31	80	23.30	4.32	2.76**

** $p<.01$.

Initially the data was dichotonized in terms of gender. The difference between the mean overall and specific factor mental hygiene scores of males and females was analysed by applying t-test. In Table18.1 the calculated 't' Value=2.76 is significant at 0.01 Level = 158. Hence,

Ho_1 is Rejected. It can be said that there is a significant mean difference between overall Mental Hygiene Scores of male and female subjects. The male T.B. patients scored significantly higher than the female T.B. patients.

Persual of the t values for six different factors of mental hygiene, shows that the mean scores of the male T.B. patients were higher than that of the females of all the 5 dimensions. The t values for four factors, *i.e.* perception of reality, integration of personality, positive self-evaluation, group oriented attitudes were significant ($p<.01$) However, the difference ($t = .166, p>.05$) was not found to be significant in case of environmental mastery.

Table 18.2 : The T.B. Patients' Age and Their Mental Hygiene t-test (N =160)

Factors of Mental Hygiene	*Below 34 Yrs. Patients*			*Above 34 Yrs. Patients*			*t-Value*
	N	*M*	*SD*	*N*	*M*	*SD*	
1. Perception of reality	85	4.50	1.46	75	4.80	1.48	1.30
2. Integration of personality	85	5.30	1.48	75	6.20	1.12	4.29**
3. Positive self-evaluation	85	3.10	1.25	75	4.95	1.35	8.80**
4. Group oriented attitudes	85	4.36	1.27	75	5.10	1.50	3.36**
5. Environmental mastery	85	3.20	1.02	75	3.90	1.05	4.38**
6. Overall MH scores	85	23.97	3.44	75	25.13	4.14	1.98*

*P <.05, **P≤.01.

In order to study the relationship between age and mental hygiene scores, the sample was dichotomized into two groups, *i.e.* below 34 years and above 34 years. Comparison between the overall MH score revealed a significant difference ($t = 1.97, p<.05$) between the subjects of the two groups. Further comparison on the individual dimension showed a significant difference on four dimensions while that on perception of reality ($t = 1.30, p>.05$) was not significant.

Table 18.3 : The T.B. Patients' Area and Their Mental Hygiene t-test (N = 160)

Factors of Mental Hygiene	*Rural T.B. Patients*			*Urban T.B. Patients*			*t-Value*
	N	*M*	*SD*	*N*	*M*	*SD*	
1. Perception of reality	106	3.05	0.97	54	3.85	0.90	5.00**
2. Integration of personality	106	5.40	0.72	54	5.88	0.79	3.69**
3. Positive self-evaluation	106	4.25	0.82	54	5.01	0.84	5.42**
4. Group oriented attitudes	106	3.85	0.96	54	3.10	0.95	4.68**
5. Environmental mastery	106	3.83	0.99	54	3.96	0.87	0.86
6. Overall MH scores	106	23.86	4.35	54	24.99	2.76	2.02*

* P<.05, ** P ≤ 0.01.

Further comparison was made between the M.H. scores of subjects from Rural and Urban areas. Here again the sample was divided into two groups in term of area and the difference between the mean scores were analysed. As in case of gender, the differences in mean overall M.H. scores and those on four dimensions, except environmental mastery ($t = 0.86, p>.05$) were found to be significant.

Table 18.4 : Statistical Analysis of Mental Hygiene Inventory Scores (for Six Factors) of Male and Female T.B. Patients (Lungs and Brain, N = 160)

Factors of Mental Hygiene	*Lungs T.B. Patients*			*Brain T.B. Patients*			*t-Value*
	N	*M*	*SD*	*N*	*M*	*SD*	
1. Perception of reality	100	3.60	1.00	60	3.10	0.97	3.13**
2. Integration of personality	100	4.71	1.02	60	4.50	1.00	1.23**
3. Positive self-evaluation	100	5.09	1.10	60	4.37	1.05	4.00**
4. Group oriented attitudes	100	5.20	1.19	60	4.60	0.99	3.33**
5. Environmental mastery	100	4.49	1.25	60	3.[illegible]0	1.01	3.00**
6. Overall MH scores	100	24.98	4.10	60	23.68	3.90	2.00*

* $P \leq 0.05$, ** $P \leq 0.01$.

Lastly, in order to compare the difference between the M.H. of lung and brain & stomach T.B. patients, the mean scores of the subjects suffering from the two type of T.B. were computed and analysed. Here the difference in the overall M.H. Score ($t = 2.00$, $p < .05$) was found to be significantly and the mean score of the lung T.B. patients was higher. Further comparison between the scores on the individual dimensions revealed significant differences on all dimensions except integration of personality. Here again, mean scores of the lung patients were found to be consistently higher.

From the present findings it can be concluded that the male T.B. patients experience greater degree of overall mental hygiene as compared to the female T.B. patients.

The male T.B. patients scored significantly higher on perception of reality, integration of personality, positive self-evaluation and group oriented attitudes than the female T.B. patients. There exist non-significant mean difference between the male T.B. patients and the female T.B. patients and their MH factor environmental mastery.

Above 34 yrs. old patients experience greater degree of overall mental hygiene as compared to below 34 yrs. old patients. Above 34 yrs. old patients scored significantly higher on integration of personality, positive self-evaluation, group oriented attitudes and Environmental mastery than below 34 yrs. old T.B. patients. There non-significant mean difference exists between above 34 yrs old patients and below 34 yrs old patients factor of mental hygiene for perception of reality. The urban T.B. patients experience greater degree of overall mental hygiene as compared to the rural T.B. patients. The urban patients scored significantly higher on perception of reality, integration of personality and positive self-evaluation than the rural patients. This indicated significant mean difference between the rural patients and the urban patients and their MH factor group oriented attitudes. There was non-significant mean difference between the urban patients and the rural patients and their MH factor environmental mastery. The lungs T.B. patients experience greater degree of overall mental hygiene as compared to the brain & stomach T.B. patients. The lungs patients scored significantly higher on perception of reality, positive self-evaluation group oriented attitudes and environmental mastery than the brain & stomach patients. There revealed non-significant mean difference between the lungs patients and the brain & stomach patients and their MH factor integration of personality.

Thus these results show that gender, area, age and nature of T.B. in TB patients is related to mental hygiene scores, where male, older and brains stomach T.B. patients had better mental hygiene.

REFERENCES

Akhani, P., Rathi, N. & Nath, P. (2003). Correlation Study of Mental Health and Personal Values of Hostilities and Day Scholars, *Praachi Journal of Psycho-cultural Dimensions, 19*, 99-104.

Bhatt, D.J. & Gida, G.R. (1992). "*Mental Hygiene Inventory*," unpublished *Manual*, Department of Psychology, Saurashtra University, Rajkot (Guj).

Kasinath, H.M. (2003). Interactive Effect of Mental Health School Adjustment and SES on Academic Achievement, *Indian Journal of Psychometry & Education, 34*, 159-164.

Khan, R.H. (2003). Importance of Teacher's Mental Health in promoting Good Mental Health of Children, *Indian Journal of Psychometry & Education 34*, 93-95.

Jagdish & Yadav, S. (1999). Relationship Between Home Deprivation and Mental Health Among School Students, *Indian Journal of Psychometry & Education, 30*, 35-38.

Latha (2002). Psychological Risks for Coronary Heart Disease (CHD), A Case-Control Analysis, *Journal of the Indian Academy of Applied Psychology, 28*, 125-130.

Mishra, P.C. & Somani, H.R. (1993). Occupational Stress in Relation to Mental Health of Supervisors, *Indian Journal of Behaviour, 17*, 1-5.

Kothari, S. (2003). *A Study of Mental Hygiene of T.B. Patients M.A. Level Dissertation*, Department of Psychology, Saurashtra University, Rajkot (Guj.).

Nakum, N. (1995). *A Study of Mental Hygiene of Patients of Rajkot Cancer Hospital, M.A. Level Dissertation*, Department of Psychology, Saurashtra University, Rajkot-360 005.

Ojha, S. (2002). Social Anxiety and Mental Health of Handicapped, *Praachi Journal of Psycho-cultural Dimensions, 18*, 27-31.

Schultz, D.P. & Schultz, S.E. (2004). *Psychology and Work Today,* Delhi : Pearson Education India Branch.

Sharma, S. & Palit (1991). *National Mental Health Programme*, A progress report 1982-90, New Delhi : The Directorate General of Health Services.

Vidyasagar (1971). *Innovations in Psychiatric Treatment at Amritsar Hospital Report on a Seminar on The Organization and Future Needs of Mental Health Services*, New Delhi : World Health House.

Verma, K. & Ashthana M. (1993). "Mental Health of Cancer Patients," *Psychology in Progress, 1*, 1-5.

19

Personality Differences Among School Children of Various Medium of Instruction in Gujarat State

L.R. Yagnik & Arvind S. Shah***

Language is a great gift to mankind. No one, except human being can read or write language. Without language there would be no books to read, no papers to write, no lectures to endure. In absence of language each of us would live in a largely solitary and isolated world, unable to communicate or receive any information.

In world more than 4,000 languages are spoken, only about 300 are in regular use, in written form and fewer than 100 of these have significant written literature. India, with over 1,000 languages and more than dozen scripts, acknowledges fourteen official regional languages, but not exclusively local and state government, in politics and education. Hindi has status of National language, but English is widely used in government, politics, commerce, industry and education.

Child learns language at home. After home, the school is considered to be second, because of its influence on the development of child's personality. The school is the chief contenting and supplementing institution in which children develop sound mental heath and good personality. The school is charged with providing experience to develop the total individual through self actualization, human relationship, economic efficiency and civic responsibilities. School experiences are designed to enhance growth and development, stimulate learning and develop good behaviour patterns. According to Carroll (1964) the school has two functions :

1. To make its instructional programme positive and to use disciplinary measures which are constructive, so that emotional and other maladjustment may be prevented rather than caused.
2. To identify these children who are maladjusted so as to provide adequate remedial treatment to them.

---

*Prof. & Head. Department of Psychology, Sardar Patel University, Vallabh Vidyanagar-388120.
**Lecturer in Psychology, A.S.C. Mahila Arts College, Mehsana.

Heredity and environment are the main factors of growth and development. The root of ability distribution undoubtedly lies in hereditary innate endowment, but educational environment is also a necessary condition for nurturing the latent potentialities given by heredity. The very definition of talent makes it clear that talent is an ability in a specific field which is capable of high functioning under training without timely, identification and proper training.

Early studies (Hildreth,1938) tried to relate giftedness with personality and had found that gifted children are self-confident, independent and emotionally more stable. Genius has been also found to be related with Psychopathological disturbances. (Witty and Lehman, 1930; Lange, 1931; and Krestschmer, 1931). A few studies have tried to explore the relationship between science and personality characteristics, Vahista (1982) studied personality differences among family reared and institution reared boys, girls. Chaliha (1997) studied personality pattern of 60 mentally retarded persons with CPQ test.

The environment provided during childhood lays foundation for their personalities. The way the children are brought up determines not only their own future but also of their parents, community, nation and mankind. The child needs sympathetic ears to which he can pour out his troubles and loving heart that makes him feel always welcome. Parents give love, care. It is well known that children deprived of parental love, care and security usually face economic, psychological and social problems. These problems may lead them to depression, frustration, insecurity, anxiety, and personality imbalances.

When child enters the school, he or she has many problems. What happens to the beginning of pupil depend upon the personal resources he brings to school, the values of the culture, as transmitted by school and the behaviour of teacher and media of instruction.

There are many types of schools in India. Growth of Indian schools in number is surprising. In 1950-1951 there were only 13596 upper primary schools and in 2001 - 2002 there were 219626 schools. The schools are providing education for different subjects, for example English Medium Schools, Government Schools of small villages, Agricultural schools and the Schools providing training for Army, Navy and Air Force.

These days the influence of English language has an attentive value. It is a prestige language. Most of the parents prefer English Medium schools for their children. These children who do not want to study in English Medium schools, but by the pressure of their parents seek admission to the English Medium schools experience difficulty in communication because of the pressure from authorities. Anand (1971) compared English Medium students and found the former to be significantly superior in verbal intelligence and achievement.

On the other hand there are a lot of students in Gujarati medium but they actually want to study in English medium. The fee structures in these English Medium Schools are actually a burden to the poor parents. It is necessary to get a chance to every student to study as per wish. The medium difference separates our generation from one extreme to another.

So to study the difference in personalities of these students will give an insight to parents of both kinds of students, especially the parents who force their children to study in a particular medium. In this study the investigator made an attempt to investigate the effects of school environment as per the medium and training on the personality structure of both English and Gujarati medium school going students.

Accordingly, the study was carried with the following objectives :

1. To study the personality characteristics of English medium school students.
2. To study the personality characteristics of Gujarati medium students.
3. To study the personality differences between English Medium boys and girls and Gujarati Medium boys and girls.
4. To compare the difference in girls & boys of different medium schools. Following hypotheses were formulated :
   1. There would be no difference in personality among students of English medium and Gujarati Medium in 14 personality factors.
   2. There would be no difference in personality among boys and girls of English and Gujarati medium students.
   3. There would be no difference in personality among the English medium boys and girls & Gujarati Medium boys and girls of secondary schools.

METHOD

Design

A 2 × 2 factorial design was used to measure personality differences in English and Gujarati Medium students.

Medium of Instruction	*Sex*		*Total*
	A_1 *(Boys)*	A_2 *(Girls)*	
English Medium (B_1)	200	200	400
Gujarati Medium (B_2)	200	200	400
Total	400	400	800

Sample

In initial stage a sample of 1000 students, comprising 500 girls and 500 boys was taken randomly from 8th standard in various schools in some districts of Gujarat, *i.e.* Mehsana, Ahmedabad, Bhavnagar and Surat. It was necessary to have huge sample to cover the variables of gender and Medium of instruction. Ultimately a final sample of 800 students was taken for the final analysis.

Tools

Children's personality questionnaire (Porter & Cattle, 1975) Form A was used to find out personality differences between English and Gujarati medium boys and girls students. The CPQ is one of the personality questionnaires developed by Institute of Personality and Ability Testing (IAPT) for different age group in U.S.A. The CPQ yields a generic assessment of personality by measuring 14 distinct dimensions, which have been found by psychologists to assess total personality. In this study Gujarati version of CPQ was used. Reliability was found by test-retest method. The test-retest reliability of each factor reported by author were as follows : Factor A : (0.59), Factor B : (0.72), Factor C : (0.67) Factor D : (0.67), Factor E : (0.67), Factor F : (0.70), Factor G : (00.66), Factor H : (0.58), Factor I : (0.72), Factor J : (0.59), Factor N : (6.70), Factor 0 : (0.60), Factor A3 : (0.061) and Factor A4 : (0.58).

Procedure

Every student was given Child personality questionnaire (CPQ) form A, along with the answer sheet. Although simple and clear instructions were printed on the cover page of test booklet, the investigator gave clear instructions with demonstration in 8th standard classroom, The student was instructed to give frank and honest answers in describing himself. Each student was instructed to write his name, class and age on the answer sheet. The questions of the test were provided with alternatives. The students were told to choose proper answer and cross on the separate sheet. Students were specifically told that no answer should remain unanswered. If students were puzzled about procedure to answer they were guided. Each student was given enough time to read and answer the questions.

Investigator who made sure that each question was answered and given only one of the alternative answers, collected the completed answer sheets. The collected answer sheets were scored as per key given in the manual.

The scoring of CPQ was done with the help of scoring stencils. The results of the 800 students have been arranged in 2 × 2 factorial research design and technique of two way analysis of variance was used in order to examine main as well as the interaction effects. Subsequently, another statistical technique termed least significance difference (L.S.D) was applied to find out significant differences between two means in specific groups of students of two main variables sex and medium of instruction. All these results have been presented in various tables and discussed in the following section.

RESULTS AND DISCUSSION

The obtained results have been shown in Table 19.1

(1) Factor—A (Reserved v/s outgoing)

The mean score of boys was higher than that of girls and the differences in both groups was statistically significant ($F = 12.67$), while the mean score of English medium students was higher than the of Gujarati medium students and 'F' ratio was also found to be significant at 0.01 level. Therefore, English medium students and boys are more outgoing, and sociable than Gujarati medium students & girls respectively.

(2) Factor—B (Less Intelligent v/s more intelligent)

The girls were found to be more intelligent than boys and F ratio 31.69 was found to be statistically significant at 0.01 levels. As far as the medium variable is concerned the Gujarati medium students were found to be more intelligent than that of English medium students and F ratio 31.63 was found to be statistically significant at 0.01 level.

(3) Factor - C (Emotionally less stable v/s emotionally stable)

The mean score of boys was higher than the girls. The F ratio 37.52 was found to be statistically significant at 0.01 level, while the mean score of English medium students was higher than girls and the F ratio 5.93 was found to be statistically significant at 0.01 level. This shows that the students of English medium school and boys were found to be more emotionally stable.

Table 19.1 : Showing the Value of All F Ratio for Gender & Language Variable on Fourteen Personality Factors

Source of Variable	*DF*	*Factor A*	*Factor B*	*Factor C*	*Factor D*	*Factor E*	*Factor F*	*Factor G*	*Factor H*	*Factor I*	*Factor J*	*Factor N*	*Factor O*	*Factor Q3*	*Factor Q4*
		F	*F*	*F*	*F*	*F*	*F*	*F*	*F*	*F*	*F*	*F*	*F*	*F*	*F*
Main effect															
Sex (A)	1	12.67**	31.69**	37.52**	9.25**	38.69**	12.55**	8.80**	38.75**	74.14**	78.76**	39.27**	7.13**	74.71**	23.78**
Language (B)	1	7.89*	31.65**	5.93**	2.88*	12.13**	8.28**	9.07**	1.23	3.36**	5.05*	43.76**	22.25**	3.60*	34.53**
Interaction Effect															
A × B	1	0.08	4.36*	4.40*	19.52**	9.25**	2.59*	0.8	1.23	2.42	5.71	3.41	7.21**	2.40	5.03

* Significant at 0.01 level.

** Significant at 0.05 level.

(4) Factor - D (Phlegmatic temperament v/s excitability)

The mean score of boys was higher than that of girls with a significant F (9.25) which indicates that boys are more impatient, demanding and overactive than girls, while English medium students were more excitable, impatient, demanding, overactive than students of Gujarati medium which shows that Gujarati medium students are phlegmatic, deliberate and inactive. (F = 2.88)

(5) Factor - E (Submissiveness v/s ascendance)

The boys obtained high mean score than mean score of girls, which indicates that boys are more assertive, independent, aggressive and stubborn than girls. The F ratio 38.69 was found to be significant at 0.01 level. Regarding second variable medium of instruction F ratio 12.13 is significant at 0.01 levels. English medium students have higher mean score (M = 5.90) than students of Gujarati medium. Therefore, English medium students are more assertive, independent, aggressive and stubborn than students of Gujarati medium.

(6) Factor - F (Sober v/s happy-go-lucky)

The boys obtained higher score on this trait and therefore, tend to be cheerful, active, talkative, carefree than girls. The F ratio 12.55 is significant on 0.01 levels. English medium students had higher mean score than Gujarati medium students on factor 'F'. Which indicates that English medium students are happier-go-lucky, heedless gay and enthusiastic than students of Gujarati medium with significant F ratio (8.28) at 0.01 level.

(7) Factor - G (Expedient v/s conscientious)

On factor 'G' higher mean of boys indicates that the boys are more conscientious, persevering, staid and rule-bound than girls. F ratio of 8.80 is significant at 0.01 level. English medium students have stronger superego strength than students of Gujarati medium. F (9.07) value is significant.

(8) Factor - H (Shy v/s venturesome)

The mean score of boys was higher than that of girls, and F value (38.75) is significant. This indicates that boys are more venturesome, socially bold, inhibited, and spontaneous than girls. The F for medium of instruction (1.23) is found to be insignificant at 0.05 level, indicating no significant difference in Factor H in English & Gujarati medium school.

(9) Factor - I (Tough-minded v/s tender minded)

Boys are more tender minded, dependent, over protected and sensitive than girls. The mean score was higher than that of girls with F ratio of 74.14, which is significant at 0.01 level. The students of English medium are more tender minded, dependent, over-protective and sensitive than Gujarati medium students as the mean score of English medium students was higher than Gujarati medium. The F value was 2.45, which is significant at 0.01 level.

(10) Factor - J (Zestful v/s reflective)

The mean score of girls was higher than that of boys. A significant F (78.70) which indicates that girls are more doubting, obstructive, individualistic, reflective, restrained and unwilling to act than boys, while boys are more vigorous, go readily with group, zestful and willing to act than girls. The students of English medium had higher mean score than Gujarati medium. F ratio 5.08 is significant at 0.05 level.

It means that the students of English medium are more doubting, obstructive, individualistic, reflective, internally restrained, and unwilling to act than Gujarati medium students.

(11) Factor N (Forthright v/s shrewd)

The mean score of boys was higher than that of girls with F ratio 39.27, that is significant at 0.01 level. This indicates that boys are more shrewd, calculating, worldly, penetrating than girls, while girls, are more forthright, natural, artless and sentimental than boys English medium students are more forthright natural, artless and sentimental than students of Gujarati medium (F = 43.76, significant 0.01 level).

(12) Factor - O (Placid v/s apprehensive)

The mean score of boys on factor O was higher than girls (4.96). F ratio of 7.13 is significant at 0.01 level. It shows that boys are more apprehensive, warring, depressive and trebled than girls, while girls are self assured, placid, secure, and serene. The English medium students had higher mean score than girls, (4.54) which indicates that English medium students are more apprehensive, warring, depressive, and troubled than Gujarati medium students.

(13) Factor Q3 (Undisciplined self-conflict v/s controlled)

The mean score of boys was higher than that of girls with significant F ratio 74.71 at 0.01 level, which indicates that boys are more controlled, socially precise, self-disciplined, and compulsive than girls.

The difference in second main variable of medium of instruction is significant at 0.05 level (F= 3.60), which shows that English medium students are more controlled, socially-precise, self-disciplined and compulsive than students of Gujarati medium.

(14) Factor - Q4 (Relaxed v/s tense)

Boys are tenser, driven, over wrought, fretful than girls as the mean score of boys was higher than that of girls with F ratio of 23.78, which is significant at 0.01 level.

English medium students had higher mean score than Gujarati medium students. A significant F (34.54) at 0.01 level indicates that English medium students are more tense, driven and overwrought, as well as fretful than Gujarati medium students.

Thus the boys are found to be more outgoing, emotionally stable, assertive, dominant, happy-go-lucky, venturesome, tender minded, apprehensive, conscientious, controlled, tense, while girls are found to be more intelligent, emotionally less stable, sober, shy, forthright and phlegmatic. The students of English medium were found to be more sociable, emotionally stable, excitable, cheerful, moralistic, tender minded and shrewd, than the students of Gujarati medium. The students of Gujarati medium were found to be more intelligent, assertive, shy, reflective than the students of English medium.

REFERENCES

Anand, C.L. (1971). *The Study of the Effect of Socio-economic Environment and Medium of Instruction on the Mental Abilities and Academic Achievement of Children in Mysore State*, A Ph.D. Thesis, submitted in University of Mysore.

Carroll, H.A. (1964). *Mental Hygiene : The Dynamics of Adjustment*, New York : Prentice Hall.

Chaliha-Mala (1997). The comparative study of personality patterns of normal and Mentally retarded children, *Indian Journal of Psychometry and Education, 27*, 87-92.

Hildreth, G. (1938). Characteristics of young gifted children, *Journal of Genetic Psychology, 53*, 287-311.

Krestschmer, E. (1931). *The Psychology of Man of Genius,* New York, Harcourt, Brace.

Lange-Eichbaum W. (1931). *The Problem of Genius,* London, Kagan Paul.

Vashista, K.C. (1982). *Personality Differences among Family Reward for Boys & Girls,* Ph.D. Thesis, submitted at Kurukshetra University, Kurukshetra.

Witty, P.A., and Lehman H.C. (1930). Instability and genius : same conflicting opinions, *Journal of Abnormal & Social Psychology, 24*, 486-497.

20

Mental Health of Cash-Crop Farmers and Non-Cash-Crop Farmers

*P.V. Rasal**

The modern life is full of a variety of confusions, tensions & complications. Individuals face many ups and downs at different developmental stages in life. The increasing irregularity, competition and workload are the causes of disharmony, whereas for good quality of life, we need an order and harmony. It is the psychological well being, happiness and harmony that account for our mental health. And mental health is the essence of life. Therefore, mental health has become an important issue for the researchers.

The increasing population has led to behavioural, emotional and interpersonal problems, (Wig, 1979) which affect our mental health. The literature indicates that Rasal (1998) studied the mental health of migrated people. Positive job attitude has been shown to improve the performance, & mental health, whereas negative job attitudes lead to a sense of insecurity and psychosomatic symptoms (Dolke, 2000). Marital disruption is also a precursor for poor health (Wade, and Pevalin, 2004). Gender and age also have been found to influence mental health (Kim, 2003). Socio-economic status influences our mental health, poverty and unaffordable housing leading to poor mental health, (Parks, Nelson, 1998; Hudson, 2005).

India has agro-based economy. About 70% population depends on agriculture in India. Agriculture also provides employment to around 65 to 69% of the total workers. Farming is the backbone of Indian economy. But there are various problems for farmers. Farmers have behavioural, emotional, social, financial, educational and health problems. Due to these problems the mental health of farmers is deteriorating day by day. Now-a-days urbanization is increasing fast, so the outlook of the common people about farmers is not positive. The government policies are also not for the farmers. So they are in pendulam position. They have various problems in their life. Cash-crop farmers and non-cash-crop farmers are the mainly two types of farmers. Cash-crop farmers are the irrigating farmers and they take the

* Head & Reader, Dept. of Psychology, Niphad College, Nasik, Maharashtra.

crop by commercial view. They grow the crops like cotton, onion, sugar cane, grapes, groundnuts etc. They cultivate fertile land and have their own permanent water system. The non-cash-crop farmers are non-irrigating farmers. They grow the crops like food grains and they are totally dependent on monsoon. They are totally dependent on nature, rainfall. So they do not have any surety about any crop. They are always worried. Farmer men, women and their family members generally face anxiety due to uncertainty of rainfall, accidental change of atmosphere, increasing prices of pesticides, seeds, fuel, problems of labour, problem of marketing, govt. policies etc. Thus they are always under tension. Now-a-days how to maintain mental health is the problem of every-body. In view of the problems being faced by farmers, mental health is one of the most important problem among them.

Therefore, in the present research an attempt has been made to find out whether cash-crop farmers and non-cash-crop farmers differ for their mental health and the level of various problems, with the following objectives :

1. To study the importance of mental health of cash-crop farmers and non-cash-crop farmers.
2. To study the level of various problems between cash-crop farmers and non-cash-crop farmers.

For this following hypotheses were formulated :

1. The mental health of cash crop farmers would be better than the mental health of the non-cash-crop farmers
2. The levels of various mental health problem in terms of personal, emotional, financial, educational, security etc. would be lesser amongst the cash crop farmers as compared to non-cash-crop farmers.

METHOD

Design

A two group design was employed to compare the mental health of cash and non-cash crop farmers.

Sample

Researcher selected 50 farmers out of which 25 were cash-crop farmers and 25 were non-cash-crop farmers at Nashik District in Maharashtra. The investigator used the incidental sampling method for data collection.

Tools

1. To measure the mental health of cash-crop farmers and non-cash-crop farmers, mental health scale by C.G.D. Deshpande (1991) adapted by A.S. Borse (1995) was used.
2. Second tool for data collection was interview technique. For interview investigator prepared structured open-ended questionnaire.

Procedure

Having selected the relevant sample the Ss were contacted individually. Rapport establishment was necessary in order to get accurate information on the various aspects of personal life, *i.e.* personal, emotional, financial, feelings of security etc. The confidentiality was assured and the Ss were given the mental health questionnaire. (Desh Pande, 1991). These Ss were now again made to sit comfortably and asked the questions in the prepared interview schedule. The answers given by Ss at length were recorded. Now the scoring of the answers to Deshpande's questionnaire was done. Regarding the interview, the responses were analysed in term of percentages.

RESULTS AND DISCUSSION

't' test was used to see whether there is a significant difference between cash-crop farmers and non-cash-crop farmers. Table 20.1 depicts those results.

Table 20.1 : Showing the Differences between Cash-crop Farmers and Non-cash-crop Farmers for Their Mental Health

Cash-Crop Farmers N=25		Non-Cash-Crop Farmers N=25		't'
X	SD	X	SD	
32.64	5.92	24.06	4.38	5.83*

* P<0.01.

Table 20.1 shows that the mean score of cash-crop farmers was 32.64 with S.D. of 5.92. The mean score of non-cash-crop farmers was 24.06 and SD was 4.38. The obtained t value was 5.38 which was statistically significant. The hypothesis in this regard that, the mental health of cash-crop farmers would be better than non-cash-crop farmers has proved. So the obtained results indicated that there was statistically significant difference between cash-crop farmers and non-cash-crop farmers for their mental health.

Table 20.2 : Showing the Percentage Level of Various Problems Between Cash-crop Farmers and Non-cash-crop Farmers

Problem	*Cash-Crop Farmers*	*Non-Cash-Crop Farmers*
Personal	Average 50%	High 60%
Social	Low 32%	Average 50%
Emotional	Average 50%	High 65%
Financial	Low 27%	High 70%
Education	Low 30%	Average 50%
Security	High 60%	Average 50%
Bad Habits	Average 50%	Low 32%
Health	Low 40%	High 55%

Table 20.2 shows the levels of personal, social, emotional, financial, education, security, bad habits and health. According to the percentage of cash-crop farmers they are having high level of security, average level of personal emotional problems and bad habits, and low level of social, financial, education and physical health problem. While non-cash-crop farmers are having high level of personal, emotional, financial, and physical health problems, average level of social problems, education and security and low level of bad habits.

It was observed that there is difference of level of various problems between cash-crop farmers and non-cash-crop farmers.

As the term non-cash-crop farmers indicates, that there is a total dependence on the nature as a means of cultivation. This population lacks the capacity to fight the natural calamity, if any. This is a very strong source of anxiety. Besides this, these farmers never earn as much through the farming as the non-cash-crop farmers. It is already established that economic insecurity leads to many personal, social and emotional problems leading to insecurity and physical health. That's how there might have been a significant difference between the mental health of cash & non-cash-crop farmers. The results are congruent with Hudson (2005) which indicate that low SES may lead to even depression. In his study, unemployment, poverty and housing unaffordability were correlated with a risk of mental illness.

REFERENCES

Hudson, G. (2005). Socio-economic Status and Mental Illness : Tests of the social causation and selection hypotheses, *American Journal of Orthopsychiatry, 75,* 224-230.

Kim, A. (2003). Correlation of mental health problems with psychological constructs in adolesence, *International Journal of Nursing Student, 40*, 115-24.

Parks, J. & Nelson C.H. (1998). The investigation of stress in resource dependent communities : the effect of rapid socioeconomic changes on mental health service use, *International Journal Circumpolar Health, 57,* 432-8.

Rasal, P.V. (2004). Mental health and quality of life of migrated labours, *Asian Journal of Psychology and Education*, 27.

Wade, T.J. & Pevalin D.J. (2004). Marital transitions and mental health, *Journal of Health and Social Behaviour, 45,* 155-70.

Wig, N.N (1979). Mental health and population growth, *Indian Journal of Psychiatry, 21,* 12-33.

21

Does your Status Make you well? Socio-Economic Status and Well-Being

Radheyshyam * **& *Rajbir Singh*** **

Several terms are prevalent for the concept of well-being in the psychological literature. Quite often terms like general well-being, subjective well being, happiness, and satisfaction from life have been used interchangeably (Easterlin, 2001). Diener who has worked quite extensively in this area, in a review article (Diener, Suh, Lucas & Smith, 1999) has stated that subjective well-being is a general area of scientific interest rather than a single specific construct. It is a broad category of phenomena that include people's emotional responses, domain satisfaction and global judgements of life satisfaction. Each of the specific constructs needs to be understood in its own right. The components often correlate substantially, suggesting the need for higher order factors (Stones & Kozma, 1985). Four major components of subjective well-being, *viz.*, pleasant affect, unpleasant affect, life satisfaction and domain satisfaction have been reported (Diener *et al.*, 1999). The component of pleasant affect consists of joy, elation, contentment, pride, affection, happiness and ecstasy whereas unpleasant affect consist of guilt, shame, sadness, anxiety, worry, anger, stress, depression and envy. Life satisfaction comprises of desire to change life, satisfaction with current life, satisfaction with past and future and significant other's view of one's life, whereas, domain satisfaction contains work, family, leisure, health, finances, self and one's group. For the present study general and subjective well-being are taken as one and the same and happiness as a separate phenomenon though considered to be a strong correlate of well-being.

Wilson (1967), a pioneer in this area, reported that a majority of people avow positive level of happiness (and also by Diener & Diener, 1996; Headey & Wearing, 1988) and most people report that their well-being varies between slightly satisfied and very satisfied, and between slightly happy and very happy. Wilson (1967) concluded that happy people are young, healthy, well-educated, well-paid, religious, married persons with high job morale of either

*Reader, Department of Psychology, M.D. University, Rohtak.
**Professor & Head, Department of Psychology, M.D. University, Rohtak.

sex and of any level of intelligence. Since then a number of studies have been conducted and Wilson's conclusions have been re-examined and several predictors such as subjective satisfaction, income, age, gender, race, employment, education, marriage and family, social class and social contacts, activities and personality have been reported (Diener *et al.*, 1999, Diener, Suh & Oishi, 1997; Headey & Wearing, 1989; Diener, 1984) to influence well-being significantly. An exhaustive review of all these is beyond the scope of this article, however, a brief review related to socio-economic status and related factors is presented here.

Education, employment/occupation, wealth/income, race and social class etc. have been reported to be as broad indicators of SES (Tello, Jones, Bonnizzato, Mazzi, Amaddeo & Tansella, 2005; Frelick, 2004; Wagstaff & Watanabe, 2003). Studies have indicated an association between indicators of SES and health and well-being. For example, Subramanian, Kim and Kawachi (2005) examined the individual level determinants of self-rated health and happiness as well as the extent of community level covariation in health and happiness. They reported a strong income and education gradient for self-rated poor health and unhappiness. Luo and Waite (2005) emphasized the role of childhood (*i.e.* parental) SES and adult SES for health and well-being of an individual.

The relationship between income, an important constituent of SES and well-being has been analysed in several different ways. First, relation between personal income of individuals and well-being has been reported (Veenhoven, 1993) to be significant yet the co-efficient of correlation were small. Seidliz and Diener (1993), too reported a weak ($r=0.12$) correlation between income and well-being. Haring Stock and Okun (1984) found it to be around 0.17 whereas Easterlin (2001) reported $r = 0.20$. On the contrary, Clark and Oswald (1994) in a sample from British population, did not find any relation between income and well-being. Secondly, when SWB of people from wealthy and poor nations was compared, persons of wealthier nations reported higher SWB than persons in poor countries (Easterlin, 1974; Silver, 1980) but this effect was weaker than within-country differences (Diener, 1984) Moreover, Gross National Product (GNP) per capita was found to correlate substantially ($r=.50$) with life satisfaction across 39 countries (Diener *et al.*, 1993). Third, when change in income is considered, the relationship of income and well-being becomes less clear and confusing. Freedman (1978) reported that income has an effect only at extreme levels of poverty, but once the basic needs are met income is no longer influential. Recent studies (Diener *et al.*, 1999; Diener & Suh, 1997) taking U.S. data, revealed that beyond a point increase in income does not lead to increase in well-being of its people. Thus, the relation between income and well-being is complex and when one tries to explain, it becomes still more complex.

Relationship between education and SWB has also been reported (Campbell, 1981) to be significant, yet small (Diener, *et al.*, 1993). On the basis of meta-analysis of studies relating to education and well-being, Witter, Okun and Haring (1984) reported a median effect size of .13 and this median size did not differ significantly for measures of life satisfaction (.15), morale (.15), quality of life (.13) or happiness (.12). Veenhoven (1994) reported that education is highly related to well-being for individuals with lower incomes and in poor countries. Infact part of the relation of education and well-being may be mediated by other variables such as income and occupational status (Campbell, 1981; Witter *et al.*, 1984). At times higher education may even lead to distress as Clark and Oswald (1994) found educated unemployed subjects in greater degree of distress than uneducated unemployed ones.

Racial differences in well-being have also been reported (Andrews & Withey, 1976; Freudiger, 1980) such that Blacks scored lower than Whites on measures of SWB. Diener (1984) reported that these effects were not universal and when factors like age, education, urbanicity, income and marital status were controlled the Black-White difference was quite small. Though there is a lack of studies, however, caste and class—which are the important factors in determining one's social status in Indian society may have effect on one's well-being also.

Employment has been reported as a strong correlate of subjective well-being even when income differences were controlled (Campbell, Converse & Rodgers, 1976). Job satisfaction has been found to have a modest (r=0.44) correlation life satisfaction. Employment/occupation/work may be related to SWB because it provides an optimal level of stimulation that people find pleasurable (Csikszentmihalyr, 1990). Haring, Stock and Okun (1984) on the basis of a meta-analysis of related studies, reported that work (full-time, part-time or not employed) was significantly related to SWB though at a low level.

Aforesaid review suggests a potent role of several indicators of socio-economic status in various indicators of well-being (subjective well-being, general well-being, happiness) separately instead of taking global SES scores or overall socio-economic status. In a country like India where large disparities in income, employment material possessions and land holding exists in addition to social class variations which influence one's social and economic position, study of relationship of SES and well-being would help us in understanding its concept and dynamics of relationship.

Objectives

- To study the relationship of Socio-economic status and well-being.
- To identify the role of SES in predicting one's state of well-being.

METHOD

Design

To fulfill the objectives of the study a correlational study design was used.

Sample

300 subjects of both sexes from general population were selected from rural and urban (in and around Rohtak) areas following non-random incidental sampling procedure. To give adequate representation to people belonging to various social classes, people of general class(G),

Table 21.1 : Demographic Features of the Sample (N=300)

Sex	Male = 151	Female = 149
Area of Residence	Rural = 151	Urban = 149
Marital Status	Married = 230	Unmarried =70
Social Class	General=185, O.B.C.=61, SC=54	
Qualification	Illiterate = 43, Matric = 102	
	Senior Sec. = 44, Graduate = 61	
	Post Graduate and above = 50	

officially backward class (OBC) and scheduled caste (SC) categories, were selected. Majority of the subjects were married (n=230). The sample consisted of both literate (n=257) and illiterate (n=43) subjects. Age of the sample ranged from 18 to 81 years with a mean of 36.93 (SD = 13.05) years. The demographic features of the sample are given in Table 21.1.

Tools Used

Measures of well being : PGI general well-being scale (in Hindi) by Verma and Verma (1989) a 20 item standardized measure was used. The items are to be endorsed in 'Yes' 'No' format and scored as one and zero, respectively. Thus, the total score may range from 0 to 20.

Subjective well-being Inventory—Subjective well-being inventory (in Hindi) developed by Sell and Nagpal (1992) is a forty (40) item measure. The items are to be endorsed on a three point scale, 'very much', 'to some extent' and 'not so much' a weightage of 3, 2,1, is given for positive items and reverse of it in case of negative items. The total score may range from 40-120. It yields three scores *viz.* the positive affect score (range 19-57), negative affect (termed as absence of negative affect in this study considering the direction of scores) score (range 21-63) and composite score (range 40-120). The reliability and validity of the inventory are well established.

Happiness—A single item measure of happiness was administered to all subjects. The question was, "Keeping last one month in mind, how do you rate your own state of happiness?" It was to be rated on a five point scale. 1 complete unhappy, to 5 completely happy. Such a single item measure of well-being, happiness and/or life satisfaction have been used quite extensively (Easterlin, 2001; Veenhoven, 1983) with acceptable reliabilities and validity.

Socio-economic Status—Socio-economic status of subjects was measured by using Socio-economic-status scale (Singh, Shyam and Kumar, 2004). It is applicable to subjects belonging to both rural and urban areas. It takes care of all the indicators of a person's social and economic status in present day circumstances.

Procedure

The study was conducted by administering all the measures individually in the form of structured interviews by paid trained investigators (PG and Doctoral students of Psychology, M.D. University, Rohtak) under the supervision of the authors. First of all, verbal consent of the respondent was taken and then interview (structured) was conducted. Questions relating to general information and happiness were asked, it was followed by SES related questions, and then well-being measures were administered. Scoring was done as described above and following the procedure as described in the test/scale manuals.

Besides measures of central tendency and variability, Pearsons product moment correlation was calculated to examine the relationship between SES and scores on well-being measures. To identify the role of SES in determining well-being of subjects, regression co-efficients were calculated for its indicators, separately.

RESULTS AND DISCUSSION

Results of the study have been described objectivewise in two sections/parts. In the first part relationship of SES with indicators of well-being is described whereas, in the second part results of regression analysis are given. The means and SD's of scores on various measures are given in Table 21.2 alongwith coefficients of correlations.

Table 21.2 : Intercorrelation Matrix (N=300)

	SES	*WB*	*P. Affect*	*N. Affect*	*Happiness*	*Composite subjective well-being*
SES	1.00					
WB	0.19**	1.00				
P. Affect	0.20**	0.48**	1.00			
N. Affect	0.30**	0.56**	0.62**	1.00		
Happiness	0.24**	0.47**	0.31**	0.41**	1.00	
$\bar{X}$	67.53	13.52	44.15	49.08	3.20	91.94
SD	29.46	5.66	7.54	8.03	1.11	15.66

*Significant at .05.

**Significant at .01.

On PGI general well-being scale the obtained mean score was 13.52 with an SD of 5.66 whereas the mean of the original sample of normal P.G. students, was 10.43 (S.D. 5.62) and graduate students, 9.45 with S.D. = 8.12 (Verma, Dubey and Gupta, 1983).

Subjective well-being inventory of Sell and Nagpal (1992) gives three scores, composite, positive affect and absence of negative affect. The composite scores were 91.94 (SD = 15.66) though it is slightly higher than the mean composite score of 90.80 (SD = 9.20), of Sell and Nagpal's sample in 1992 yet it did not differ significantly ($t = 0.92$, $df = 418$, $p > 0.05$). Mean positive affect scores of the present sample was 44.15 (SD = 7.54) whereas 42.90 (SD 4.60) for Sell and Nagpal's study. These mean scores differed significantly ($t = 2.05$, $df = 418$, $p < 0.05$). The mean absence of negative affect score of the present study (mean = 49.08, SD = 8.03) was slightly higher than that of Sell and Nagpal's study (mean = 47.90, SD = 5.10) yet the difference was non-significant ($t = 1.78$, df 418, $p > 0.05$).

Thus, over a period of about thirteen (13) years there seems to be an appreciable change in the living conditions of people in general however, there was no appreciable change in the overall well-being of the people (Composite and negative affect scores) except that in positive affect where there was a significant increase in positive affect of the sample. Mean happiness score of the subjects was 3.20 (SD = 1.11) and it indicate that the average happiness level of the sample was little bit higher than the mean of 5 point scale, *i.e.* to say happiness status in the sample was moderate. The mean score on SES scale was 67.53. (SD = 29.46). It happens to be a typical average middle class with a percentile of 51 in respect to scale norms.

Inter-correlation matrix showing coefficients of correlation between SES and measures of well-being is given in Table 21.2. It is evident from the coefficients that SES correlated positively and significantly though moderately with score on PGI general well-being score ($r = 0.19$, $p < 0.1$). Subjective well-being inventory (SBI) gives three scores *viz.*, positive affect, absence of negative affect and the composite score. Since the composite score is only the sum of scores on positive and absence of negative affect, it was not taken up for further analysis. SES scores correlated positively and significantly with positive affect ($r = 0.20$, $p < 0.01$), and absence of negative affect ($r = 0.30$, $p < 0.01$) components of SWBI, however, the size of the coefficients was moderate (Table 21.2). Similarly SES and self-reported level of happiness correlated significantly ($r = 0.24$, $p < 0.01$) and the direction was positive. In general, higher the SES, greater was the happiness.

The second objective of the study was to identify the role of one's socio-economic status in predicting his or her state of well-being. For this scores on measures of well-being *viz.* PGI general well-being scale, positive and absence negative affect scores on SWBI and self-reported level of happiness were regressed on socio-economic status scores; Statistics are given in Table 21.3. Simple regression equation in score from along with the percent contribution of SES in dependent variables have been described in Table 21.4.

Table 21.3 : Summary of Simple Regression in SES ($\bar{X}$ = 67.53); (DV= Dependant Variable; R= Multiple Correlation Coefficient; $\bar{X}$ = Mean; b = Regression Coefficient; k - constant)

Dependent Variables	$\bar{X}$	*R*	*R2*	*b*	*k*
1. Well being	13.52	0.19	0.04	0.0036 ± 0.01	11.12 ± 0.81
2. Positive affect	44.75	0.30	0.09	0.078 ± 0.01	38.89 ± 1.04
3. Absence of negative affect	49.08	0.23	0.05	0.062 ± 0.02	44.89 ± 1.13
4. Happiness	3.20	0.23	0.05	0.0085 ± 0.002	2.63 ± 0.16

Table 21.4 : Simple Regression Equations and Contribution of SES in Dependent Variables

DV	$\bar{X}$	*Simple Regression Equation* *b* ($\bar{X}$ *SES*) + *K*	*% Contribution of Existing SES in DV*
Well-being	13.52	0.036 (67.53) + K 2.43 + 11.12	17.98
Positive affect	44.15	0.078 (67.53) + K 5.27 + 38.89	11.93
Absence of negative affect	49.08	0.062 (67.53) + K 4.19 + 44.89	8.53
Happiness	3.20	0.0085 (67.53) + K 0.57 + 2.63	17.81

SES came out to be a significant ($F = 10.63$, df 1,298, $p < 0.01$) predictor of well-being scores (PGI well-being scores) accounting 4 percent of variance. The regression coefficient was 0.036 with an SE of 0.01. It indicates that one unit increase in SES scores add only 0.036 in general well-being. Existing SES contributed toward 18% of the existing psychological well-being. SES also turned out to be the significant predictor of positive affect ($F = 30.43$, df =1, 298, $p < 0.01$) and absence of negative affect ($F = 16.26$, df =1,298, $p < 0.01$) components of SUBI accounting 9 and 5 per cent of the total variance, respectively (Table 21.3). The regression coefficients were 0.078 and 0.062, respectively, for positive and absence of negative affect (Table 21.3). SES contributed toward 11.93% and 8.53% of all affects. Socio-economic status was also a significant ($F = 15.58$, df =1,298, $p < 0.01$) predictor of self-reported level of happiness accounting 5 per cent of the total variance. The regression coefficient was 0.0085 ± 0.002 (Table 21.3). It point toward the contribution of SES in self reported level of happiness that half a scale value (on five point scale), *i.e.* 17.81% of the existing happiness was due to existing SES (Table 21.4).

Findings of the study are in agreement with those of Subramanian, *et al.* (2005) and Luo and Waite (2005) reporting associations between SES and well-being. The size of the coefficients of correlation was more or less similar to that reported by Haring *et al.* (1984) and Easterlin, (2001) between income and well-being but greater than that of 0.12 as reported by Seidliz and Diener (1993) and contrary to those of Clark and Oswald (1994). The moderate size, significant and positive association between SES and indicators of well-being can be explained in terms of Diener, *et al.* (1999) and Diener and Suh (1997) proposition that increase in a person's income beyond a certain level does not lead to increase in well-being and happiness. The population under study could perhaps came at the lower side of income compared to U.S. per capita income. Secondly, a sizeable section of the sample belonged to joint families where the pleasure and pains are shared. The contribution of SES in predicting one's state of well-being and happiness was less (*e.g.* about 3% for general well-being; 9 % for positive affect, 5% for absence of negative affect and 4% for self-reported level of happiness) also seems to support the studies cited above. Although, separating the component of constant (other unknown variables) and taking the role of existing SES in the sample, it can be conducted that about 20% of one's well-being was due to one's socio-economic status. It is much greater a role than revealed by western studies. Since global SES was used in the present study while indicators of SES had been implicated in the existing literature, findings were not simply comparable. Moreover, results attest to their validity/generality in the sense that four measures of well-being were used and potency of SES as significant predictor has been replicated. It is to add that the measures correlated significantly (positively and highly $r = 0.31$ to 0.62) among themselves (Table 21.2). Even single item measure of happiness correlated with other three measures of PGI general well-being (Varma and Verma, 1989); positive affect and absence of negative affect of SWBI (Sell and Naglal, 1992).

Higher status provides one with opportunities and means for job, elation, contentment etc. (Positive effect) and also protects one from anxiety, worry, stress etc. (*i.e.*, absence of negative affect), thus one feels happy or be in a state of happiness more often. Ultimately, you are well.

REFERENCES

Andrews, F.M. and Withey, S.B. (1976). *Social Indicators of Well-being*, New York : Plenum Press.

Bradburn, NM. and Caplovitz, D. (1990). *Reports of Happiness*, Chicago : Aldine.

Clark, A.E. and Oswald, A.J. (1994). Unhappiness and Unemployment, *Economic Journal, 104*, 648-659.

Campbell, A. (1981). *The Sense of Well-being in America : Recent Patterns of Trends*, New York : McGraw-Hill.

Campbell, A., Converse, P.E. and Rogers, W.L. (1976). *The Quality of American Life*, New York : Russell Sage Foundation.

Csikszentmihalyi, M. (1990). *Flow : The Psychology of Optimal Experience*, New York : Harper Perennial.

Diener, E. and Suh, E. (1997). Measuring quality of life : economic, social and subjective indicators, *Social Indicators Research, 40*, 189-216.

Diener, E.; Suh, E.M.; Lucas, R.E. and Smith, H.L. (1999). Subjective well-being : Three decades of progress, *Psychological Bulletin, 125*, 276-302.

Diener, E. (1984). Subjective well-being, *Psychological Bulletin*, *95*, 542-575.

Diener, E. and Diener, C. (1996). Most people are happy, *Psychological Science*, *7*, 181-185.

Diener, E., Gohm, C., Suh, E. and Oishi, S. (1998). Do the effect of marital status on subjective well-being vary across cultures? c/f. Ed. Diener, *et al.* (1999). Subjective well being : Three decades of progress, *Psychological Bulletin*, *125*, 276-302.

Diener, E., Sandvik, E.' Seidlitz, L. and Diener, M. (1993). The relationship between income and subjective well-being : relative or absolute? *Social Indicators Research*, *28*, 195-223.

Diener, E., Suh, E.M. and Oishi, S. (1997). Recent findings on subjective well-being, *Indian Journal of Clinical Psychology*, *24*, 25-41.

Easterlin, R.A. (1974). Does economic growth improves the human lot? in (P.A. David, and M.W. Reder, Eds.) Nations and Households in Economic Growth: Essays in honour of Moses Abramovitz, New York : Academic Press.

Easterlin, R.A. (2001). Income and happiness : Towards a unified theory, *The Economic Journal*, *111*, 465-484.

Eaton, W.W. and Kessler, L.G. (1981). Rates of symptoms of depression in a national sample, *American Journal of Epidemiology*, *114*, 528-538.

Freedman, J. (1978). *Happy people : What happiness is, who has it and why,* New York : Hascourt Brace Jouvanovich.

Frelick, R.W. (2004). SES discrepancies and Delaware cancer death rates, *Delaware Medical Journal*, *76*, 103-139.

Freudiger, P.T. (1980). Life satisfaction among American women (Doctoral Dissertation, North Texas State University, 1979), *Dissertation Abstracts International*, *40*, 6438A.

Glenn, N.D. (1975). The contribution of marriage to the Psychological well-being of males and females, *Journal of Marriage and Family Relations*, *37*, 594-600.

Gove, W.R. and Shin, H. (1989). The psychological well-being of divorced and widowed men and women, *Journal of Family Issues*, *10*, 122-144.

Gove, W.R., Hughes, M. and Style, C.B. (1983). Does marriage have positive effects on Psychological well-being of the individual? *Journal of Health and Social Behaviour*, *24*, 122-131.

Gurin, G., Veroff, J. and Feld, S. (1960). *Americans View their Mental Health*, Ann Asbor : University of Michigan, Survey Research Centre.

Haring, H.M.; Stock, W.A. and Okun, M.A. (1984). A research synthesis of gender and social class as correlates of subjective well-being, *Human Relations*, *37*, 645-657.

Headey, D. and Wearing, A. (1989). Personality life events and subjective well-being : Towards a dynamic equilibrium model, *Journal of Personality and Social Psychology*, *57*, 731-739.

Headey, B. and Wearing, A. (1992). The sense of relative superiority – Central to well-being, *Social Indicators Research*, *20*, 497-516.

Kurdek, L.A. (1991). The relations between reported well-being and divorce history, availability of a proximate adult and gender, *Journal of Marriage and Family Relations*, *53*, 71-78.

Luo, Y. and Waite, L.J. (2005). The impact of childhood and adult SES on physical, mental and cognitive well-being in later life, *Journal of Gerontology* , *60*, 593-510.

Mastekassa, A. (1992). Marriage and well-being : Some evidence on selection into marriage, *Journal of Marriage and Family Relations*, *54*, 901-911.

Morczek, D.K. and Kolarz (1998). The effect of age on positive and negative effect : A developmental perspective on happiness, *Journal of Personality and Social Psychology*, *75*, 1333-1349.

Seidlitz, L. and Diener, E. (1993). Memory for positive and negative events : Theories for the differences between happy and unhappy persons, *Journal of Personality and Social Psychology*, *64*, 554-684.

Sell, H. and Nagpal, R. (1992). *Assessment of Subjective Well-being : The Subjective Well-being Inventory (SUBI)*, New Delhi : WHO, Regional Office for South East Asia.

Shmotkin, D. (1990). Subjective well-being as a function of age and gender : A multivariate look for differentiated trends, *Social Indicators Research*, *23*, 201-230.

Silver, M. (1980). Money and Happiness? Towards "Eudiamonology" *Kyklos*, *33*, 157-160.

Singh, R., Shyam, R. and Kumar, S. (2004). *Belief in Heredity/Environment in Relation to Social Perception*, Report of U.G.C. Major Research Project, M.D. University, Rohtak.

Stones, M.J. and Kozma, A. (1985). Structural relationship among happiness, *Psychological Bulletin*, *67*, 294-306.

Subramanian, S.N., Kim, D. and Kawachi, I. (2005). Covariation in the socio-economic determinants of self-rated health and happiness : A multivariate multi-level analysis of individuals and communities in the U.S.A., *Journal of Epidemiology Community Health*, *59*, 664-669.

Tello, J.E., Jones, J., Bonnizatto, P.; Mazzi, M., Amaddeo, F. and Tansella, M. (2005). A Census-based Socio-Economic Status (SES). Index as a tool to examine the relationship between mental health services use and deprivation, *Social Science Medicine*, 25.

Veenhoven, R. (1993). *Happiness in Nations, Subjective Appreciation of Life in 56 Nations 1946-1992*, Rotterdam : Erasmus University.

Veenhoven, R. (1994). *Correlates of Happiness : 8, 736 Findings from 603 Studies in 69 Nations, 1911-1994*, Unpublished Manuscript, Esasmus University, Rotterdam : The Netherlands.

Verma S.K. and Verma, A. (1989). *Manual for* PGI *General Well—being Measure*, Lucknow : Ankur Psychological Agency.

Verma, S.K., Dubey, B.L. and Gupta, D. (1983). General well-being scale–some correlates, *Indian Journal of Clinical Psychology*, *10*, 299–304.

Wagstaff, A. and Watanabe, N. (2003). What difference does the choice of SES make in health inequality measurement? *Health Economics*, *12*, 885-890.

White, J.M. (1992). Marital status and well-being in Canada, *Journal of Family Issues*, *13*, 390-409.

Wilson, W. (1967). Correlates of avowed happiness, *Psychological Bulletin*, *67*, 294-306.

Witter, Okun, M.A., Stock, W.A. and Haring, H.M. (1984). In Diener, Ed. *et al.* (1999). Subjective well-being : Three decades of progress. *Psychological Bulletin*, *125*, 276-302.

22

Parental Attitudes and Well-Being of the Wards in Rural and Urban Haryana

Rajesh Kumar** & *Promila Batra***

The children and their development has always been an important concern for researchers. There has been an upsurge in the researches on this crucial and the vital social issue during last two decades. This interest has evoked and enhanced not only because such research is a means of understanding the child development but also because it is a means of developing the best future citizens. The child development has a wide range of concern and impact *i.e.* from infants to adolescence, and from adolescence to adulthood. The well-being, even at later stages of life, depends upon the childhood experiences. Adolescence has been considered to be a period of stress and storm (Freud, 1958; Bloss, 1962). Actually, the transition from childhood to adulthood entails dramatic developmental changes with impact upon adolescents' health and their well-being (Offer, Howard, Schonert and Ostrov, 1991). Negative effect increases at this stage (Larson and Lampman-Petraitis, 1989) and the sensitivity to environmental stressors, like conflict, also increases leading to higher levels of distress (Larson and Ham, 1993). As a result the number of people seeking professional help increases although more at an informal level (Feldman, Hodgson, Corber and Quinn, 1986; Offer, *et.al.*, 1991).

To reduce this stress, and need of help as well as to enhance the well-being it is important to understand the family environment. Many theories indicate that the behaviour of a child is determined by the environment (Hull, 1943, 1951, 1952; Lashley, 1923; Skinner, 1938,1967, 1981; Tolman, 1925; Watson, 1925). Our primary group is the family and in that too the first experiences are with the mother and the father. The children, when born are precious human being who if nurtured, and protected adequately develop healthy and sociable attitudes towards them, others and life. This will lead to positive well-being, but the *vice-versa* has a devastating effect. Poor family relationships may lead to a lower self-esteem, poor social relationship, lack of empathy, drug addiction or delinquency and homicide (Gabarine, 1976). It may cause

*Research Scholar, Department of Psychology, M.D. University, Rohtak (Haryana), India.
**Professor, Departments of Psychology, M.D. University, Rohtak (Haryana), India.

depression, generalized anxiety, adjustment problems, emotional and thought disturbances, helplessness, and dependency, poor school performance, aggression and the like, thus reducing the well-being of any individual. This indicates that the family relationship has a vital role in determining the development of a child.

Studies in each sphere of development, *i.e.* physical, mental, emotional, or cognitive, play or academics, indicate that the childhood experiences play an important role in determining our behaviour and even personality. The child starts developing the concept of 'Good me', 'bad me' and 'not me', very early in life, which carries life long impacts on individual's behaviour.

Keeping this in mind it was decided to compare the family relationships of adolescents with parents in rural and urban families.

METHOD

Design

Two-groups design, having one group of rural and another of urban adolescents was employed. But since the score of both the groups were obtained on three types of relationship, the scores were distributed in the following format of factorial.

Family Relationships

Background	*Acceptance*	*Concentration*	*Avoidance*
Rural			
Urban			

Sample

A total of 90 subjects were taken up, 45 from the rural areas and 45 from the urban areas. The age range of the Ss was 16 to 24 years and they were selected randomly. The urban sample belonged to various cities in Haryana, whereas the rural sample belonged to different villages of Haryana.

Tools

Family Relationship Inventory by Sherry and Sinha (1977) was used, which is an Indian adaptation (in Hindi) of Brunken and Crites' (1964) Family Relationship Inventory. The inventory consists of 150 items related to relationship with parents, *i.e.* the mother and the father. It helps in discriminating the individuals who feel emotionally accepted, over protected (concentrated) or rejected (avoided) by their parents. In other words it measures the parental attitude, as reported and felt or experienced by their children.

Procedure

Having selected the Ss randomly, they were given the FRI and Response Sheet. A very close rapport was established with each subject. They were contacted individually and explained the purpose of the study in detail. As the required information was very personal, there was every possibility that the Ss may hide their responses and tend to show off a positive relationship being employed by their parents. Therefore, they were told about the practical implications of this piece of research. They were also assured of a strict and complete confidentiality to enhance the possibility of being accurately revealing. Now they were instructed in the following manner :

"There are some statements in the inventory. You have to put (√) mark in the column of 'True' if the statement suits you and if it does not suit you put (√) mark in the column of 'False'. Please try to do the work quickly. Your responses will be kept confidential."

Then the subjects did their work and the inventory was taken back. The scoring was done with the help of scoring keys.

RESULTS AND DISCUSSION

As already mentioned the obtained scores were distributed to form a 2x3 factorial design. Two-way ANOVA was employed, and F-values and the level of their significance have been shown in Table 22.1.

Table 22.1 : Showing the F-values and Significance Level of the Groups

Source of Variance	*F- values*
Between Parental Attitudes	207.01**
Between Rural-Urban Background	11.99**
Interaction	3.93*

** P ≤ .01, * P ≤ .05.

Table 22.1 clearly indicates that the F-values for both, the parental attitude and rural-urban dimension were significant at .01 level. Since F-values do not reveal that which of the groups significantly differed, Duncan's Range Test (DRT) was employed as post-hoc analysis technique and the results have been summarized in Table 22.2.

Table 22.2 : Showing the Mean Scores of Rural and Urban Population on Acceptance, Concentration and Avoidance Towards their Children and the Summary of DRT. Whereas P< .05

Avoidance Rural	*Avoidance Urban*	*Concentration Rural*	*Concentration Urban*	*Acceptance Rural*	*Acceptance Urban*
13.02	16.80	19.53	21.13	32.64	38.04

P ≤ .01.

The Table 22.2 clearly indicates that the urban parents avoid their children significantly more than the rural parents, indicating towards a poorer family relationship in urban families. Both rural and urban parents concentrate equally on their wards, as there is no significant difference between rural concentration and urban concentration means. For acceptance, the rural family group mean is significantly lesser than the urban family group mean. This indicates a poor relationship amongst rural families, as compared to the urban families as acceptance is the most wanted attitude. Studies indicate that the attitude of acceptance is the one that is required for a complete growth and full development (Batra, 2000).

Before discussing the impacts of having this poor relationship, another significant fact revealed by results and worth mentioning is a positive finding. The score on the acceptance is high in both the rural and the urban parents and is significantly higher than the other four combinations of rural avoidance, urban avoidance, rural concentration, and urban concentration. The minimum score for both the groups is on avoidance. The score on concentration for both the groups is significantly higher than avoidance and significantly lesser than acceptance.

The avoidance, which was found to be minimum in both the groups according to Roe (1957), characterizes the disposition of parents who either neglect or reject the child. They are withdrawn when the child approaches them, and spend a little time with the child. Besides this overt rejection, they may generate a general atmosphere by unconcern for the child's welfare by active dominance, excessive demands, and conspicuous hostility. It is really good that the score on this attitude for both the groups is minimum.

Unfortunately the parent rejection jeopardizes normal security feelings, undermines the child's self-esteem and induces feelings of helpless and frustration, which can permanently disable the child in his adjustment. Among young children who feel rejected enuresis, feeding difficulties, nail biting and other nervous mannerism are common. Aggression, cruelty, lying, seeking attention, praise, unnecessary help and showing off are some of the characteristics (Roe, 1957), which are indicative of poor well-being.

These parents frequently in their rejection behave as if they are over protecting and act dominantly. The results of various studies compiled by Baumrind are the best yard stic for understanding the impacts of these relationships. Baumrind (1967, 1971, 1978 & 1989) has clearly indicated the authoritarian parents develop a conflicted, irritable, fearful, apprehensive, moody, unhappy, easily annoyed, passively hostile, aimless, sulky and unfriendly personality that is vulnerable to stress. This indicates that urban children are facing a total environment that is meant for leading them towards poor well-being.

The second kind of attitude, *i.e.* concentrated refers to the parents who are actually over protective. This over protection is through restriction upon their efforts to explore the environment. Parents place heavy demands upon them, without realizing the capabilities of the children and set too rigid and unrealistic goals for them. According to Roe (1957) this leads to over dependency in the children. Their characteristic pattern is manifested by a low ego strength, aspiration and frustration tolerance. Such children exhibit withdrawing relations, lack emotional control and openly refuse responsibility. They seem to be afraid to grow up, they have low confidence, low self-esteem, poor self-concept and are easily influenced by others (Schaffer, 1989). Thus concentration also provides an environment that may cause poor well-being. On this dimension, no significant difference existed between the rural and urban population. Thus both of the kinds of population are equally vulnerable to the development of poor well-being, through concentrated parents. However, the score on concentration in both urban and rural population was lower than the acceptance.

Regarding the third kind of parental attitude *i.e.* Acceptance, the rural parents showed significantly low acceptance for their wards than the urban parents. The parental acceptance means when the parents realistically accept the capabilities of the child and the realistic goals are set for the children. Such parents may impose discipline, but are never too restricted, nor are they just too permissive. They are indeed very flexible and supporting. According to Roe (1957) the accepted child is generally better socialized, cooperative, friendly, loyal, emotionally and cheerful. Such children are proving to have high and positive well-being.

Accepting parents are called the authoritative parents. Baumrind (1967, 1971, 1978 & 1989) concluded that authoritative parents by far are the best as they develop their wards as energetic, friendly, self reliant, self controlled, cheerful and friendly, cooperative with adults, purposive and achievement oriented who cope very well with stress. Unfortunately, the significant low score of the rural population on acceptance indicates that rural population does not grow up in a family environment that is suitable for leading to high levels of well-being.

The F-value for interaction was also significant at .05 level this indicates that the interaction between parental attitude and rural-urban background is significant.

To conclude and sum up the results, the picture is certainly poorer but not that poor in the villages of Haryana regarding the family relationship. On one of the negative dimension, *i.e.* concentration, the two groups did not differ significantly. On avoidance, *i.e.* another negative dimension, rural parents were better. But on acceptance the rural parents have been found to be worse than the urban parents, which will certainly impede the exposure and growth of one's potentialities and personalities in the villages. A positive observation is that both the groups scored maximum on the best and most required attitude, *i.e.* acceptance. Thus the rural population, during their developmental stage is being devoid of the total healthy family environment that is required for healthy and positive well-being. Therefore, the interventions be made to create an awareness amongst the parents about the importance of 'acceptance' and 'not to avoid' their wards. However, the study indicates that the need to learn acceptance is more in rural areas than the urban areas in Haryana, whereas the need to learn not to avoid is more important in urban areas of Haryana, whereas the need to learn not to avoid is more important in urban areas of Haryana.

REFERENCES

Batra, P. (2000). *Gender Discrimination in the Families.* A paper presented in the seminar on Human and woman rights, M.D. University, Rohtak (Haryana), India.

Baumrind, D. (1967). Child practices anti-ceding three patterns of pre-school behaviour, *Genetic Psychology Monographs, 75*, 43-88.

Baumrind, D. (1971). Current patterns of parental authority, *Developmental Psychology Monographs, 4,* 4-12.

Baumrind, D. (1978). Parental disciplinary patterns and social competence in Children, *Youth and Society*, 9, 239-276.

Baumrind, D. (1989). Rearing competent children. In W. Damon (ed). *Child Development Today and Tomorrow*, San Francisco : Jossey-Bass.

Bloss, P. (1962). *On Adolescence*, New York : Free Press.

Brunken, R.J. & Crites, J.O. (1964). An inventory to measure the parental attitude variables in Roe's theory of vocational choice, *Journal of Counseling Psychology, 11*, 3-12.

Feldman, W. Hodgson, C., Corber, S., & Quinn, A. (1986). Health concerns and health related behaviours of adolescents, *Canadian Medical Association Journal, 134*, 489-493.

Freud, A. (1958). Adolescence, *Psychoanalytic Study of the Child, 13*, 255-278.

Gabarine (1976). Ecological Correlate of Child Abuse : The Impact of Socio-Economic Stress on Mother, *Child Development, 47*, 178-185.

Hull, C.L. (1943). *Principles of Behaviour : An Introduction to Behaviour Theory,* New York : Appleton-Century-Crofts.

Hull, C.L. (1951). *Essentials of Behaviour,* New Haven : Yale University Press.

Hull, C. L. (1952). *A Behaviour System,* New Haven : Yale University Press.

Larson, R. & Ham, M. (1993). Stress and "storm and stress" in early adolescence : The relationship of negative events with dysphoric affect, *Developmental Psychology, 29,* 130-140.

Larson, R. & Lampman-Petraitis, C. (1989). Daily emotional stress as reported by children and adolescents, *Child Development, 60,* 1250-1260.

Lashley, K.S. (1923). The behaviourists interpretation of consciousness, *Psychological Review, 30,* 237-272.

Offer, D., Howard, H.I., Schonert, K.A., & Ostrov, E. (1991). To whom do adolescents turn for help? Differences between disturbed and non-disturbed adolescents, *Journal of the American Academy of Child and Adolescent Psychiatry, 30,* 623-630.

Roe, A. (1957). Early determinants of vocational choice, *Journal of Counseling Psychology, 4,* 212-217.

Schaffer, D.R. (1989). *Developmental Psychology : Childhood & Adolescence,* Pacific Grove, Brooks & Cole.

Sherry, G.P., & Sinha, J.C. (1977). *Family Relationship Inventory (FRI),* Agra : National Psychological Corporation.

Skinner, B.F. (1938). *The Behaviour of Organism : An Experimental Analysis,* New York : Appleton-Century, Crofts.

Skinner, B.F. (1967). In E.G. Boring and G. Lindzey (Eds.), *A History of Psychology in Autobiography,* New York : Appleton-Century, Crofts.

Skinner, B.F. (1981). Selection by consequences, *Science, 213,* 499-504.

Tolman, E. (1925). Behaviourism and purpose, *Journal of Philosophy, 22,* 36-41.

Watson, J.B. (1925). *Behaviourism,* New York : People's Institute.

Weiss, A.P. (1925). *A Theoretical Basis of Human Behaviour,* Columbus, Ohio : Adams.

23

Impact of Socio-economic Status on the Choice of Game in Sports

Rameshwari Devi*[*] & R. K. Bhatia[**]

Sports today are much more than a simple recreation or play. These have definite rules, roles and behaviours which have been established formally and traditionally. Sports require extensive preparation to fulfil the requirements of structured time, space and goal. Robinson and Sarvin (1969) have shown that sports participation in general is positively correlated with psychological well being and that people who are active in a variety of ways in such activities tend to report a higher degree of emotional well being, life satisfaction and happiness.

Sports participation and sports efficiency are influenced by a variety of factors. A careful observation of the statements of experts who have mentioned various reasons for sports participation indicates that the interest can be bound in the initial stage, to the individual himself. The urge and drive to participate in the sports comes out from the individual himself, either out of his own interest or by the influence of others. Various other factors may be there to sustain that interest, to continue that participation and to excel and reach the peak performance level in sports.

The literature has also revealed that social agents such as peers, parents, teachers and coaches have significant impact on sports participation (Almarif and Muhammad, 1986; Applebee, 1993; Passer, 1987;). Many studies have suggested that birth order, community, and opportunities may also influence sports participation (Mixon, 1992; Stone, 1996).

Parents are the first and usually the most direct source of outside influence on the athlete. Parental influence will differ depending upon varied things, as for example, the section of the country they are from, socio-economic situations, race, religion, intelligence, education, family background and personal experience with athletes (Muthuraman, 1992; Ravi, 1990).

There are so many socio-psychological factors like attitudes, motives, audience or spectators, self concept, intelligence socio-economic background, achievement, motivation,

[*]Reader in Physical Education, M.D. University, Rohtak.
[**]Deptt. of Physical Education, Kurukshetra University, Kurukshetra.

adjustment etc., which influence the participation and performance of sportsmen in competitive sports (Banerjee, 1990; Cratty, 1967; Hutton, and Johnson, 1960; Johnson, Massicotlee and Markan, 1989; White, 1975) .

The total environment which is responsible for the performance of the child involves work place, school, home, community, and recreational pursuits. The total environment which influences one's sports performance is also greatly affected by socio-economic factors which have created many distinct classes in the society. Due to this some get best things and facilities and some get none or are forced to compromise with the minimum.

The socio-economic status of the group and the status of an individual in his group influence competitive and cooperative behaviour. An individual from lower class competes for different reasons and the different factors than those motivating people in the middle and upper economic group, influencing the well being of the players.

Therefore, the present problem was formulated "A Study of University Sports Participants in relation to their Socio-Economic Status" for investigation.

METHOD

Sample

575 male sports participants of intervarsity level belonging to Haryana state were selected as subjects for this study. The intervarsity sports participants who have represented their respective Universities namely M.D. University, Rohtak, Kurukshetra University, Kurukshetra and Chaudhary Charan Singh Agriculture University, Hissar, either during academic year 1997-98 & 1998-99 or both the years were included in the selected population. These subjects have represented the team of Athletics, Badminton, Basketball, Cricket, Football, Handball, Hockey, Kabbadi, Kho-Kho, Table Tennis, Volley Ball, Tennis, Weightlifting, Gymnastics, Judo, Boxing or Wrestling were in the age range of 17 to 25 yrs.

The sample from each university was selected on the basis of stratified random sampling technique.

Tool

Socio Economic Status scale by Kapoor and Kochar (1984) was used to asses the Socio Economic Status of each player.

Procedure

Administration of SES is very simple. Before giving the SES questionnaire, the investigator explained the purpose of performing the study. This scale seeks information about respondent's family and their members. The subjects were requested to give exact information about their families and the confidentiality was assured. There are different possible answers for each of the question included in the scale. The subjects were to select only one answer for each question which suited them most and tick mark (√) against it. However, in case of question 10 they were to put a cross or tick mark for each of the items present in their house.

RESULTS AND DISCUSSION

The number of players representing each game was calculated SES wise. The results have been shown in Table 23.1.

Table 23.1 : Showing the Distribution of the Sample Selected for the Study in Each Game

Sl. No.	*Name of Games*	*High SES*	*Middle SES*	*Low SES*	*Grant Total*
1.	Athletics	6	15	19	40
2.	Badminton	7	8	3	18
3.	Basketball	10	15	11	36
4.	Cricket	20	16	12	48
5.	Football	12	22	20	54
6.	Handball	10	12	14	36
7.	Hockey	13	15	20	48
8.	Kabbadi	6	18	20	36
9.	Kho-Kho	4	8	12	24
10.	Table Tennis	7	6	5	18
11.	Tennis	10	5	1	16
12.	Volleyball	8	13	15	36
13.	Gymnastic	4	7	5	16
14.	Weightlifting & Best Physique	4	19	12	35
15.	Boxing	4	16	14	34
16.	Judo	6	18	20	44
17.	Wrestling	4	15	17	36

The Table 23.1 indicates that out of seventeen games only in two games *i.e.* Cricket and Tennis, the representation was more from the higher SES.

The difference in the number of participants in different groups was assessed by employing Chi-square test. The results have been shown in Table 23.2.

Table 23.2 : Showing the Value of Chi-Squares

Sl. No.	*Name of Games*	*Chi-Square*
1.	Athletics	6.66*
2.	Badminton	2.34
3.	Basketball	1.63
4.	Cricket	2.0
5.	Football	2.44
6.	Handball	0.66
7.	Hockey	1.62
8.	Kabbadi	6.0*
9.	Kho-Kho	4.0*
10.	Table Tennis	0.33
11.	Tennis	7.63*
12.	Volleyball	1.75
13.	Gymnastic	0.87
14.	Weightlifting & Best Physique	9.66*
15.	Boxing	7.29*
16.	Judo	7.70*
17.	Wrestling	8.16*

* Significant.

The table indicates that the representation from high SES was significant for tennis but not for cricket. Thus tennis seems to be a game of elite class.

Further the higher representation from middle. SES was for Basketball, Football, Kabbadi, Gymnastics, Weightlifting, and Boxing (Table 23.1). Chi-square value for Kabbadi, Weightlifting and best physique and boxing was significant (Table 23.2), indicating a higher representation from middle class. But the chi-square value for basketball, football, and gymnastics was not significant. Kabbadi, weightlifting and boxing are the games of strong bodies. Although there are many studies indicating no difference in the physical strength of low, middle and high SES (Karuppaian, 1990; Stockhill, 1991; Taddonip 1992), yet in the Indian scenario, no doubt the under nutrition amongst poor leads to physically weak bodies thus leading towards an inability to play such games.

Muthuraman (1992) studied and revealed that in Tamilnadu the representation in Kabbadi was from low and may be very low SES. But in Haryana, Kabbadi also seems to be a popular game for the population of middle class. The reason for less representation from high SES could be the negative attitude of high SES population towards physical education (Charles, and Eskinner, 1998; Evan, 1993; Ravi, 1990) towards such games.

Low SES population represented the athletics, handball, hockey, kho-kho, volleyball, judo, and wrestling (Table 23.1). Chi-square value for handball, hockey and volleyball was not significant (Table 23.2) whereas the representation of Low SES subjects in athletics, judo, wrestling and kho-kho was significant. This significant participation in athletics, judo, wrestling and kho-kho is indicative of high physical energies in Low SES. Therefore, it seems that choice is not determined by the energy levels, but it is perhaps a matter of attitude and interest (Applebee, 1993). The attitude of both the parents and the player is important. Exposure to games and opportunity could be the other factors affecting the choice of sports. According of Qureshi (1987) the community area where the players hail profession of their parents and the income of parents are important factors determining the selection of game and also the performance. Karuppaian (1990) found that some people growing in poverty bidden society play the games, which incur less expenditure. Accordingly the games like tennis cannot be afforded by anyone else than the people of high SES.

This study is clearly indicative of the fact that the choice of game most probably, was not determined by any lack of interference with the physical development. Clearly, it must have been the lack of facility as well as the lack of exposure that determined the choice of game to be taken up. Actually lack of exposure does not allow the interest in the game to develop during childhood. Later when the interests develop, the subjects do not get these required facilities to develop the skills for learning a game to represent at higher levels of competitions. In fact by this time they have already developed a lack of perceived ability. That's how the population of lower and middle SES are deprived in choosing an appropriate game as their career. It is recommended on the basis of interpretations of this data in the light of earlier studies, that the government must take steps to provide equal opportunity to the population of each level of SES, by providing maximum facilities to the students at school level. This will lead towards a wider exposure about various developments of healthy interests, a more accurate attitude and a more suitable choice of game thereby enhancing the well being of subjects.

REFERENCES

Almarif, L. and Muhammad, Y. (1986). Personal motives and sociological factors related to participation in specific sports by teenagers in Baghdad-Iraq, *Dissertation Abstracts International, 45, 1682-1684.*

Applebee, A.C. (1993). The relationship of values, attitudes and interests to participation in interscholastic athletics among selected American, Indian youth, *Dissertation Abstracts International, 44,* 103-A.

Banerjee, Samuel (1990). Parent's Fault, *The Tribune,* Nov. 5.

Charles, B.J. and Estinner A. (1988). Attitudes Towards Required Physical Education in University & Colleges, *Dissertation Abstracts International, 35,* 31-35.

Cratty, A., and Bryant, J. (1967). *Social Dimensions of Physical Education,* Engle wood cliffs, N.J. Prentice Hall.

Evans, E. E. (1993). Attitudes of gifted middle school students towards physical education in connection to public schools, *Dissertation Abstracts International, 44,* 427-436.

Johnson, W.R.; Hutton, D.C. and Johnson, B.J. (1960). Personality traits of some champion athletes as measure by two projective test. *Roreshach and H-T-P Research Quarterly, 25,* 484-485.

Kapoor and Kochar (1984). *Questionnaire on Socio-Economic Status Scale,* Published by National Psychological Centre, Agra.

Karuppaian, T. (1990). The socio-economic status of the Tamil Nadu University men players during the Academic year 1989-90 and their performance in games and sports. *Unpublished Master's Thesis,* Alagappa University.

Massicotlee, D.R.G. and Markan, P. (1985). Prediction of vol. 2 Max from 'The running performance in the children aged 10-17 years', *Journal of Sports and Physical Fitness, 25,* 10-17.

Mixon, L.B. (1992). An analysis of attitudes pertaining to equality of opportunity to play sports and sports engagement of 5th and 8th grade students in an inner City, Urban and Suburban setting, *Disseration Abstract International, 42* : 10, 139-142.

Muthuraman (1992). Socio-economic status of Tamil Nadu high and higher secondary schools district level Kabbadi players during the academic year, 1989-90. *Unpublished Master's Thesis,* Alagappa University, Karaikudi.

Passer, M.W. (1987). Children in sports, Participation Motives and Psychological Stress, *Quest, 33,* 231-234.

Ravi, (1990). The socio-economic status of the Tamil Nadu University women players during the academic year 1989-90 and their performance in the games and sports. *Unpublished Master's Thesis,* Alagappa University.

Robinson, P. and Sarvin, T.R. (1969). A preface to the psychological analysis of Self, *Psychological Review, 59*; 11-22.

Stockhill, J.L. (1991). A Study of junior high school boys physical fitness scores as related to the families socio-economic status, size and type of occupation, *Completed Research in Health, Physical Education and Recreation, 25,* 72-75.

Stone, W. J. (1996). The influence of race and socio economic status on physical performance, *Completed Research in Health, Physical Education and Recreation, 44,* 10-16.

Taddonip, D.A. (1992). A comparison of physical fitness of public school students from economic deprived areas with national norms, *Dissertation Abstracts International, 43,* 1375-1378.

White, A.J. (1975). The inter-relationship between measures of Physical fitness and measures of self concept of selected, Mississipi state university male students, *Dissertation Abstract International, 397,* 412-415.

24

Gender Differences in U.S.H.A. Well-Being Among Irulas of Nilgiris District, Tamil Nadu, South India

*R. Roja Ramani**, *R. Babu** & *R. Balakrishnan***

The primary concern of all is to be healthy. Hippocrates (*ca.*460-377 B.C), the father of western medicine is of the view that "health" depends on a state of equilibrium among the various factors that govern the operation of the body and the mind; the equilibrium in turn is reached only when a man lives in harmony with his external environment (Nachimuthu, Dhanalakshmi, Balakrishnan, 2004). In pursuance of these principles of health *viz.*, body, mind in harmony with environment, health was conceptualized as an integrated well-being of body, mind, and spirit (Taub, 1996) in a person in dynamic partnership with his family, community, society and the infinite universe christened as the concept of Universal Supreme Health For All, U.S.H.A. for short (Balakrishnan, 2000a, b; 2003).

An outline of the scheme of U.S.H.A. well-being in terms of concerns and conditions that promote well-being is given in Table 24.1.

Table 24.1 : An Integrated Scheme of the Concerns and the Necessary and Sufficient Conditions for U.S.H.A. Well-being

Primary U.S.H.A. concerns	*Conditions that promote U.S.H.A well-being*				
Physical well-being	Nutrition	Hygiene Safety	Exercise	De-medication	De-addiction
Mental well-being	Happiness	Kindness and empathy	Learning	Self-esteem	Ethics
Spiritual well-being	Harmlessness	Awareness	Lovingness	Faith and devotion	Transcendence and joy

*M. Sc. students, Department of Psychology, PSG College of Arts and Science, Coimbatore - 641 014.
**Head of the Department of Psychology, PSG College of Arts and Science, Coimbatore - 641 014.

The U.S.H.A orientation comprising all the above fifteen factors of USHA well-being in a person enables him to view that his own and the universal health is dependent in all glory on each other. And that healthy people have an unique U.S.H.A. force within them that keeps them to remain at peace with themselves, as also in harmony with universe (Balakrishnan, 2000b), and so they remain naturally stable in health and well-being unless interrupted by forces adverse to U.S.H.A. orientation in them and in the universe which will get manifested in people in the form of deformity, disability, disorder, disease-acute or chronic, organ defect or finally as death, or the universal environment will face degradation and depletion of its natural resources.

A recent study on U.S.H.A., health of male and female medical college students (Balakrishnan, 2004) shows that in both the sexes, the U.S.H.A physical well-being was related to De-medication, De-addiction, Exercise, Nutrition, Hygiene and Safety; their mental well-being was connected to the factors of Learning, Self-esteem, Ethics, Happiness, Kindness and Empathy; and for their spiritual well-being, the contributing factors were found to be Faith and Devotion, Awareness, Harmlessness, Lovingness, Transcendence and Joy. In another study (Balakrishnan and Babu, 2004) of women undergraduate students in Arts, Science and Commerce faculty, it was found that they have the health beliefs (what they think as "true" health) bearing on De-medication, Kindness and Empathy, Harmlessness, Transcendence and Joy, Awareness and Happiness. The health practices of them were found to revolve around Self-esteem, Hygiene and Safety, De-addiction, Lovingness, Learning and Nutrition. Health is an important concern for both tribal and modern people. To our knowledge, no study has examined the effect of gender and well-being among Irulas of Nilgiris district, Tamil Nadu, South India, who are living in natural habitat. Hence, in the present study an attempt was made to investigate the physical, mental and spiritual well being of Irulas, a majority tribal community of Nilgiris District, Tamil Nadu and south India. Thus the aim of the study was :

To determine the gender differences in the U.S.H.A dimensions of well-being among Irulas. For this following hypothesis was formulated.

There exists no significant gender difference between the mean scores on the physical, mental and spiritual sub-dimensions of U.S.H.A. well-being among male and female Irulas.

METHOD

Design

A two independent group design was used. One group comprised of male Ss and another group comprised of female Ss.

Sample

30 male and 30 female Irulas were selected at random for this study from the villages using an incidental sampling technique; their age ranged from 40-55 years. Irulas are the majority aboriginal tribe of Nilgiris District (Jakka, 1986). Their history goes back to more than 500 years of existence in the District. Their original habitations were in and around the reserved forests of Nilgiris. They always live in the altitudes of 2500 to 3000 feet of MSL. Their approximate population in Nilgiris district is around 20,000. And there are around 5000 people in the adjoining district of Coimbatore. They are spread over the Eastern slopes of Nilgiris. They have a genetic problem of Sickle Cell Anaemia. They are short statured.

These people are mainly agricultural labourers. They work only three or four days in a week. Either of the husband and wife goes for work. In a very few families both the husband and wife may be working for their living. Their family consists of five or six people. Drinking of milk is a taboo in the tribe. They generally lead a life eating traditional food like ragi, thinai and maize; eating meat or chicken is an occasional feature (Ramasamy, 2004). The sites of the present study are located in Kolikarai and Kunjapanai villages in the Kotagiri Taluk of Nilgiris District—a tribal district in the state of Tamil Nadu, South India.

Tools

To ascertain the U.S.H.A. physical, mental and spiritual well-being among Irulas the U.S.H.A. questionnaire in its Tamil version developed and validated by Balakrishnan (2002) was used. The questionnaire contains 45 items spread into 15 sub-dimensions of U.S.H.A. well being on the physical, mental and spiritual well-being.

Procedure

The individuals were contacted individually and after a rapport establishment, the U.S.H.A. questionnaire was read out item by item by the investigator to the sample and questionnaire responses of the sample were recorded. In order to analyse the data collected the following statistical techniques were used *(i)* mean *(ii)* standard deviation (S.D), and *(iii)* "t"-ratio.

RESULTS AND DISCUSSION

Table 24.2 : Mean, SD and 't' Ratio of the Five Aspects of U.S.H.A. Physical Well-being Scores of Male and Female Irulas

Dimensions	*Sex*	*N*	*Mean*	*SD*	*SE*	*'t' ratio*
Nutrition	M	30	1.00	0.51	0.20	4.00**
	F	30	1.60	0.68		
Hygiene and safety	M	30	0.30	0.45	0.20	0.35
	F	30	0.23	0.72		
Exercise	M	30	0.90	0.63	0.22	1.36
	F	30	0.60	0.82		
De-medication	M	30	2.20	0.70	0.22	2.73**
	F	30	1.60	0.71		
De-addiction	M	30	0.80	0.77	0.22	2.27**
	F	30	1.30	0.66		

** $P < .01$.

The data given in Table 24.2 show that there are significant gender differences in the U.S.H.A. physical well-being factors of Nutrition, De-medication and De-addiction among Irulas. Female Irulas compared to their counterparts are more nutrition conscious, and de-addiction oriented. However, male Irulas are more de-medication oriented compared to their counterparts. There are no significant gender difference in the physical well-being dimensions of Hygiene and safety and Exercise. Thus, the findings of this study support the null hypothesis only as regards Hygiene and safety and Exercise factors of U.S.H.A. physical dimensions of well-being but rejects the hypothesis bearing on Nutrition, De-medication and De-addiction. They feel that their children and spouse should be fed with good food, the former for their growth and development and the latter to remain physically strong and addiction-free. The higher level of De-medication consciousness among male Irulas compared to their counterparts lends credence for this concen of being oriented towards physical well-being just like their counterparts. The similarity in Hygiene scores obtained by the sample of this study shows that both the male and female members of the community have concerns that they must keep their houses and surroundings clean. The absence of the gender difference in Irulas and a low score on the Exercise factor of U.S.H.A. physical well-being suggests that there are no traditional practices of doing formal exercises in this tribal community. May be it is not required, since both males and females walk miles together to reach other villages.

Table 24.3 : Mean, SD and 't' Ratio of the Five Aspects of U.S.H.A. Mental Well-being Scores of Male and Female Irulas

Dimensions	*Sex*	*n*	*Mean*	*SD*	*SE*	*'t' ratio*
Happiness	M	30	2.20	0.63	0.23	3.04**
	F	30	1.50	0.99		
Kindness & empathy	M	30	2.00	0.52	0.29	0.00
	F	30	2.00	0.52		
Learning	M	30	1.60	0.71	0.21	0.00
	F	30	1.60	0.69		
Self esteem	M	30	2.30	0.64	0.22	3.64**
	F	30	1.50	0.80		
Ethics	M	30	2.40	0.76	0.22	0.00
	F	30	2.40	0.72		

** $P<.01$.

Table 24.3 shows that there are significant gender differences in the U.S.H.A. mental well-being dimensions of Happiness and Self-esteem and no significant gender difference in Kindness and Empathy, Learning and Ethics partially support the null hypothesis of this study. Indeed male Irulas compared to their counterparts are more Happy and high on Self-esteem. It may be that male Irulas do indulge in more funny things, daily peeking at the troubles of others so they can make their own difficulties seem lighter or even insignificant by comparison, or indulge in quiet moments and communication with themselves that keep them feel more balanced, and confident about life. The absence of gender differences in Kindness and Empathy, Learning, and Ethics may be interpreted to mean that Irulas are not violent or arrogant people. There are no curious interest in learning among both the sexes, and ethics followed by both the males and females are common.

As can be seen in Table 24.4 that there is only one significant gender difference in the U.S.H.A. Spiritual well-being dimension *viz.*, Transcendence and joy on which females scored higher, and in the remaining dimensions of Harmlessness, Awareness, Lovingness, Faith and devotion there are no significant gender differences. These findings provide partial support to the null hypothesis of this study. Taken together these findings it can be concluded that Irulas are generally harmless and spiritually aware people who have the potentials to see the uniqueness in everything, appreciate this and yearning to merge with everything. It is a great revelation that female Irulas of this study, compared to their counterparts, have more tendency to take joys and sorrows in good strides.

Table 24.4 : Mean, SD and 't' Ratio of the Five Aspects of U.S.H.A. Spiritual Well-being Scores of Male and Female Irulas

Dimensions	*Sex*	*n*	*Mean*	*SD*	*SE*	*'t' ratio*
Harmlessness	M	30	1.80	0.82	0.22	0.00
	F	30	1.80	0.69		
Awareness	M	30	1.50	0.76	0.22	0.90
	F	30	1.30	0.73		
Lovingness	M	30	2.80	0.63	0.21	1.43
	F	30	2.50	0.67		
Faith and Devotion	M	30	1.90	0.72	0.22	0.00
	F	30	1.90	0.70		
Transcendence and Joy	M	30	2.30	0.69	0.20	2.00*
	F	30	2.70	0.54		

* $P<.05$.

Future studies of gender role and health may examine the U.S.H.A. life style of these people who live in different parts of India so as to shed light on them otherwise IRULAS would remain in IRUL (a Tamil word for "Darkness"). Also, in order to help circumvent their health problem bearing on Sickle Cell Anaemia, the utility of Indian system of medicine *viz.*, Unani, Siddha, Homeopathy and Ayurveda, U.S.H.A. ISM for short, may be studied for their curative value.

REFERENCES

Balakrishnan, R. (2000a). *Universal Supreme Health for All : A New Millenium Promise.* Paper presented at the fifth Annual Conference of the Psycholinguistic Association of India, Bharathiar University, Coimbatore, 19th to 21st February, 2000.

Balakrishnan, R. (2000b). *U.S.H.A. : Human Nature for Environmental Care.* Paper presented at the National Conference on "Eco-friendly Technologies for Sustainable Development," Department of Environmental Science, PSG College of Arts and Science, Coimbatore, 27th to 29th March, 2000.

Balakrishnan, R. (2002). *Universal Supreme Health for All Questionnaire* (unpublished), Department of Psychology, PSG College of Arts and Science, Coimbatore.

Balakrishnan, R. (2003). *Points to view : Universal Supreme Health for all Questionnaire.* Paper presented at the National Conference on "Challenges and response : Psychology of integration" held at Bharathiar University, Coimbatore, February 27th to March 1st, 2003.

Balakrishnan, R. (2004). *Universal Supreme Health for All Life Style : A Study of Medical College Students.* Paper presented in the National Seminar on "Recasting communicational strategy to health for all in India," Department of the Communication, Madurai Kamaraj University, Madurai 25th, 26th March, 2004.

Balakrishnan, R. & Babu, R. (2004). *Health Beliefs and Behaviour among Final Year Undergraduate Women in Arts, Science and Commerce Faculty,* Paper presented at the National Seminar on "Recent Advances in Statistical Methodologies and Applications" Department of Statistics, Bharathiar University, Coimbatore, 18th and 19th March, 2004.

Chidambaranlingam, A. & Balakrishnan, R. (2004). *Empathy and Effective, Interpersonal, Perceiving and Responding.* Paper presented at the national seminar on "Communication and Media : Challenges and Responses", Department of Sociology, Madurai Kamaraj University, Maduari, 29th and 30th January, 2004.

Jakka, P. (1986). *Child Development among the Irulas of the Nilgiris*, Uthagamandalam : Tribal Research Centre.

Nachimuthu, P., Dhanalakshmi, V. & Balakrishnan, R. (2004). *Gender Differences in U.S.H.A. Well-being among Post-Graduate Students*. Paper presented at the UGC National Seminar on "Stress and Coping Strategies." Department of Psychology, Annalmalai University, Annamail Nagar, 23rd and 24 the March 2004.

Ramasamy, K. (2004). Personal communication dated 12.5.2004 on *Short Profile of Irula Tribes of Nilgiris, Kotagiri* : Chief Medical Officer of Nilgiri Adivasi Welfare Association.

Taub, E. (1996). *Seven Steps to Self Healing*, London : Dorling Kindersley.

25

Deprivation of Food Items and Academic Achievement of Young Girls

*Rumki Gupta**

Health is an asset to a person in all stages of life. For this reason every one needs better health care. To maintain better health, it is necessary to supply basic resource *i.e.*, proper nutritious food. Food is also an important part of life and living. It is essential component for human growth and development. For normal human development, assured supply of regular food in adequate quantity and quality is essential. But food costs money. Therefore, a child who belongs to a low income family may not receive proper nutrition.

The concept of deprivation needs to be mentioned here. Townsend (1979) has defined deprivation as the absence of resources that prevent individuals participating fully in the customary behaviours and activities enjoyed by wider society. This problem of deprivation is more in rural communities due to inequality in the patterns of housing, benefit uptake etc. (Clake, Milbourme and Thomas, 1994; Shucksmith, Roberts, Scott, Chapman and Canway 1996; Chapman, Phimister Shucksmith, Upward and Veratoscane (1998). It has been revealed from literature review that deprived environment has negative effects on many aspects of development including intellectual aspect. It has been established that recurrent lack of food may result in malnutrition over time and that even mild to moderate malnutrition can be a developmental risk factor for children (Brown and Pollit, 1996; Pollitt, Golub, Gorman, Grantham, Levitsky a Schurch, Strupp, and Wachs 1996). It is also revealed that the deprivation during the first five years of life is more detrimental than deprivation experienced during late childhood or adolescence. This deprived condition hinders the ability of the individuals to acquire a healthy diet and parents' reduced financial resources are the causes of not being able to meet daily need for food. Infant health is extremely important in regard to the cognitive and social components of school readiness because problems at this age may lead to problems in the school years. In the case of school going child, the chance of success in

*Psychologist, Psychology Research Unit, Indian Statistical Institute, Kolkata, 700108.

academic life is brighter when the child arrives the school as physically and mentally healthy (Novello, 1991). It may be noted from the previous works that undernutrition can limit a child's ability to grasp basic skills and diminish overall learning potential (Center on hunger and poverty, 1998). Household food deprivation was negatively related to certain test and achievement scores for elementary school children (Alaimo, Olson and Frongillo, 2001) .

Review of the literature provokes to think one salient question, do male and female children receive equal opportunities at home and at school? Even in the twenty first century, according to the traditional belief, parents pay more attention towards their male children than the females. They contribute additional benefits of the household in the case of boys and try to enhance prospects for marriage in the case of girls. Gender discrimination with respect to food and other amenities are also very common .

The aim of the present investigation is to focus on the level of deprivation with respect to food among girls at the Madhyamik level, and to study the impact of deprivation on intelligence and achievement of girls and boys.

METHOD

Sample

The students who appeared in Madhyamik examination conducted by the West Bengal Board of Secondary Education (WBBSE) constituted the target population for the study. The schools under WBBSE were distributed among 16 districts. Four schools (2 boys and 2 girls) were selected randomly from each of the districts with a total of 64 schools. Out of these schools, 1338 students (723 girls and 615 boys), having Bengali as medium of instruction, comprised the sample for this study.

Tools

Prolonged Deprivation Scale (PDS) : The translated Bengali version of PDS of Misra and Tripathi (1977) was administered on all the students. It has 95 items with five response categories indicating "very low degree of deprivation"(1) to "very high degree of deprivation"(5) for each item. PDS has 15 areas. A total deprivation score (tdp) was obtained through summing up the scores in the 15 areas. 'Food' is one of the important areas of prolonged deprivation and this area refers to food habits and food stuffs. Items, such as, eating habit, types of meals indicating their nutritive value etc. are included in this area. Four food related items were presented to the students. A total food deprivation score (Tfd) was obtained through summing up the scores of four food related items.

Raven's Progressive Matrices : Level of intelligence of the students was gathered through Raven's Progressive Matrices (1938). It measures the capacity to apprehend meaningless figures, see the relations between them, conceive the nature of the figure completing each system of relations presented, and, by so doing, develop a systematic method of reasoning. It consists of 60 items divided into five sets of 12. A person's score on the scale is the total number he solves correctly through the series (5 sets) indicating non-verbal intelligence.

Measures of Academic Achievement : The marks obtained by the student in their Madhyamik examination was considered as the academic achievement score. "Madhyamik" is the final examination of the students reading in tenth grade under the WBBSE.

Procedure

The Ss were selected randomly in two groups of boys and girls from Madhyamik Vidyalayas. These students wore given the Prolonged Deprivation Scale and Raven's Progressive Matrices. The Ss were contacted individually, a rapport was established and responses were recorded. The Achievement score at Madhyamik level was obtained from School Records. Now the scores were put to analyses as given in the results and discussion portion.

RESULTS AND DISCUSSION

Most common descriptive statistical techniques such as mean, standard deviation and t statistics have been used in this study. It is evident from the results that the average level of deprivation in food items of the girl students was below the middle of the range (3.0). To explore the association, multiple regression of four food items on intelligence and academic achievement was determined and factor analysis of food items have also been carried out to see the differential importance of food items.

Responses of students in food items were given on a five point scale. Maximum possible score on any food item is five and minimum possible score is one. Five indicates high deprivation and one indicates low level of deprivation. Reasonably, range of total of food items is 4-20. Similarly, high score in PDS indicates high level of deprivation in general. It is evident from the results that the average level of deprivation in food items of the girl students was below the middle of the range (3.0) and this indicates that girl students do not suffer severely from deprivation of food items. It is likely that, girls those reach up to the highest level of Secondary Education (Class X) are relatively from advantaged section of the society. Similarly, average level of deprivation in food items of boys are consistent with the girls (Table 25.1). However, it is to be noted that boys were more deprived than that of girls. The difference of mean was statistically significant at .01%. It may be due to the fact that girls from relatively more socio-economically sound families are entitled to reach the said level of education.

Table 25.1 : Mean, SD and t values of Girls and Boys Students

	Girls			*Boys*			
Variable	*Mean*	*SD*	*Range of Items*	*Mean*	*SD*	*Range of Items*	'*t*'
f_1	1.39	0.74	1—5	1.81	0.99	1—5	.57
f_2	1.89	0.82	1—5	2.22	1.00	1—5	.60
f_3	2.26	1.03	1—5	2.71	1.13	1—5	7.50**
f_4	1.85	0.70	1—5	2.17	0.87	1—5	7.34**
Tfd	7.39	2.46	4—20	8.91	3.00	4—20	10.86**
Tdp	215.65	31.79	95—475	234.02	36.03	95—475	9.83**
Intelligence	32.63	13.14	0—60	34.94	10.99	0—60	3.50**
Aca.Ach.	50.87	13.83	0—100	51.28	13.22	0—100	.56

Note : Tfd means total of four food items, tdp means total deprivation.

** P <.01.

In the case of intelligence and academic achievement, boys scored higher than that of girls and differences were statistically significant. Differential importance of food items in food intake of girls has been explored by factor analysis of four food items (Table 25.2).

Table 25.2 : Sorted Rotated Factor Loadings Pattern

Item No.	*Factor 1*
f_2	0.823
f_3	0.805
f_1	0.775
f_4	0.540
VP	2.218

It is evident from Table 25.2 that more than 55% of the variance of four food items has been explained by one factor. No other factors have been extracted. In other words, all food items are considerably related in unidimensional space. Maximum loading is .823 (item no.2 *i.e.*, f_2) . Item no. 2 was related to daily intake of varieties of food items which is the most dominant among all other items. The second important item (item no. 3 *i.e.*, f_3) was also similar in nature to the item no. 2 (varieties of nutritive materials). Third important item was the item no. 1 *i.e* f_1 which relates to the availability of sufficient food in daily life. It appears that the least dominant factor (item no. 4 *i.e.*, f_4) was related to a non-essential material for girls students. Association between food items (f_1, f_2, f_3 and f_4), total prolonged deprivation (tdp), intelligence and academic achievement have been examined by multiple regression technique.

Multiple regression of four food items and total deprivation on intelligence is given below.

$$\text{Intelligence} = -4.28\, f_1 + 0.68\, f_2 + 1.48\, f_3 + 0.16\, f_4 - .11\, \text{tdp} + 57.63 \quad \text{.... (1)}$$

Coefficients of f_1, f_3 and tdp were statistically significant in the equation above. Corresponding Multiple T was .36 which is also statistically significant at 1% level. Considerably, large coefficient of f_1 is evident in equation 1. Similarly, Multiple regression of above independent variables (4+1) on academic achievement is as follows :

$$\text{Aca. achievement} = -3.53\, f_1 + 0.94\, f_2 - .13\, f_3 + 1.83\, f_4 - .16\, \text{tdp} + 85.89 \quad \text{...(2)}$$

Regression coefficients of f_1, f_4 and tdp in equation 2 and Multiple R were significant at 1% level.

It may be concluded that varieties of food items are relatively more important in case of food intake of girls of Madhyamik students. On the other hand the extent of availability of sufficient food in daily life is the best predictor of intelligence. Similarly, the availability of adequate food is the most effective predictor of academic achievement.

REFERENCES

Alaimo, K., Olson, C.M. & Frongillo, E.A., Jr. (2001). Food insufficiency and American School aged children's cognitive, Academic and Psychosocial Development, *Pediatrics*, *108*, *1*, 44-53.

Brown, J.L. & Pollitt, E. (1996). Malnutrition, poverty and intellectual development, *Scientific American*, *74*, 38-43 .

Center on hunger and poverty (1998). Statement on the link between Nutrition and Cognitive Development in Children, Waltham, MA : Center On Hunger and Poverty.

Chapman, P., Phimister, E., Shucksmith, M., Upward, R., & Veratoscane, E.(1998). *Poverty and Exclusion in Rural Britain : The Dynamics of Low Income and Employment*, Joseph : Rowntree Foundation.

Clake P., Milbourme, P., & Thomas C. (1994). *Lifestyles in Rural England : a report to the department of the environment*, the Economic and Social Research Council and the Rural Development Commission.

Misra, G. and Tripathi, L.B. (1977). *Manual for Prolonged Deprivation Scale*, National Psychological Corporation : Agra.

Novello, A.C. (1991). Healthy children ready to learn : The Surgeon General's initiative for children, *Journal of School Health, 61*, 359-360.

Pollitt, E., Golub, M., Gorman, K., Grantham-McGregor, S., Levitsky, D., Schurch, B., Strupp, B. & Wachs, T. (1996). A reconceptualization of the effects of undernutrition on children's biological, psychosocial and behavioural development, *Social Policy, 10*, 1-21.

Raven, J.C. (1938), *Guide to Using Progressive Matrices*, London : H.K. Lewis.

Shucksmith, M., Roberts D., Scott D., Chapman P. & Canway E. (1996), Disadvantage in rural areas, *Rural Research Report, 29*, Rural Development Commission.

Townsend, P. (1979). *Poverty in the U.K. : A Survey of Household Resources and Standards of Living*, Harmondsworth, Penguin.

26

Relationship Between Socio-economic Status and Well-Being

Savita Arya[*] *& Neelam Arya*[**]

A few years ago the concept of health as being more than the absence of disease was relatively new in research literature. But now health has become widely accepted as a state of general well-being that includes both physical and psychological components (Wheeler & Myake, 1992). This is also reflected in the statement of the World Health Organization that health is "a state of complete physical, mental and social well-being and is not merely the absence of disease and infirmity. Emmons & Kings (1998) have mentioned that health and general well-being are conceptually related. There are three conceptual terms related to well-being, *viz.* general well-being, psychological well-being and subjective well-being.

General well being refers to the harmonious functioning of the physical as well as psychological aspects of the personality, giving satisfaction to the self and benefit to the society. The person reporting low well-being means that he/she is not having complete and harmonious functioning of the whole personality in relation to the physical and mental health. Diener & Diener (1996) and Lykken & Tellegen (1996) defined general well-being as the subjective feeling of contentment, happiness, satisfaction with life experiences and of one's role in the world of work, sense of achievement, utility, belongingness and no distress, dissatisfaction or worry etc.

Psychological well-being is a malleable concept which is concerned with an individual's feelings about his daily experiences. These feelings extend from negative state such as stress, worry or unhappiness to more positive states which are not simply states of absence of worry or unhappiness but are states which are related to sound mental health and include favourable self-esteem and success (Warr, Cook and Wall, 1979). Jhoda (1958) has also stated that such feelings may range from negative mental states or psychological strains such as anxiety,

*Lecturer, Govt. College of Education, Chandigarh.
**Research Scholar, Deptt. of Bio-Sciences, MDU, Rohtak.

depression, frustration, emotional exhaustion, unhappiness and dissatisfaction to a state which has been identified as positive mental health of joy, happiness, satisfaction and the like.

Subjective well-being (SWB) is an abstract superordinate construct causing the affective reactions of individuals to their life experiences along a positive-negative continuum (Okun,1987). Subjective well-being has been operationalized (Okun, Melichar & Hill,1990) by indicators of happiness, moral and life satisfaction. Diener, Suh, Lucas & Smith (1999) stated that subjective well-being is a general area of scientific interest rather than a single specific construct and is a broad category of phenomena that include people's emotional responses, domain satisfaction and global judgments of life-satisfaction.

Diener, Sandvik, Seidlitz & Diener (1993) have found a positive correlation between income and subjective well-being but Clark & Oswald (1994) did not find a statistically significant effect of income in a representative sample from Britain. Smith & Razzel (1975) found that the effects of income often led to an increased level of distress. Thus, even positive changes in income may result in more stress, mitigating the positive effects of wealth on well-being. Recently Dinear *et al.* (1999) in a review article have reported that over the years there is a linear increase in the income in America but did not find any increase in the well-being scores. Therefore, there appears to be a lack of consistency in the findings over the relationship between income and well-being. Bradley and Corwyn (2002) reveled that for children, SES influences well being at multiple levels including both family and neighbourhood. Its effects are moderated by children's own characteristics, family's characteristics and external support systems. Evans, Kantrowitz and Eshelman (2002) found that elderly residents of higher quality homes, independent of multiple demographic factors (*e.g.* income, gender), feel more attached to their home, which in turn, appears to account for the relation between housing quality and positive effect of well being. Gorden, Savage, Lahey, Goodman *et al.* (2003) highlighted ways in which match and mismatch between family and neighbourhood income may encourage positive and negative social comparisons and may influence youths' ablity to participate in social networks and enriching resources. Bookwalter and Delenberg (2004) found that important differences exist among groups based upon their economic status. For the poorest quartiles, transportation and housing play the most important role in determining well being while for richest quartiles sanitation, water, energy, education and health are relatively more important.

SES is the position that an individual or family occupies with reference to the prevailing average standards of cultural possession, effective income, material possession and participation in group activity of the community. Social status can be thought of as a continuous variable as economic factors play an important part in determining the social status, it is better to label this variable as indicating their socio economic status. It is very important to clarify the relationship between SES and well-being. Therefore, the study was conducted with following objective in mind.

To determine the relationship between Socio-Economic Status and Subjective Well Being.

It was hypothesized that there would be significant positive correlation between Socio-Economic Status and Subjective Well-Being.

METHOD

Design

A single group correlational study was conducted. A sample of 60 male and female teacher students doing B.Ed. course at Chandigarh were selected on random basis. The age range of the respondents was 20 to 29 years. There were 30 males and 30 females in the sample.

Tools

Subjective Well-being Inventory (SUBI): Subjective Well-being Inventory designed to measures feelings of well being or ill being as experienced by an individual or a groups of individuals in various day to day life concerns by Sell and Nagpal (1992) was used. It consists of 40 items and 11 factorial dimensions : General Well Being—Positive Affect (GWB-PA), Expectation—Achievement Congruence (EAC), Confidence in Coping (CC), Transcendence (Trans), Family Group Support (FGS), Social Support (SS), Primary Group Concern (PGC), Inadequate Mental Mastery (IMM), perceived ill health (PIH), Deficiency in Social Contacts (DSC), General Well Being—Negative Affect (GWB-NA).

Socio-Economic Status Scale Questionnaire (SESSQ-Urban) : The SESSQ by Kapoor and Prajapati (1998). This questionnaire apart from objective components, gives weight to psychological indicators also. The SESSQ seeks information about following eleven component variables : parental occupation, father or guardian education, father or guardian monthly income, house type, household materials possession, books, magazines, cultural sub factors in SES, education of Testee's brothers and sister, level of aspirations, social prestige, belief in caste.

Procedure

Present investigation was conducted to determine the relationship between Socio-Economic Status and the Subjective Well-being. For this purpose Socio-Economic Status Scale Questionnaire and Subjective Well-being Inventory were administered. The respondents were requested to answer frankly and honestly since the information provided by them was to be kept confidential and would only be used for research purposes. Instructions regarding each test were explained at the time of administration. First of all SESSQ of Kapoor and Prajapati was administered to target sample. After completion of SESSQ scoring was done according to the weights assigned to each item. Secondly SWBI was administered to the same sample and scored by attributing the values to response categories of different dimensions. The obtained data were now tabulated and statistically analyzed.

RESULTS AND DISCUSSION

The objective of the investigation was to study the relationship between Socio-Economic Status and Subjective Well-being. For this purpose Pearson's coefficient of correlation was calculated. Table reveals that the coefficient of correlation between socio-economic status and different dimensions of well being is .68, which is significant at .01 level. A positive significant correlation between SES and well being indicates that, higher the SES, higher the well being of the individuals. On the basis of results, it can be concluded that socio-economic status is significantly correlated with various dimensions of subjective well being. Thus the hypothesis that there would be significant positive correlation between socio-economic status and subjective well-being is confirmed.

Findings show consistent linkages between socio economic status and well-being. It is evident that socio economic status is a major determinant of subjective well being. The findings of study are clearly in agreement with a number of earlier studies. Diener *et al.* (1993) and Bradley *et al.*(2002) have also reported that financial support is positively associated with well-being.Studies of Brickmen, Coates, and Janoff (1978) have also reported that low income/ financial reports have been found to be related with poor well-being/poor mental health. In a review article, Diener *et al.* (1999) reported that subjective well-being is not related with income. Yadav (2001) has found that social financial support is one major determinant of general well being among the aged, citing the example of United States where there has been a linear increase in the income of the American people (from 1946 to 1990) but subjective well-being scores remained stable. The present findings clearly reveal that general well being is related with social and financial support and thus has implication for the policy planning and welfare schemes for the people, in the sense that while designing welfare schemes, to maintain and enhance their well-being, attention should be focused on providing social and financial support.

REFERENCES

Bookwalter, J.T., & Delenberg, D. (2004). Subjective well-being and house-hold factors in Africa, *Social Indicators Research, 65*, 333-353.

Bradly, R.H. & Corwyn, F. (2002). SES Child Development, *Annual Review of Psychology, 53*, 371-399.

Brickman, P., Coates, D.K. & Janoff, B.R. (1978). Lottery and accident victims : is happiness relative? *Journal of Personality and Social Psychology, 36*, 917-927.

Clark, A.E. & Oswald, A.J. (1994). Unhappiness and Unemployment, *Economic Journal, 104*, 648-659.

Diener, E. & Diener, C. (1996). Most people are happy, *Psychological Science, 7*, 181-185.

Diener, E., Sandvick, E., Seidlitz, L. & Diener, H. (1993). The relationship between income and subjective well-being : Relative or Absolute? *Social Indicators Research, 28,* 195-223.

Diener, E., Suh, E.M., Lucas, R.E. & Smith, H.L. (1999). Subjective well-being : Three decades of process, *Psychological Bulletin, 125*, 276-302.

Emmons, R.A. & King, L.A. (1998). Conflict among personal strivings : Immediate and long terms implications for psychological and physical well-being, *Journal of Personality and Social Psychology, 54*, 1040-1048.

Evans, G.W., Kantrowitz, E., & Eshelman, P. (2002). Housing quality and psychological well-being among elder population, *Journal of Gerontology, 57*, 381-383.

Gordon, R.A., Savage, C., Lahey B.B., Goodman, S.H. *et al.* (2003). Family and neighbourhood income : additive and multiplicative associations with youth's well-being, *Social Science Research, 32*, 191-219.

Jahoda, M. (1958). *Current Concepts of Positive Mental Health*, New York : Basic Books.

Kapoor, S.D. & Prajapati (1998). *Socio-Economic Status Scale Questionnaire (SESSQ-Urban),* New Delhi : Psycho-Centre.

Lykken, D., & Tellegan, A. (1996). Happiness is a stochastic phenomenon, *Psychological Sciences, 7*, 186-189.

Okun, M.A. (1987). Life satisfaction. In G.L. Maddox (Ed)., *Encyclopaedia of Aging*, New York : Springer.

Okun, M.A., Melichar, J.F. & Hill, M.D. (1990). Negative daily events, positive and negative social ties and psychological distress among older adults, *Gerontologist, 30*, 193-199.

Sell, H. & Nagpal, R. (1992). *Assessment of Subjective Well-being : The Subjective Well Being Inventory* (SUBI), New Delhi : WHO.

Smith, S., & Razzell, P. (1975). *The Pools Winners*, London : Caliban Books.

Warr, P.B., Cook, J.D. & Wall, T.D. (1979). Scale for the measurement of some work attitudes and aspects of psychological well-being, *Journal of Occupational Psychology, 52*, 129-148.

Wheeler, L. & Myake, K. (1992). Social comparison in every day life, *Journal of Personality and Social Psychology, 62*, 766-773.

Yadav, S. (2001). *General Well-being Amongst Institutionalized and Non-Institutionalized Aged Subjects.* Unpublished Ph.D. Thesis, submitted at Maharshi Dayanand University, Rohtak.

SECTION—IV

Health in Organizational Perspective

27

Role Efficacy and Motivation

*Archana Upadhyay** & *A.P. Singh***

Research related to role efficacy has clarified the utility of motivation for the enhancement and growth of organizations. The concept of role efficacy has become an important issue in the "research agenda" of scholars. In recent years a number of studies have explored the relationship of role efficacy with several psychological variables in the field of organizational behaviour (Pareek, 1980, 1987; Pandey, 1992, 1995, 1997). However, very little researches have examined the mechanism through which motivation influences performance.

Despite differences in terminology and measurement most studies have realized the importance of role efficacy in organizational set-up (Pareek, 1980, 1987, 1993; Pandey, 1992, 1995; Pethe and Chaudhari, 2000). Role efficacy as a frame work for understanding the interaction of individual with their roles and resultant outcomes has generated increasingly greater interest in the last two decades. It is defined as the perception of greater opportunity on the job. The concept of role efficacy in the Indian context was proposed by Pareek (1980). He has taken this concept from the model of incentive developed by Porter and Lawler (1968).

According to Pareek, if organizations assist individuals in defining their roles and if individuals are willing to share this concern through appropriate strategies, it may be possible to increase effectiveness in the work place. Role efficacy refers to the extent to which people feel pleasantness and comfort to perform their roles. It is defined as the likelihood of the perception of greater opportunity on the job (Pareek, 1987).

In the context of role perception the concept of in-role behaviour and extra-role behaviour need to be examined. It can be explained in terms of organizational citizenship behaviour (Organ, 1990) which is a basic factor behind the concept of role efficacy. The boundary between in-role and extra-role can be defined on the basis of "job breadth" (Morrison, 1994). The greater an employee's job breadth the more activities he/she will define as in-role.

*Dept. of Psychology, Banaras Hindu University, Varanasi.
**Professor, Dept. of Psychology, Banaras Hindu University, Varanasi.

In recent years a number of studies have explored to establish the relationships between role efficacy with personal and organizational dimensions. With regard to personal dimensions, role efficacy has a high and positive relationship with internal locus of control, intra-persistive coping styles (solving the problems by one's own efforts), Cattell's cyclothemia (broadly speaking people orientation), surgence (broadly speaking extraversion) adventurousness (broadly speaking outgoing tendency), general satisfaction, role satisfaction, job satisfaction and quality of work-life (Sen, 1982; Surti, 1983; Gupta and Khandelwal, 1988). Role efficacy has negative relationship with externality and role-stresses as well as total role stress, impressive coping style, Cattell's dominance and Machiavalianism, alienation and defensiveness (Sen, 1982; Surti 1983; Singhala, 1985). It has several forms of correlation with age, experience, number of children and age of children (Sen, 1982; Surti, 1983).

On the organizational dimensions, role efficacy has an important moderating influence on dependent purposeful job behaviour and independent variables such as demographic factors, organizational climate and role stress (Das, 1984). Increased work-related tension has a negative correlation with overall role efficacy. Personal attributes and job demographics also have an impact on role efficacy (Sayeed, 1995). Operational and administrative roles, as well as stations of posting have also been found to have moderating impact on the role efficacy of police-officers in Ireland (Moran, 1986). Conducive environment results in effective leadership which ultimately influences the role-efficacy of organizational members and their productivity (Sayeed, 1992). Sayeed (1995) reported strong linkage between role efficacy and appropriate structure of position power/task structure.

Role efficacy was also reported to play role in preventing rail accidents caused by motor-man in Central and Western railways (Pandey, 1995). It was found to bring about positive changes in performance, interpersonal relations and overall job behaviour of the supervisors.

Motivation

Importance of motivation for enhancing role efficacy is well known. As Pareek (1987) proposed that motivating organizational roles depends on understanding, measuring and controling the role attributes that can enhance individual contribution to organizational growth and effectiveness.

Motivation is an area that has received the greatest attention in contemporary literature. Studies on worker motivation have in the past two decades dominated the social scientific productions of Western scholars.

Motivation is an area that is very important for both, *i.e.* scholars as well as managers. A great deal of research literature written by scholars and practitioners alike, highlight both the theoretical and practical utility of motivational techniques adopted by managers in improving performance at work. Yet importance of motivation for enhancing role efficacy is well known. But inspite of being a focal point, these studies are insufficient and need further attention. In contemporary literature. Sen (1982) reported positive relationship between role efficacy and functional aspects of six motivational aspects, namely, achievement, influence, extension, control, affiliation and dependency. But the importance of motivation in organizational set-up has not been well established in the contemporary literature. Research reveals that motivation directly influences effectiveness (Singh, 1997). Motivation is helpful in enhancing organizational citizenship behaviour (Chan and Drasgow, 2001).

Motivation also works as mediating factor in predicting relationship of personality and job performance (Barrick, Piotrowski and Stewart, 2002).

To obtain some more scientific information an attempt has been made through this study to sort out additional evidence on motivation and role efficacy relationship.

Following hypotheses were formulated for further understanding :

1. Employees who score higher on motivation are likely to have higher role efficacy in comparison to those employees who score low on motivation.
2. Motivation is likely to be positively related to role efficacy.

METHOD

Sample

The subjects of this study were 170 technical grade railway employees working in Varanasi Cantt. Their ages ranged from 30 to 62 years and all were the male subjects.

Tools

1. Role Efficacy Scale

To measure organizational role efficacy, Role Efficacy Scale (RES), developed by Pareek (1980) was used. It has three dimensions namely role making, role centering and role linking. The first dimension consisted of self-role integration, productivity, creativity and confrontation factors, each factor having two items. Each item presented alternative statements. A score of +2 is assigned to positive statements.

A score of +1 is assigned for negative statements. This dimension had a maximum of 16 and a minimum of -8 score. The second dimension—namely role centering consisted of centrality, influence and personal growth factors. Each factor having two pre-weighted statements had three positive useful and negative alternatives; the dimension had six items and maximum scores of 12 and a minimum of -6. The third dimension, role linking comprised inter role linking, helping relationship and super-ordination factors. Each factor had two pre-weighted alternative statements. The dimensions had a maximum of 12 and a minimum of 6 scores. The total scores on these three dimensions constituted role efficacy score. Inter correlations between the total role efficacy and its constituent factors ranged between 0.32 to 0.72 for group A (Role Making) between 0.37 to 0.67 for group B (Role Centering) and between 0.19 to 0.72 for group C (Role Linking).

2. Motivational Analysis in Organization (Behaviour) MAO (B)

For the assessment of motivation, Motivational Analysis of Organization (Behaviour) questionnaire developed by Pareek (1997) was used. Motivation is studied in terms of achievement, affiliation, influence, control, extension and dependence in the twelve areas namely orientation, interpersonal relationship, supervision, managing problems, managing mistakes, managing conflicts, communication, decision making, trust managing, risk taking, innovation and change.

The behaviour of an employee or a manager can be explained in terms of the six motives but it can be analyzed more accurately from the perspective of approach (positive) or avoidance (negative) infected by hope for success or fear of failure. Therefore, to properly explain the behaviour of an employee in a work-setting, Operating Effectiveness Quotient (OEQ) is calculated for each motive. OEQ has been recommended as a viable strategy for bringing change in the behaviour of employees after they scored their responses and calculated their OEQ for different motives. Group profiles of OEQ for six motives through two modes are recommended to be used for developing organizational strategies to improve group profiles, as also for developing individual strategies to increase employees' OEQ for various motives.

The test-retest reliability for each motivational dimension ranged from 0.17 to 0.44.

Procedure

Questionnaires were administered to subjects in small groups. The importance of accurate response was stressed and subjects were assured of anonymity of their responses. After obtaining all the responses, scoring was done as per the manuals and scores were put to statistical analyses. Perarson's correlation, t-test and stepwise MRA predictions were employed.

RESULTS AND DISCUSSION

Table 27.1a: Pearson's (r) Correlation Coefficient Between the Scores of Various Dimensions of Motivation and Overall Role Efficacy (N=170)

Variable	*Achievement*	*Affiliation*	*Influence*	*Control*	*Extension*	*Dependence*	*Total Motivation*
Role Efficacy	0.376**	0.306**	0.298**	0.370**	0.170	0.287**	0.455**

**P<0.01.

It is evident from the result (Table 27.1a) that in general role efficacy (RE) was found to be significantly positively correlated with all the dimensions of motivation (achievement, affiliation, influence, control, dependence) as well as total motivation. This relationship was non-significant in case of extension only.

Table 27.1b: Pearson's (r) Correlation Coefficient Between the Scores of Various Dimensions of Role Efficacy and Overall Motivation (N=170)

Variable	*Role Making*	*Role Centering*	*Role Linking*
Over All Motivation	0.262**	0.014	0.329**

**P<0.01.

These findings are further confirmed through the results given in Table 27.1b that displays, correlation coefficient between various dimensions of role efficacy namely role making (RM), role centering (RC), role liking (RL), and overall motivation. The results of this table reveal that overall motivation was found to be significantly positively correlated with role making and role linking but not with role centering.

These results are further confirmed through the comparison of high and low groups of motivation formed on the basis of quartile (above 75 as high and below 25 as low motivation).

Table 27.2 reports the significance of difference (t) on dimensions, of overall RE, RM, RC and RL obtained by high and low motivation groups. The findings indicate that high motivational group scored significantly higher on role making ($t = 3.39, P<0.01$) role linking ($t = 4.17, P<0.01$) and overall role efficacy ($t = 6.20, P<0.01$). However, the difference between mean scores of role centering, for high and low motivation groups was found to be non-significant.

Table 27.2 : Significance of Difference on Mean Scores of Overall Role Efficacy and Its Dimensions between High/low Motivation Groups

Variables	*High Motivation Group (N=43)*		*Low Motivation Group (N=42)*		*t*
	Mean	*S.D*	*Mean*	*S.D*	
Role making	56.68	11.96	48.02	11.51	3.39**
Role centering	59.74	14.37	59.24	12.67	1.68
Role linking	64.46	9.71	54.68	11.84	4.17**
Over all role efficacy	60.80	7.34	51.62	6.23	6.20**

**P<.0.1.

To assess strongest motivational predictors step-wise multiple regression analysis was also computed. The results have been presented in Table 27.3.

Table 27.3 : Summary of Step-wise MRA Prediction of Various Dimensions of Motivation when Overall Role Efficacy is Treated as Criterion (N=170)

Variables	*Regression Coefficient*	*Standardized Coefficient*		*t*
Achievement	0.145	0.376		5.25**
Control	0.108	0.257		3.52**
Multiple R	R^2	ΔR^2	df	F
0.376	0.147	14.1	1,168	27.58**
0.442	0.195	5.4	1,167	20.25**

** P<0.01.

A perusal of table 27.3 reveals that in step-wise regression first entered variable is achievement and it predicts 14.7% ($F_{1,168}$ = 27.58 $P<0.01$) variance. The second variable which entered in the regression is control and it predicts 4.7% ($F_{2,167}$ = 20.25, $P<0.01$) variance.

Table 27.1a displays correlation coefficient (Pearson r) between various dimensions of motivation, and overall role efficacy. The correlation coefficient between these variables was computed to determine the extent to which the criterion and predictor variables are related. It is evident from the results that out of 7 correlation coefficients 6 correlations (85%), *i.e.* between overall motivation as well its dimensions (achievement, affiliation, influence, control, and dependence) and total role efficacy, have been found to be significant in the predicted direction. The magnitude of the correlation coefficient ranged from 0.170 to 0.455. (Table 27.1) Significant relationship has not been obtained for extension.

Table 27.1b recorded correlation coefficient (Pearson's r) between overall motivation and various dimensions of role efficacy (RM, RC, and RL). Results of this table indicate that out of 3 correlation coefficient (66.66%) 2 are significant and its magnitude ranged from 0.014 to 0.329. Significant relationship has not been obtained on the dimension of role centering. The positive relationship between motivation and role efficacy reveals the fact that employees have positive thinking for their present job. It is well known that Indian Railways is the biggest public sector organization and it provides several motivational techniques to enhance effectiveness of the employees such as opportunity for promotion, monetary benefits, job security, housing facility, travelling facility etc. These findings, that role effectiveness is related to motivation are in agreement with the bulk of literature on the topic (Sen, 1982; Surti, 1983; Das, 1984; Pareek, 1987; Singh, 1997; Mishra, Bhardwaj and Pestonjee 1999).

The positive relationship between overall motivation and its dimensions with overall RE and its dimensions provide similar results which are consistent to the hypothesis proposed by Vroom (1964), Porter and Lawler (1968), Lawler (1971), Singh (1997) and that certain activities can enhance effectiveness of the employees by raising the level of subordinates work motivation. Due to feelings of political powerlessness and lack of opportunity in decision making role centering has been less valued by the employees. A similar finding has been reported by Pandey (1997).

Table 27.2 presents the results of mean and standard deviation of study variables between high and low motivation groups. It is evident from the results that high motivational group had significantly higher scores on overall role efficacy as well as on role making and role linking, but significant difference was not obtained on the dimension of role centering. Lack of close contacts with management provide least chance of participation in decision making and lack of redesigning could be the possible causes of non-significant relationship on dimension of role centering. Our findings are consistent with previous literature which reveals that a considerable amount of research evidence supports the view that holding the ability constant for most jobs, highly motivated workers perform at significantly higher rates than do unmotivated employees (Vroom,1964; Porter and Lawler, 1968; Lawler, 1971).

As stated in review of literature that working environment (Ghosh and Gupta, 1992) promotion, salary (Bhargava and Kalkar, 2000) and allocating the job to the subordinates work as important motivators for the employees (Turner and Lawerence, 1965; Hackman and Lawler, 1971).

Thus, the findings of the present study confirm the hypotheses 1 and 2 to a large extent.

The results of step-wise regression analysis reveal that amongst the six motivational variables achievement is the strongest predictor. A similar finding has been obtained by Pandey (1997).

In conclusion, the results of this study have provided additional information on the relationship of role efficacy and motivation in specific context of technical grade railway employees. The results obtained in this study do demonstrate the need for extensive studies of the effects of motivation on workers response to role efficacy.

The results of this study are based on a limited number of technical grade employees, therefore one can not generalize the findings unless the study is replicated on wider sample and the organizations. Advanced organisational development programme namely job enrichment, job redesigning, job enlargement could be used to enhance role efficacy particularly for lower occupational level personnel, especially for the purpose of rebuilding the job.

REFERENCES

Barrick, M.R., Piotrowski, M. & Stewart, G.L. (2002). Personality and job performance : Test of the mediating effects of motivation among sales representatives, *Journal of Applied Psychology, 87,* 43-51.

Bhargava, S. & Kalkar, A. (2000). Prediction of job involvement, job satisfaction and empowerment from organizational structure and corporate culture, *Psychological Studies, 45*, 43-50.

Chan, K.Y. & Drasgow, F. (2001). Toward a theory of individual difference and leadership : Understanding the motivation to lead, *Journal of Applied Psychology, 86*, 481-494.

Das, G.S. (1984). *Purposeful Job Behaviour and Its Determinants*, Bombay : National Institute of Bank Management.

Ghosh, P.K., & Gupta, P.K. (1992). Efficacy of employee's Directors in State Bank of Indore : A Case Study, *Indian Journal of Industrial Relations, 27*, 413-418.

Hackman, J.R. & Lawler III, E.E. (1971). Employee reaction to job characteristics, *Journal of Applied Psychology, 55*, 259-286.

Gupta, P. & Khandelwal, P. (1988). Role efficacy and organizational identification among professional groups, *Productivity, 29*, 31-37.

Lawler, E.E. (1971). Relationship between job satisfaction and some aspects of job, *Dissertation Abstract*, 33-74.

Mishra, P.K., Bhardwaj, G. & Pestonjee, D.M. (1999). Motivational climate and role stress : An experience with Indian Air Traffic Controllers, *Indian Journal of Industrial Relations, 35*, 185-197.

Moran, P.J. (1986). *The Development of the Role of Grade Superintendents in the Face of Social Change, Implications for Training and Retraining*, Unpublished Master thesis in Education, Manchester University.

Morisson, E.W. (1994). Role definition and organizational citizenship behaviour : The importance of the employee's perspective, *Academy of Management Journal, 37*, 1543-1567.

Organ, D.W. (1990). The motivational basis of organizational citizenship behaviour. In L.L. Cummings and B. M. Staw (Eds.) *Research in Organizational Behaviour*, pp. 12, 43–47 : Greenwich, CT : J AI.

Pandey, A. (1992). Employees occupation as moderator of role efficacy–A pilot study, *Indian Journal of Applied Psychology, 29*, 87-93.

Pandey, A. (1995). *Prevention of Accident through Role Efficacy Development in Driving Personnel on Indian Railways*. Paper presented in the safety conference in staff college, Vadodara.

Pandey, A. (1997). Motivational analysis of organisational behaviour : An experience with Rail Engine Drivers, *Indian Journal of Industrial Relations, 31*, 193-210.

Pareek, U. (1980). Role Efficacy Scale. In J. W. Pfeiffer., & J.E. Jones (eds.), *The 1980 Annual Handbook for Group Facilitators*, pp.100-195 : San Diego, California University.

Pareek, U. (1987). *Motivating Organizational Roles, Role Efficacy Approach*, Jaipur : Rawat.

Pareek, U. (1993). *Making Organisational Role Effective*, New Delhi : Tata McGraw Hill.

Pareek, U. (1997). *Training Instrument for HRD*, New Delhi : Tata McGraw Hill.

Pethe, S., & Chaudhari, S. (2000). Role efficacy dimension as correlates of occupational self-efficacy and learned helplessness, *Indian Journal of Industrial Relations, 35*, 505-517.

Porter, L.W. & Lawler, E.E. (1968). *Managerial Attitude and Performance*, Irwin : Homewood, III.

Sayeed, O.B. (1985). Job stress and role making behaviour, relationship between job-stress and role efficacy dimension, *Managerial Psychology, 6*, 35-37.

Sayeed, O.B. (1992). Role making behaviour, organizational priorities and managerial situational control, *Indian Journal of Industrial Relations, 27*, 346-361.

Sayeed, O.B. (1995). Participation in problem solving groups : A role efficacy approach, *Productivity, 36*, 119-127.

Sen, P.C. (1982). *A Study of Personal and Organizational Correlates of Role Stress and Coping Strategies in Some Public Sector Banks.* Unpublished Doctoral Dissertation in Management, Gujarat University, Ahmedabad.

Singh, R. (1997). The work motivational strategies used by central government officers : Relationship to effectiveness indicators, *Indian Journal of Industrial Relations, 32,* 309-327.

Singhala, Y. (1985). *Managing Frustration for in Organising Role Efficacy at Work as well as Home.* Paper presented in the IFTDO World Conference, Stockholm, Sweden.

Surti, K. (1983). *Role Stress and Coping Styles of Working Women,* Doctoral Dissertation in Psychology, Gujarat University, Ahmedabad.

Turner, A.N. & Lawrence, P.R. (1965). *Industrial Jobs and the Worker,* Boston : Harvard University,

Vroom, V.H. (1964). *Work and Motivation,* New York : Wiley.

28

Police Stress and Stressors : A Study Amongst Police Personnels

Radheyshyam & Sunita Siwach***

Modern living has brought with it not only innumerable means of comfort but a plethora of demands also that tax a person's body and mind. Stress is the awareness of a demand which exceeds the coping ability of an individual. Going beyond the individual level to the organizational level, it is said that some degree of stress is common to each and every profession but policing is certainly a profession, which demands more from the individual and exert more stress and pressure on the person. Few occupations require employees to face the kind of dangerous situation that police officers may encounter as part of their daily routine. This constant exposure of police officers to physical danger puts them in a state of continual conflict between their instinctual tendency to avoid hazard and their obligation to face the risks. Moreover, their continuous observation of incidents of injury and death only serves to reinforce this conflict.

The strain and pressure under which the police and paramilitary officials work, gets expression in various forms may that be normal or deviant. Mishra (2005) reported that there has been an alarming rise in the Boarder Security Force (BSF) jawans committing suicides and shooting colleagues and sometime even to family members, in a fit of rage or frustration. Elaborating, further, he said that on an average over 30 cases of suicide and as many angry shootouts takes place in a year. Not only this, stress, also gets expressed in the form of various physical and psychological disturbances such as sore muscles, an upset tummy, headache, high rate of heartbeat, diarrhoea, sweating from hands, dry mouth, restlessness and fatigue. Psychological signs are characterized by warring nervousness, feeling of sorrow, anger or feeling pressed for time (Vaishnavi, 1999).

*Reader, Department of Psychology, M.D.University, Rohtak.
**Head, Department of Psychology, M.K.J.K. Mahavidyalaya, Rohtak.
Authors wish to acknowledge their sincere thanks to BPR&D, Ministry of Home Affairs, GOI for providing financial support for the study.

Stressful life events, stress and strain have been found to be associated with high incidence of certain psychological disturbances *e.g.* anxiety, depression, coronary heart disease, hypertension, migraine, chronic headache, post-transmatic stress disorder etc. (Comer, 1992; Carson, Butcher and Mineka, 2000). In a study in Punjab Police, Singh and Mohan (1997) found high level of mental stress among Punjab Police personnels. They said that the high level of stress is adversely affecting their professional, physical and psychological well-being. They further observed that because of continuous and high level of stress, the police officials are getting prone to depression, alcoholism, anxiety, post-transmatic stress disorder etc. A variety of stressors such as frustration, conflicts, pressures, life events, daily hassles etc. have been identified (Comer, 1992; Carson *et al.*, 2000; Asnani, Singh and Javed, 2004). A sizeable body of literature has been developed over the years, that has examined police stress from a variety of perspectives. Clinton (1981) discussed stress and pointed out that there are four types of stressors *(i)* external, *(ii)* internal, *(iii)* individual, and *(iv)* task related. Smith (1982) found characteristics of the police organization and its administration as a source of stress among police personnel. Police officials perceived the criminal justice system as a source of frustration and found the public attitude towards the force as hostile. Kroes and Gould (1979) in an empirical study of job stress in policemen found lack of administrative support as a potent source of stress. Cooper (1982) examined the sources of stress among 200 British supervisory officers working at various ranks and found work overload, lack of personal recognition, frustration, autocratic management as prominent stressors. Quantitative work overload, underload, lack of control over the job (Frankenhaeuser and Gardell, 1976) excessive task demands and long working hours (Landy and Trumbo, 1976), role ambiguity and excessive role responsibilities (Arsenault and Dolan, 1983) have been reported as significant stressors amongst the police personnels. Fatigue emanating from job, separation from family, not being able to attend important domestic work have been reported as perennial sources of stress (Mishra, 2005) among the police officials. Harsh living and working conditions, inhospitable environments and differences with colleagues and seniors over various matters may perhaps further aggravate the situation.

Thus personal familial and organizational factors account for most of the stress and strain in the police officials. These stressors may work differently for officials working at different levels of organizational hierarchy (Yadav, 1995). Therefore, it has become a major challenge before the health professionals to help the police organization to identify the major and prominent sources of stress on police and help them in managing it. Keeping this in mind, present study was designed to assess and compare the level of police specific stress along with the identification of chronic job stressors in police officials working at different levels of organizational hierarchy.

METHOD

Design

To fulfill the objectives of the study a multigroup design (three groups) was used. Police officials working at different levels of organizational hierarchy were classified and included in three groups.

Sample

Present study was conducted on a sample of 300 police personnel selected by multistage, stratified, non-random purposive sampling procedure. The police officials working at different ranks *e.g.* Constables and Head Constables were taken as Subordinate group (Group I), Assistant Sub-Inspector, Sub-Inspector and Inspectors were taken in non-gazetted officers group (Group II) and those working as Dy. Superintendents of Police, Superintendents of Police and Additional Commissioners of Police and Deputy Commissioners of Police were taken in the gazetted officers group (Group III). The sample was drawn from Haryana, Punjab, Rajasthan, Delhi, and Uttar Pradesh states. The sample was selected from police officials at police training institutions of states as well as from those posted in the field (rural and urban areas as well).

Average age of the officials in group I, II and III was, 30.95 (S.D. 1.48), 40.45(S.D. 2.44) and 43.43 (S.D. 1.42) years respectively. Age range of the total sample was 20-55 years with a mean of 38.05 years (SD = 2.61 years). On the job experience ranged from 2-35 years with a mean of 13.46 years (1.92 years).

Tools

Following tools were used :

1. Police specific stress : was measured by administering police specific stress questionnaire (Savery Souter and Weaver, 1993). The questionnaire used in the present study included 13 items such as "my job tends to directly affect my health". Subscribed by a five point scale ranging from strongly agree (SA), agree (A), Undecided (U), to disagree (D) and strongly disagree (SD). A score of 4 was given to strongly agree and 0 to strongly disagree. Total score ranged from 0-52.
2. Chronic job stressors : For measuring chronic job stressors the following scales were used :
   - (i) *Neglected Family Life (NFL)* : Three items (such as, I feel guilty about leaving my children when I go to work) developed by Frone and McFarlin (1989) were used to measure the extent to which the respondents felt they are neglecting the family due to work. The items were subscribed by a five point scale strongly agree (score 4) to strongly disagree (score 0) and thus the score ranged fro 0-12, higher score indicating more feeling that they are neglecting their family.
   - (ii) *Job Boredom (JB)* : Four items developed by Frone and McFarlin (1989) subscribed by five point scale with a score of 4 to strongly agree (SA) and 0 to strongly disagree (SD), were used for measuring job boredom, score ranged from 0-16 with high score indicating more job boredom.
   - (iii) *Qualitative Work Overload (QWL)* : A three item scale from Michigan organizational questionnaire (Seashore, Lawler, Mirvis and Common,1982) was used to assess the respondents perception of having too much work to do. The items were subscribed by five point scale with a score of 4 to strongly agree and 0 to strongly disagree and total score ranged from 0-12. High score indicate more workload.
   - (iv) *Noxious Physical Environment (NPE)* : Four items developed by Frone and McFarlin (1989) were used to assess the respondents perception of whether their physical work environment exposed them to dangerous equipments and situations. Scale points and scores as described above *(ii)* high score indicating greater perception that their work put them in hazardous situation.

(v) *Communication Quality (CQ)* : Three items adapted from the International Communication Association (ICA) Audit (Goldhaber and Rogers,1979) and Modeled after a measure used by Frone and Major (1988) were used to assess the extent to which respondents perceived that their immediate boss clearly communicated job expectations. Scale points and scores as described above *(iii)* Higher score indicate better communication.

(vi) *Praise (PR)* : Two items adapted from International Communication Audit (Goldhaber and Rogers, 1979) were used to assess the extent to which respondents were recognized and praised for outstanding work. Item were subscribed by five point scale and score ranged from 0-8 with higher score indicating higher praise.

(vii) *Procedural Justice (PJ)* : Four items developed by Frone and McFarlin (1989) were used to assess the extent to which organizational policies and procedures were perceived to be faire and/or unfair. Items were subscribed on a five point scale with score ranging from 0-16. Higher score indicate better procedural justice.

(viii) *Decision Latitude (DL)* : was assessed by six items subscribed on a five point scale, developed by Frone and McFarlin (1989). Score ranged from 0-24 with high score indicating better decision latitude.

(ix) *Distributive Justice (DJ)* : was assessed by a five item scale developed by Prince and Mueller (1986). The extent to which the respondents perceived the rewards as fair, or unfair was assessed by it and score ranged from 0-20, high score indicate better distributive justice.

(x) *Role Ambiguity (RA)* : was assessed by five item scale from organizational role stress scale (Pareek, 1983). Score ranged from 0-20 and high score indicate greater role ambiguity.

(xi) *Role Conflict (RC)* : was assessed by five item scale from organizational role stress scale (ORS by Pareek, 1983). It was used to assess the respondent's perception of having conflicting demands or expectations, placed on them by others. Scores ranged from 0-20, high score indicate more role conflict.

Procedure

The respondents were administered the tools uniformly under similar testing conditions. Scoring was done as per the scoring guidelines and procedure. Results were analyzed by one way ANOVA followed by Duncan's post-hoc test. Pearson's Coefficient of Correlation was also calculated and multiple regression (Stepwise) was done to identify the chronic job stressors.

RESULTS AND DISCUSSION

The first objective was to assess the level of police stress in police officials and to compare the stress of police officials working at different level of organizational hierarchy. The mean (SD) stress scores (PPS) are given in Table 28.1. The mean stress score were 42.96 (S.D.= 6.44), 38.84 (S.D.=6.45) and 36.72 (S.D.=5.83) for the gazetted, non-gazetted and subordinate police officials respectively. These mean scores were found to be significantly different ($F = 25.81$, $p < 0.01$, df, 2, 297) from each other (Table 28.2). Post-hoc comparison by Duncan's test revealed (Table 28.1) that the gazetted officers had higher stress than both the non-gazetted and subordinate police officials. The non-gazetted official also scored significantly higher on stress scale than the subordinates. This shows that there is an increase in police specific stress with rise in police organizational hierarchy. This may perhaps be due to the greater accountability media scrutiny, political pressure, public pressure at the gazetted officers level. Non-gazetted officers' work in between the gazetted officers and lower level officials and are in a way sandwiched between them and thus experience more stress. The findings of the study are in agreement with those of Burke (1994) and Mathur (1995) but are in sharp contrast to Yadav (1995).

Table 28.1 : Mean Scores (SD's) on Police Specific Stress and Stressors Perceived by the Police Officials in Group I (Subordinates) Group II (Non-gazetted Officers) and Group III (Gazetted Officers)

	G I (n=100)	*G II (n=100)*	*G III (n=100)*
PSS	36.72[a] (5.83)	38.84[b] (6.45)	42.96[c] (6.44)
CQ	3.11[a] (1.97)	2.81[a] (2.13)	4.15[b] (2.64)
OJ	2.50[a] (2.38)	2.27[a] (2.21)	1.53[b] (0.89)
QL	2.82[a] (2.40)	1.98[b] (1.84)	1.57[b] (1.09)
JBD	11.91[a] (3.19)	11.60[b] (3.35)	13.64[b] (2.00)
NFL	10.46[a] (2.13)	10.39[a] (2.03)	11.02[b] (1.47)
NPE	11.55 (3.51)	12.14 (3.57)	12.26 (2.26)
PJ	2.54 (2.27)	2.30 (2.27)	2.01 (1.15)
PR	2.39 (1.61)	2.40 (2.38)	2.41 (1.27)
QWL	9.83[a] (2.79	9.87[a] (2.25)	10.57[b] (1.94)
RA	11.56[a] (3.39)	11.62[a] (4.28)	13.57[b] (2.45)
RC	11.27[a] (3.48)	11.90[a] (4.33)	12.80[b] (2.36)

Subscripts a, b and c shows significant mean comparison by Duncaon's post-hoc test.

Table 28. 2: Summary of ANOVA for Police Specific Stress (PSS) and Stressors in the Three Groups of Police Officials

(df=2,297)

Variables	*Between MS/ Within MS*	*F*
Police Specific Stress (PSS)	1006.77/39.01	25.81**
Communication Quality (CQ)	48.09/5.13	9.38**
Distributive Justice (DJ)	25.69/5.69	4.51*
Decision Latitude (DL)	40.60/5.93	6.85**
Job Boredom (JBD)	120.84/8.46	14.28**
Neglected Family Life (NFL)	11.92/3.62	2.29*
Noxious Physical Environment (NPE)	14.44/10.07	1.43
Procedural Justice (PJ)	7.04/3.89	1.81
Praise (PR)	0.01/3.81	0.00
Quantitative Work Overload (QWL)	17.32/5.53	3.13*
Role Ambiguity (RA)	180.57/12.17	14.83*
Role Conflict (RC)	59.13/12.16	4.86**

* $P \leq 0.05$, **$P \leq 0.01$.

** Significant at 0.01 level.

To compare the police officials working at different levels of police organizational hierarchy in their perception of chronic job stressors. One way ANOVA was done for the significance of mean differences and results are given in Table 28.1 (Means and S.D.'s) and Table 28.2 (F values). Out of the eleven chronic job stressors measured in the study, the police officials (Group I, Group II and Group III) differed significantly on eight, *i.e.* communication quality (CQ), distributive justice (DJ), decision latitude (DL), job boredom (JB), neglected family life (NFL), quantitative work over load (KWL), role ambiguity (RA) and role conflict (RC) (Table 2). Mean scores of the three groups *viz.*, subordinates ($\overline{X}$ 3.11), non-gazetted ($\overline{X}$ 2.81) and gazeted ($\overline{X}$ = 4.15) police official on perceived communication quality were significantly ($F = 9.38$, $p < 0.01$, df 2,297) different (Table 28.1). Post-hoc comparison by Duncan's test revealed that the gazetted officers perceived the communication quality better than the non-gazetted and subordinates, whereas, the subordinate officials did not differ from non-gazetted officials (Table 28.1). The three groups of police officials differed on perceived distributive justice ($F = 4.51$, $p < 0.05$, df 2,297). The subordinate and non-gazetted police officials perceived the distributive justice better than the gazetted officers (Table 28.1). The perceived decision latitude scores of the three groups differed significantly ($F = 6.85$, $p < 0.01$, df 2,297). The subordinates again perceived more decision latitude than the non-gazetted and gazetted officers. The non-gazetted and gazetted officers did not differ significantly (Table 28.1).

Subordinate, non-gazetted and gazetted police officers differed significantly ($F = 14.28$, $p < 0.01$, df 2,297) in their prescribed job boredom scores. The gazetted officers perceived their job as boring more than the non-gazetted and subordinates (Table 28.1). Similarly, there was greater degree of feelings in the gazetted police officers that due to their work their family life was neglected, they also perceived higher quantitative workload, more role ambiguity, and role conflict than both the non-gazetted and subordinates (Table 28.1 and

Table 28.3 : Coefficient of Correlation Among Chronic Job Stressors and Police Stress

	PSS	*CQ*	*DJ*	*DL*	*JBD*	*NFL*	*NPE*	*PJ*	*PR*	*QWL*	*RA*	*RC*
PSS	1.00											
CQ	0.07	1.00										
DJ	–0.19**	0.22**	1.00									
DL	–0.19**	0.35**	0.75**	1.0*								
JBD	0.36**	–0.02	–0.25**	–0.24**	1.00							
NFL	0.24**	–0.16**	0.27**	–0.28**	0.52**	1.00						
NPE	0.28**	–0.21**	–0.13**	–0.19**	0.46**	0.32**	1.00					
PJ	–0.23**	0.44**	0.61**	0.69**	0.27**	–0.22**	–0.22**	1.00				
PR	–0.07	0.56**	0.23**	0.33**	–0.15**	–0.17**	–0.16**	0.47**	1.00			
QWL	0.22**	–0.06	–0.11*	–0.15**	0.30**	0.29**	0.39**	–0.18**	–0.09	1.00		
RA	0.24**	0.15**	–0.24**	–0.19**	0.29**	0.28**	0.24**	–0. 34**	–0.27**	0.13	1.00	
RC	0.22**	–0.14**	–0.18**	–0.10	0.31**	0.20**	0.25**	–0.32**	–0.22**	0.17**	0.35**	1.00

* P ≤ 0.05 level.

** P ≤ 0.01 level.

Table 28.2). Though it sounds strange, that the officers at the higher level, who are supposed to direct their subordinates experienced more role conflict, role ambiguity, may be due to this they have experienced more stress.

The second objective of the study was to identify the significant predictors of police stress. Pearson Coefficient of Correlation between stress and the eleven chronic job stressors were calculated and are given in Table 3. Procedural Justice (–0.23), distributive justice (–0.19) and decision latitude (–0.19) were negatively related with police stress, whereas, job boredom (0.36) neglected family life (0.24), noxious physical environment (0.28), quantitative work overload (0.22), role ambiguity (0.24) and role conflict (0.22) were positively related. Though all these coefficients of correlation were low yet significant. The correlation between police stress, communication quality and praise was negligible (Table 28.3).

Table 28.4 : Model Summary of Stepwise Multiple Regression, R, R^2, Between and Within MS and F Values

	R	R^2	*Between MS/Within MS*	*F*	*df*
1.	0.36	0.13	1778.86/39.66	44.84**	1,298
2.	0.39	0.15	1036.47/38.81	26.71**	2,297
3.	0.43	0.18	823.54/37.59	21.90**	3,296
4.	0.45	0.21	703.28/36.56	19.24**	4,295

** $P \leq 0.01$ level.

1. Constant + JBD
2. Constant + JBD + PJ
3. Constant + JBD + PJ + CQ
4. Constant + JBD + PJ + CQ + NPE

Table 28.5 : Stepwise Multiple Regression of Police Specific Stress on Chronic Job Stressors (Only Significant Predictors were Taken)

X_1	*Police Specific Stress*	$\overline{X}$	*Reg. Coefficient*	*SE*
Model 1	Job Boredom	12.38	0.80	0.12
	Constant		29.56	1.53
Model 2	Job Boredom	12.38	0.71	0.12
	Procedural Justice	2.28	–0.52	0.19
	Constant		31.86	1.73
Model 3	Job Boredom	12.38	0.67	0.12
	Procedural Justice	2.28	–0.83	0.21
	Communication Quality Constant	3.38	0.56	0.17
			31.23	1.71
Model 4	Job Boredom	12.38	0.49	0.13
	Procedural Justice	2.28	–0.82	0.21
	Communication Quality Noxious Physical	3.37	0.66	0.17
	Environment	11.98	0.39	0.13
	Constant		28.46	1.92

To identify the significant predictors of police stress, multiple regression (stepwise) was done and results are given in Table 28.4 and 28.5. Four models significantly predicted police specific stress (Table 28.4 and 28.5). Job boredom turned out to be the prominent predictor of stress accounting 13% of (R^2=13) the variance. Job boredom and procedural justice together accounted 15% of variance (R = 39, R^2=0.15). When another significant predictor *i.e.* communication quality was taken up, they (job boredom, procedural justice and communication quality) accounted 18% of the variance (R=0.43, R^2=0.18). Model 4, taking job boredom, procedural justice, communication quality and noxious physical environment but together accounted maximum *i.e.* 21% of variance (with R = 0.45 R^2 = 21), (F = 19.24, $p < 0.01$) with 2 and 295 degrees of freedom (Table 28.4). The regression coefficients were 0.49, - 0.82, 0.66 and 0.39 for job boredom, procedural justice, communication quality and noxious physical environment respectively. This indicate that out of the eleven chronic job stressors only four significant predictors for police stress. Procedural justice reduces stress, whereas job boredom and noxious physical environment add to police stress. Strangely enough, communication quality was found to add to police stress. The items in the communication quality scale were related to the immediate boss, 'his being honest with the respondent, listen what the respondent has to say, and clear communication with the respondent' and the respondents might have fear that the information may leak and reach the boss, though they were clearly told that it will not, they might have not been able to give the exact response and perhaps may be the reason for this unusual direction. Job boredom and noxious physical environment add significantly to police stress. It was confirmed by the informal chat with the officials, who reported that they are not enjoying their job still they have to do it as they don't have any other option. They were also weary of the working conditions and hazardous environment they are required to work in. The finding are in agreement with those of Huvvell (1995) who reported on the basis of his study that about 56% of the police officials feeling bored out of their job and Mathur (1995) who found fear of death or injury, arresting a criminal, use of weapon, facing an ambush and antiterrorist operation as major stressors in Indian police officials.

It can be concluded that the police officials working at higher level of organizational hierarchy experience greater amount of police stress and there was increase in stress with rise in organizational hierarchy. The police officials working at different levels of police organizational hierarchy differed in their perception of various chronic job stressors. The senior police officials perceived to have better communication quality but at the same time experienced greater degree of job boredom with the feeling of neglecting the family life due to their job, perceived to be overloaded with work. They also experienced role ambiguity and role conflict. Job boredom, procedural justice, communication quality and noxious physical environment accounted variance of the police stress to the tune of 21%. The findings of the study may have implications for the police officials and the police organizations for understanding the sources of stress and consequently planning for reducing stress by eliminating the stressor or by reducing its intensity for strengthening the coping resources of the individual.

REFERENCES

Arsenault, A. and Dolan, S. (1983). The role of personality occupation and organization in understanding the relationship between job stress, performance and absenteeism, *Journal of Occupational Psychology*, *56*, 227, 240.

Asnani, V.; Singh, N.P. and Javed, A. (2004). Psychosocial stress and social support. In A. Hussain and T. Rashid (Edited) *Stress Behaviour, The Coping Strategies*, New Delhi : Friends.

Burke, R.J. (1994). Stressful events, work-family conflict, coping, psychological burnout and well-being among police officers, *Psychological Reports, 75*, 787-800.

Carson, R.C.; Butcher, J.N. and Mineka, S. (2000). Abnormal Psychology and Modern Life (11th edition) Delhi : Allyan and Bacon.

Clinton, L. (1981). Police Stress : The Empirical Evidence, *Journal of Police Science and Administration, 9*, 61-75.

Comer, R.J. (1992). *Abnormal Psychology*, New York : Freeman.

Cooper, C.L. (1982). Stress at work, *John Wiley.*

Frankenhaveuser, M. and Gardell, B. (1976). Underload and overload in working life : Outline of a multidisciplinary approach, *Journal of Human Stress, 2*, 35-46.

Frone, M.R., and McFarlin, D.B. (1989). Chronic occupational stressors, self-focused attention and well-being : testing a cybernetic model of stress, *Journal of Applied Psychology, 74*, 876-887.

Frone, M.R. and Major, B. (1988). Communication quality and job satisfaction among managerial nurses : The moderating influence of involvement, *Group and Organisational Studies,13*, 332-347.

Goldhaber, G.M. and Rogers, D.P. (1979). *Auditing Organizational Communication System : The ICA Communication,* Audit. Dvbvque, 1A : Kendal/Hunt.

Hurrell, J.J. (1995). Police work, occupational stress and individual coping, *Journal of Organizational Behaviour, 16*, 27-38.

Kroes, W.H. and Gould (1979). Job stress in policemen : an empirical study, *Police Stress, 1*, 44-46.

Landy, F. and Trumbo, D. (1976). *Psychology of Work Behaviour*, Illinois : Dorsey Press.

Mathur, (1995). Perception of police stress : An empirical study stressor and coping responses among police personnel in India, *Indian Journal of Criminology, 23*, 9-19.

Mishra, B. (2005). Fatigue takes its toll, BSF Jawan on the brink, *Times of India*, Friday, May 6, New Delhi.

Pareek, U. (1983). *Role Stress Scales Manual*, Ahamedabad : Naveen Publication.

Price, J. L., and Muller, C.W. (1986). *Handbook of Organizational Measurement,* Marsh-field, M.A. : Pitman.

Savery, L.K.; Souter, G.N. and Weaver, J.R. (1993). Stress and police officer : Some west Australia Evidences, *The Police Journal.*

Seashore, S.E., Lawler, E.E., Mirvis, P. Common, C. (1982). *Observing and Measuring Organizational Change : a guide to field practice*, New York : Wiley.

Singh, D. and Mohan (1997). *Stress in Punjab Police*, The Tribune, Chandigarh.

Smith, D. (1982). Sources and consequences of stress for the police, *American Journal of Police, 1*, 114-148.

Vaishnavi, C. (1999). Coping with stress : A strategy, *The Tribune*, May 19, Chandigarh.

Yadav, S. (1995). A study of stress and emotional problems in police personal : A research report, University of Rajasthan, Jaipur.

29

Stress State and its Effect on Task Performance, Job Involvement, and Job Satisfaction

Sandeep Kumar, Lalit Kumar Mishra**, A. P. Singh****

To study the effects of stress state upon task performance, job involvement and job satisfaction and how these effects differ as a function of personality as a mediator has been a long-standing endeavor of the scientific community. Researches have examined the stress-performance relationship and have identified a number of factors, which may moderate this relationship, such as social support, locus of control, perceived control, trait anxiety, self-efficacy, self-control, and experience (Weaver, Morgan, Adkins-Holmes, and Hall, 1992). To date, research on stress and performance has been concerned with specific sources of stress state, in particular the context of work situation and different form of tasks.

A problem in explaining the effects of stress on performance is that such effects depend upon features of the environment (including the task) and also of the individual operator. The transactional theory of stress addresses this issue by defining the construct in terms of person environment interactions. Within the framework of a transactional model, stress states may be viewed as abstracted representations of the relation between individuals and the external demands placed upon them (Matthews, 2001). Lazarus and Folkman (1984) defined psychological stress as a case in which individuals appraise their environment as taxing or exceeding their resources and/or endangering their well being. The negative effects of stress are most likely to occur when individuals view an event as a threat and when they assess their coping skills as inadequate for handling the stressor.

*Lecturer in Psychology/Personnel Management and Industrial Relations, Department of Psychology, Banaras Hindu University, Varanasi-221005. E-mail : sk_bhu@yahoo.co.in

**Project Fellow, Department of Psychology, Banaras Hindu University, Varanasi-221005. E-mail: lalit_bhu@yahoo.co.in

***Professor, Department of Psychology, Banaras Hindu University, Varanasi-221005. E-mail: aps_bhu@yahoo.co.in

Earlier researches emphasized upon examining the physiological reactions to stress followed by an emphasis on examining coping mechanisms during stress. Although both physiological as well as behaviour oriented theorists were fascinated towards defining 'stress' and its effect, the causal relationship has never been established due to a great variety of psychological and situational determinants that precipitate it (Pestonjee, 1992). The futility of these researches led later researchers to examine this relationship taking the mediators of stress into account. A bulk of researches on personality and social support (as mediators) have failed to bring forward promising results. Researchers these days, therefore, have concentrated upon the assessment of stress-state. This is because there is a growing realization that a person's reaction to a stressful event is both complex and highly variable across individuals and events. This means that personality measures are of limited use in predicting stress reactions (Matthews, Jones and Chamberlain, 1990). It also means that experimental studies of stress using external agents such as noise fail to recognize the complexity of the stress reactions provoked with a reliable and valid measure of stress-state. Thus, a better understanding of the effects of stressors on well being and performance needs to be obtained.

Motowidlo, Packard and Manning (1988) suggested that subjective stress generates anxiety, hostility and depression, which, in turn, affect components of job performance such as tolerance for frustration, clerical accuracy, interpersonal sensitivity and altruism. Performance usually drops off sharply when stress rises to high levels (Robert, 1986). Stress has the strongest impact on aggressive actions such as sabotage, interpersonal aggression, hostility and complaints (Chen, and Spector, 1992). These types of problems from stress, in turn, are especially relevant to poor job performance, lowered level of self-esteem, and resentment of supervision, inability to concentrate and make decisions, and job dissatisfaction. These outcomes of stress can have direct cost effect on the organization. There is evidence that employees under high stress can cost their organizations in terms of money due to higher accident levels, lost time, and reduced productivity.

Broota (1993) examined the nature and extent of life stress experienced by 60 schizophrenics (30 indoor and 30 outdoor patients) and 60 normal subjects matched on age (18-65 years old), sex, education, socio-economic status, occupation and rural-urban background. It was found that indoor patients' scores were significantly higher than those of outdoor patients and normals. Latha, Bhutt and D'Sayza (1994) carried out a study on a group of 73 individuals (aged 16-65 years) who had attempted suicide, 58 depressives (aged 16-51 years) and 60 normal controls (aged 18-53 years). Findings indicated that compared to the depressives and controls, suicidal individuals reported more stressful life events, which included marital discord, conflicts with in-laws or family, problem in love, illness, death in the family and unemployment.

A chronic state of physical and emotional depletion results from excessive job demands and continuous hasseles (Shirom, 1989; Zohar, 1997). Currently more and more researchers conceive of burnout as a work-related strain that can emerge in any occupation, including management and technology (Maslach, and Schaufeli, 1993; Leiter, and Schaufeli, 1996). Research by Etzion, Eden, and Lapidot (1998) has shown that the burnout relief experienced while the job stressors were "turned off". Work family conflict and family-work conflict are associated with less work satisfaction and greater psychological distress. Strain based work interfering with family has emerged as an outcome of stress (Kelloway, Gottlieb, and Barham,

1999). The relationship between number of hours worked and burnout depends on the extent to which work schedule meet the needs of the worker, her or his partner, and their children, if any (Barnett, Gareis, and Brennan, 1999).

Srivastava (2002) in his study examined the effectiveness of "Cognitive Intervention" in prevention, mitigation and help coping with occupational stress and job and health strains in relation to employee's locus of control. The results indicated a significant decline in the degree of occupational stress and severity of psychological and somatic distress, and improvement in job satisfaction of the S's after the intervention. Comparison of intervention and control groups with regard to their job stress and consequent distress also confirmed the effectiveness of the intervention.

Chaudhry, Latif, Anjum and Rashid (2002) in their study on the sample of 172, mostly (93%) male employees of both public and private enterprises in Pakistan administered the SWS-International Survey of Stress and Mental Health, to investigate whether there are differences in the degree of stress at different organizational levels. Results showed stress in all domains. Social/situational, work and self for top executives were found to be significantly lower and support scores were significantly higher compared to employees at lower organizational levels. Consistent with this pattern, top management scores for poor mental health were found to be significantly lower and for good mental health significantly higher compared to employees at lower organizational levels.

Kao (2002) tried to explore the effects of depression on college students' well-being by testing impacts of stress, social support, self-esteem, and self-rated health status. The results revealed that significant correlations existed among depression and four chosen variables. Furthermore, multiple regression process indicated that stress and social support were significant predictors for the magnitude of depression. With high stress and low social support, the likelihood of depression magnitude increased. In addition, different supports played a significant role in depression phenomena.

It has been widely accepted that reactions to stress may lead to dysfunction of various sorts of disorders; ranging from immuno-suppression of body mechanism to psychosomatic disorders of all kinds. The specificity of a disorder, however, depends upon the exact nature types of stress, such as acute time-limited stress (*e.g.* surgery), time-bound single stressor (*e.g.* divorce), or intermittent stressor (*e.g.*, unemployment). Whatever be the nature of stress, psychologists these days are preoccupied with predicting the reactions of a stress state (time limited or long-term). In doing so, the emphasis has shifted from predicting relatively permanent stress reactions to state-dependent reaction of the individual.

To examine the above, it becomes imperative to analyze the psychological state of the individual that comprises cognitive, components. (*e.g.*, worry, task-irrelevant thoughts of self, focus of attention), emotional components (*e.g.*, mood), motivational components (*e.g.*, task effort), and connative components (*e.g.*, determination of behavioural strategy, for example, active passive glossing over, active-avoidance, passive-avoidance etc.). Put together, the emphasis in this study was to examine the concept of stress state in terms of behavioural outcomes and to predict performance change in organizational as well as social set up of an individual. Most of the researchers have dealt with the issues of stress and its deleterious effect on behavioural outcome and well being. Very few of them have tried to manipulate stress factors or stressors to bring forth changes in performance.

This seems too important since prediction of performance change may increase individual effectiveness, which in turn may have positive effect on well being. A new concept of 'energetic arousal' has been introduced. This concept is differentiated from 'tense arousal' in terms of hedonic valence of stress-state. Concepts, 'energetic arousal' and 'tense arousal' are associated to some extent with the hedonic (emotional) tone. The concept of 'energetic arousal' refers to a positive emotional state of stress; the energy arising out of it may be utilized to produce desirable change in performance.

In view of the above presumptions and facts, the following specific objectives have been laid down for the present study :

1. To find out whether there is any difference in level of pre and post task stress state due to the effect of task performance.
2. Finding out the effects of stress state on task performance.
3. Finding out the effects of stress state on job involvement.
4. Finding out the effects of stress state on job satisfaction.
5. Assessing personality (*e. g.*, extraversion, psychoticism and neuroticism) as moderator variable in the relationship of stress and performance.
6. Testing whether the stress-state measure could be used to predict performance change on simple tasks.

METHOD

Design

A before-after design was employed.

Sample

This study was conducted on the 50 underground mine workers employed in Bharat Cocking Coal Ltd., Dhanbad (Jharkhand). The subjects were convinced to participate in the study and they were not paid for their participation in this study.

Tools

The following questionnaires and tests were administered on participants of the present study :

1. *Eysenck's Personality Questionnaire-R* : This scale is an Indian adaptation of EPQ-R (Eysenck, Eysenck, and Barrett, 1985) by Dr. I. L. Singh. In this scale there are 48 questions of different dimensions of personality *i.e.* psychoticism, extraversion, neuroticism and lie score.

2. *Stress State Questionnaire (Pre task)* : This questionnaire measures stress state as predictor of future performance on simple tasks. In this questionnaire there are 90 items, which has been derived from the existing measures and from other works on stress states. The items for emotional component of the stress states are mainly based on UWIST Mood Adjective Checklist (Matthews, Jones and Chamberlain, 1990). Aston Motivation Scale developed by Matthews has also been used to assess motivational dimension of the stress state. For the assessment of cognitive dimension of stress-state items related to general assessment of style of thinking and belief about the task are also included. For the assessment

of specific intruding thoughts the items have been taken from Savason and Associates' (1986) Cognitive Interference Questionnaire (CIQ), which includes both task-relevant and task-irrelevant interference.

3. *Stress State Questionnaire (Post task)* : This questionnaire measures stress state after performing simple tasks. In this questionnaire there are 96 items, which have been derived from the existing measures and from other works on stress states. The items for emotional component of the stress states are mainly based on UWIST Mood Adjective Checklist (Matthews, Jones and Chamberlain, 1990). Aston Motivation Scale developed by Matthews has also been used to assess motivational dimension of the stress state. For the assessment of cognitive dimension of stress-state items related to general assessment of style of thinking and belief about the task are also included. For the assessment of specific intruding thoughts the items have been taken from Savason and Associates' (1986) Cognitive Interference Questionnaire (CIQ), which includes both task-relevant and task-irrelevant interference.

4. *Digit Span Task* : In this digits were presented to the participants verbally. The number of digits recalled correctly was taken as a performance measure.

5. *Stroop Colour Task* : This task is manipulated version of the task developed by Stroop. In this task we have taken 55 words, *i.e.* name of colours, which were written in different colours. The reaction time was taken as performance measure.

6. *Job Involvement Scale (Singh & Kapoor, 1984)* : This scale consists of 20 items from the following sub areas of job involvement : intrinsic motivation, attachment to work, fulfillment of organizational demand, commitment for work, internalization of organizational goals and organizational identification.

7. *S-D Employees Inventory (Pestonjee, 1973)* : There are 80 items in this inventory from the areas like job, management, personal adjustment and social relation. We have used 40-items from the job and management area. Items of the job area includes nature of work, hours of work, fellow workers, opportunities or the job for promotion and advancement (Prospect) over time regulation, interest in work and physical environment, mechanic and tools etc. and the items of the management include items from supervisory treatment. Participation, rewards and punishment, praise and blame, leave policy, favouritism, etc.

Procedure

In this study first of all the informations about the subjects were collected, *e.g.* name, age, their working conditions etc. Then the self-administering questionnaires like EPQ-R, Stress State Questionnaire (Pre and post task), Job Involvement Questionnaire, and S-D Employees Inventory were given to the subjects and their responses were taken. When the subject completed EPQ-R, the Stress State Questionnaire (Pre task) was given to the subject. Just after the completion of this questionnaire the Digit Span Task was administered on the subject. The researcher read out the number of digits of the task one by one and the subject recalled the digits. The maximum number of digits recalled by the subject was recorded as the performance score on this task. After this task Stroop Colour Task was administered on the subject. In this task there are 55 words such as Red, Blue, Green and Yellow written in different colours, *e. g.* Red is written in blue colour, Blue is written in Green colour etc. The reaction time was taken as performance measure on Stroop Colour Task. When the subject completed these two tasks, Stress State Questionnaire (Post task) was given to the subject immediately. After finishing this questionnaire S.D. Employees Inventory and Job Involvement Questionnaire was given to the subject and the subject gave his responses in these questionnaires himself. The whole process of data collection took approximately 30-60 minutes.

RESULTS AND DISCUSSION

Table 29.1 : Comparison of Pre and Post Task Stress State (Mood State) (N=50)

Mood State		*Mean*	*Std. Deviation*	*t-value*
Energetic Arousal	Pre task	24.2200	3.5530	1.034 ns
	Post task	23.5400	3.0653	
Tense Arousal	Pre task	15.8000	3.6478	1.209 ns
	Post task	16.7600	3.5025	
Hedonic Arousal	Pre task	24.0600	4.5058	.130 ns
	Post task	23.9800	3.0270	
Anger/Frustration	Pre task	9.1000	3.6547	1.569 ns
	Post task	9.8600	2.7256	

Non-significant.

The results of the significance of difference (paired comparison t-test) between mean scores of pre and post task stress state indicate that there is difference between pre and post task stress state on mood state dimension (Table 29.1) but it is not significant difference.

Table 29.2 : Comparison of Pre and Post Task Stress State (Motivation) (N=50)

		Mean	*Std. Deviation*	*t-value*
Motivation	Pre task	51.7600	9.0949	3.766**
	Post task	57.1200	8.3388	

**p< .01.

The research findings further reveal that pre and post mean scores of motivation dimension of stress state significantly differed from each other.

Table 29.3 : Comparison of Pre and Post Task Stress State (Thinking Style) (N=50)

Thinking State		*Mean*	*Std. Deviation*	*t-value*
Self Focused Attention	Pre task	14.6200	3.9222	2.864**
	Post task	16.2800	4.7339	
Self Esteem	Pre task	17.4400	3.8975	2.740**
	Post task	19.1200	3.7178	
Concentration	Pre task	20.5200	4.3857	2.293*
	Post task	19.0000	5.7888	
Control and Confidence	Pre task	14.9600	3.9947	.634
	Post task	14.4800	4.9373	

*p< .05, **p< .01, ns-non-significant.

The findings of significance of difference (paired comparison t-test) between mean scores of pre and post task stress state based on thinking style dimension (Table 29.3) further indicates significant difference between the means of self focused attention, self esteem and concentration in relation to task performance.

Table 29.4 : Comparison of Pre and Post Task Stress State (Thinking Content) (N=50)

Thinking Content		*Mean*	*Std. Deviation*	*t-value*
Task Relevant Interference	Pre task	20.2600	4.8731	1.109
	Post task	21.0600	5.0524	
Task Irrelevant Interference	Pre task	17.5200	3.6097	2.192*
	Post task	16.1800	4.9721	

*p< .05.

There is no significant difference between the means of control and confidence sub dimension of thinking style dimension. The results further indicate significant difference between the mean scores of pre and post task stress state of task irrelevant interference sub-dimension on thinking content dimension of stress state; but it is not significant on the other sub-dimension, *i. e.* task relevant interference (Table 29.4).

Table 29.5 : Comparison of High and Low Level Stress State (Mood State) and in Relation to Task Performance (N= 50)

Mood State	*Task*	*High/Low Categories of Stress*	*Mean*	*Std. Deviation*	*t-value*
Energetic Arousal	Digit Span Task	25	6.5200	.9183	1.380
		25	6.2000	.7071	
	Stroop Colour Task	25	1.5650	.2161	.000
		25	1.5650	.2632	
Tense Arousal	Digit Span Task	25	6.6400	.8602	2.521**
		25	6.0800	.7024	
	Stroop Colour Task	25	1.5003	.2331	1.977*
		25	1.6298	.2300	
Hedonic Arousal	Digit Span Task	28	6.3929	.9165	.314
		22	6.3182	.7162	
	Stroop Colour Task	28	1.6844	.1661	4.813**
		22	1.4132	.2322	
Anger/ Frustration	Digit Span Task	31	6.2258	.7620	1.483
		19	6.5789	.9016	
	Stroop Colour Task	31	1.5876	.2482	.854
		19	1.5282	.2227	

*p< .05, **p< .01.

When the significance of difference (independent sample t-test) was calculated for high and low level of stress state in relation to task performance (Table 29.5), *it* indicated significant differences on tense arousal and hedonic arousal. For energetic arousal and anger frustration sub-dimensions it was found that there were differences but they were not significant.

Table 29.6 : Comparison of High and Low Level Stress State (Motivation) in Relation to Task Performance

(N= 50)

Mood State	*Task*	*High/Low Categories of Stress*	*Mean*	*Std. Deviation*	*t-value*
Motivation	Digit Span Task	28 22	6.2500 6.5000	.8872 .7400	1.062 ns
	Stroop Colour Task	28 22	1.5844 1.5405	.2496 .2265	.643 ns

Non-significant.

Table 29.6 indicates no significant differences for high and low level of stress in relation to task performance in motivation dimension of stress state.

Table 29.7 : Comparison of High and Low Levels of Stress State (Thinking Style) in Relation to Task Performance (N= 50)

Thinking Style	*Task*	*High/Low Categories of Stress*	*Mean*	*Std. Deviation*	*t-value*
Self Focus Attention	Digit Span Task	28 22	6.2143 6.5455	.9567 .5958	1.420
	Stroop Colour Task	28 22	1.5844 1.5404	.2636 .2050	.643
Self Esteem	Digit Span Task	27 23	6.2593 6.4783	.8130 .8454	.932
	Stroop Colour Task	27 23	1.6511 1.4640	.1862 .2565	2.982**
Concentration	Digit Span Task	29 21	6.6207 6.0000	.8200 .7071	2.795**
	Stroop Colour Task	29 21	1.5830 1.5402	.2354 .2459	.623
Control and Confidence	Digit Span Task	31 19	6.9951 6.8276	1.1820 1.1077	1.340
	Stroop Colour Task	31 19	1.2839 1.3070	.3030 .3026	.704

**$p < .01$.

The significance of difference (independent sample t-test) was also calculated for high and low levels of stress state (thinking style dimension) in relation to task performance (Table 29.7). The findings reveal that there is significant difference between the mean scores only on self-esteem and concentration sub-dimension of thinking dimension of stress state.

Table 29.8 : Comparison of High and Low Level Stress State (Thinking Contents) in Relation to Task Performance (N= 50)

Thinking Contents	*Task*	*High/Low Categories of Stress*	*Mean*	*Std. Deviation*	*t-value*
Task Relevant Interference	Digit Span Task	29	6.2143	.9567	1.561 ns
		21	6.5455	.5958	
	Stroop Colour Task	29	1.5844	.2636	.998 ns
		21	1.5404	.2050	
Task Irrelevant	Digit Span Task	31	6.2258	.9205	1.483 ns
		19	6.5789	.6070	
	Stroop Colour	31	1.5636	.2745	.055 ns
		19	1.5674	.1704	

Non-significant.

There were no significant differences between the high and low levels of stress state in relation to task performance on thinking content sub dimension of stress state (Table 29.8).

Table 29.9 : Zero-order Pearson Product-Moment Correlations Between Stress State Job Involvement and Job Satisfaction (N=50)

	Stress State	*Job Involvement*	*Job Satisfaction*
Mood State	Energetic Arousal	.231	.179
	Tense Arousal	.043	–.475**
	Hedonic Arousal	.099	.677**
	Anger Frustration	.044	–.447**
Motivation		.231	.161
Thinking Style	Self Focused Attention	.448**	–.017
	Self Esteem	–.337*	.329*
	Concentration	–.108	.523**
	Control and Confidence	–.088	.420**
Thinking Contents	Task Relevant Interference	.455**	.189
	Task Irrelevant Interference	.222	–.169

*P ≤ 0.05 level (2-tailed).

**P ≤ 0.01 level (2-tailed).

Pearson's product-moment correlation was calculated to study the relationship of stress state with job involvement and job satisfaction (Table 29.9). The results indicate that there is positive correlation between the self focused attention (.448, $p<.01$) sub-dimension of thinking style dimension of stress state and job involvement. There is also positive correlation between the task relevant interference (.455, $p<.01$) sub-dimension of thinking content dimension of stress state and job involvement. There is negative correlation between self-esteem (–.337, $p<.05$) sub-dimension of thinking content dimension of stress state.

In case of job satisfaction and stress state, results of Pearson's product moment correlation reveal that there is positive correlation between hedonic arousal (.677, $p<.01$) sub dimension of mood state dimension of stress state, self-esteem (.329, $p<.05$), concentration (.523, $p<.01$)

and control and confidence (.420,<.01) sub dimensions of thinking style dimension of stress state. The results show negative correlation between the tense arousal (–.475, p<.01) and anger/frustration (–.447, p<.01) sub-dimensions of mood state dimension of stress state.

Table 29.10 : Summary of Results of Correlation Coefficients Between Personality and Task Performance (N=50)

Performance	*Personality dimension*		
	Psychoticism	*Extraversion*	*Neuroticism*
Digit Span Task	–.132	.162	–.489**
Stroop Colour Task	.213	.041	–.135

**p< .01.

The results of coefficient of correlation (Table 29.10) indicated that neuroticism is the only dimension of personality, which moderates the task performance (r=.489, p<.01) on digit span task. There is positive correlation between digit span task performance and neuroticism. The correlation coefficient between task performance on stroop colour task and neuroticism (–.135) is negative but it is not significant. There is negative correlation between reaction time (lower reaction time indicates better performance) and neuroticism.

Table 29.11: Summary of the Results of Stepwise Multiple Regression Analysis with Performance (Digit Span Task) as Criterion Variable (N=50)

Predictors Pre Task Stress State	*Multiple R*	*R Square*	*Adjusted R Square*	*df*	*F-ratio*
Self focused attention	.328	.108	.089	49	5.792*

* P ≤ .02.

The findings of the step-wise multiple regression analysis (Table 29.11) indicates that when digit span task performance was taken as criterion variable and all the dimensions and sub-dimensions of stress state were taken as predictor variables, only self focused sub-dimension of thinking style played significant role in the variance of criterion variable.

Table 29.12: Summary of the Results of Stepwise Multiple Regression Analysis with Performance (Stroop Colour Task) as Criterion Variable (N=50)

Predictors Pre Task Stress State	*Multiple R*	*R Square*	*Adjusted R Square*	*df*	*F-ratio*
Hedonic Arousal	.497	.247	.231	49	15.612*
Motivation	.638	.407	.368	49	10.876*
Concentration	.563	.317	.288	49	10.555*
Control and Confidence	.677	.458	.410	49	9.509*

* P <.01.

The results of the stepwise multiple regression analysis further indicate that when reaction time (Stroop colour task) was considered criterion variable and the stress state was taken as predictor variable, hedonic arousal sub-dimension of mood-state dimension, motivation dimension, concentration and control and confidence sub-dimension of thinking style dimension of stress state play significant role in the prediction of task performance. (Table 29.12)

The findings of the current study reveal that the data collected from the subjects is coherent with the assumptions of the normal probability curve, *i.e.* the scores on the different dimensions of the stress are normally distributed. So we can assume that approximately 50% of the population lies below mean and the other 50% of the population lies above the mean.

The basic objective of the present study was to find out whether there is any difference in level of pre and post task stress state due to the effect of task performance in underground mine workers. The research findings show that there is no significant difference between the mean scores of pre and post task stress state on mood state dimension of stress state. The findings further indicate that mean scores of pre and post task stress state on motivation dimension differ significantly. It indicates that task performance has significant role in level of stress in the underground mine workers. Further, the mean scores of pre and post task stress state based on thinking style dimension indicate significant difference between the means of self focused attention, self esteem and concentration sub-dimensions in relation to task performance. There is no significant difference between the means of control and confidence sub-dimension of thinking style dimension.

The results further indicate significant difference between the mean scores of pre and post task stress state of task irrelevant interference sub-dimension on thinking content dimension of stress state; but it is not significant on the other sub-dimension, *i.e.* task relevant interference. Some other researchers' in their study used two visual, high event rate vigilance tasks; the 'successive' task version required integration of information across trials, but the 'simultaneous' version did not. Both versions were sensitive to individual differences in task performance; consistent with their previous studies energetic arousal emerged as one of the principal components of stress state. Hence, the stress state measure allows the precise description and identification of the stress factors that are most detrimental to specific tasks.

The second objective of the study was to study the effects of high and low level of stress state on task performance and the findings indicated significant differences on tense arousal and hedonic arousal sub dimensions of stress state. For energetic arousal and anger/frustration sub-dimensions it was found that there were differences but they were not significant. The results of significance of differences further indicated no significant differences for high and low levels of stress in relation to task performance in motivation dimension of stress state. The findings further revealed that there was significant difference between the mean scores only on self-esteem and concentration sub-dimension of thinking dimension of stress state. There were no significant differences between the high and low levels of stress state in relation to task performance on thinking content sub-dimension of stress state. Evans, Allen, Taffalla and O'Meara (1996) also studied the interactive effects of multiple stressors on cognitive performance and psychophysiological indices and found negative effect of noise on concurrent and after effect performance.

The next two objectives of the research were to find out the effects of stress state on job involvement and job satisfaction. The findings indicate that there is positive correlation between the self-focused attention sub-dimension of thinking style dimension of stress state and job involvement. There is also positive correlation between the task relevant interference sub-dimension of thinking content dimension of stress state and job involvement. There is negative correlation between self-esteem sub-dimension of thinking content dimension of stress state. In case of job satisfaction there is positive correlation between hedonic arousal sub-dimension of mood state dimension of stress state, self-esteem, concentration and control and confidence sub-dimensions of thinking style dimension of stress. The result shows negative correlation between the tense arousal and anger/frustration sub-dimensions of mood state dimension of stress state.

The next objective of the study was to relate personality as moderator variable of the task induced stress state and its effect on task performance. The findings indicate that neuroticism is the only dimension, which played significant role in the performance of the task.

In this study it was assumed that after completion of the present study, the stress state measures would be studied as the predictors of the performance in different areas such as education, industries, organizations etc. The findings of the step-wise multiple regression analysis indicate that self focused sub-dimension of thinking style play significant role in the prediction of task performance. Motowidlo, Packard and Manning (1988) also suggested that subjective stress generates anxiety, hostility and depression, which, in turn, affect components of job performance such as tolerance for frustration, clerical accuracy, interpersonal sensitivity and altruism.

Thus, in view of the above discussion, it can be concluded that there are explicit differences between pre and post task stress state due to the effect of task performance; not on all but many dimensions and sub dimensions of stress state. It shows that performance also affects the stress state of subjects working in coalmines. There are also significant differences in the performance of the subjects who belong to high and low levels of stress. The correlations of stress state with job involvement and job satisfaction indicate, that job satisfaction is highly correlated with stress state in respect of job involvement. The neuroticism dimension has emerged as the major moderator of stress states in this particular study. It is also concluded that future performance of an individual can be visualized in advance with the administration of stress state questionnaire to a certain extent.

REFERENCES

Barnett, R.C., Gareis, K.C., & Brennan, R.T. (1999). Fit as a moderator of the relationship between work hours and burnout, *Journal of Occupational Health Psychology, 4,* 307-317.

Broota, A. (1993). Stress and schizophrenia, *Journal of Psychological Researches, 37,* 9-15.

Chaudhry, F.N., Latif, A., Anjum, A. & Rashid, T. (2002). *Comparison of Stress, Support and Mental Health of Employees at Five Organizational Levels in Pakistan.* Paper presented at 25th International Conference of Applied Psychology, Singapore.

Chen, P. Y., & Spector, P. E. (1992). Relationships of work stressors with aggression, withdrawal, theft, and substance use : An exploratory study, *Journal of Occupational and Organizational Psychology,* 177-184.

Etzion, D., Eden, D., & Lapidot, Y. (1998). Relief from job stressors and burnout : Reserve service as a respite, *Journal of Applied Psychology, 83,* 577-585.

Evans, G.W., Allen, K.M., Tafall, R. & O'Meara, T. (1996). Multiple stressors : performance, psychophysiological and Affective responses, *Journal of Environmental Psychology, 16,* 147–154.

Kao, Y.T. (2002). *A Study of Taiwanese College Students' Well-being : The Relationships among Depression, Stress, Social Support, Self-esteem, and Self-rated Health Status.* Paper presented at 25th International Conference of Applied Psychology, Singapore.

Kelloway, E.K., Gottlieb, B. H., & Barham, L. (1999). The source, nature, and direction of work and family conflict : A longitudinal investigation, *Journal of Occupational Health Psychology, 4,* 337-346.

Latha, K.S., Bhat, S.M., & D'Souza, P. (1994). Attempted suicide and recent stressful life events : A report from India, *Crisis, 15*, 136.

Lazarus, R. & Folkman, S. (1984). *Stress, Appraisal, and Coping*, New York : Springer Verlag.

Leiter, M. P. & Schaufeli, W. B. (1996). Consistency of the burnout construct across occupations, *Anxiety, Stress and Coping, 9,* 229-243.

Maslach, C. & Schaufeli, W.B. (1993). Historical and conceptual development of burnout. In W.B. Schaufeli, C. Maslach & T. Marek (Eds.), *Professional Burnout : Recent Developments in Theory and Research,* pp. 1-16, Washington, DC : Taylor & Francis.

Mathews, G. (2001). Levels of transaction : A cognitive science framework for operator stress. In P. A. Hancock & P. A. Desmond (Eds.), *Stress, Workload, and Fatigue,* p. 5-33, Mahwah, NJ : Erlbaum.

Mathews, G., Jones, D.M. & Chamberlain, A.G. (1990). Redefining the measurement of mood : The UWIST Mood Adjective Checklist, *British Journal of Psychology, 81,* 17-42.

Motowidlo, S.J., Packard, J.S. & Manning, M.R. (1988). Occupational Stress : Its causes and consequences for job performance, *Journal of Applied Psychology, 71,* 618-629.

Pestonjee, D.M. (1992). *Stress and Coping,* New Delhi : Sage Publications India Ltd.

Robert, A.B. (1986). *Behaviour in Organizations,* Boston : Allyn and Bacon.

Savason, I.G. *et al.* (1986). Cognitive interference : Situational determinants and trait like characteristics, *Journal of Personality and Social Psychology, 51,* 215-226.

Sedikides, C. (1992). Mood as a determinant of attentional focus, *Cognition and Emotion, 6,* 129-148.

Shirom, A. (1989). Burnout in work organizations. In C.L. Cooper and I. Robertson (Eds.), *International Review of Industrial and Organizational Psychology,* New York : Wiley.

Srivastava, A.K. (2002). *Effectiveness of Cognitive Intervention in Stress-management in Relation to Employees' Attributions.* Paper presented at 25th International Conference of Applied Psychology, Singapore.

Zohar, D. (1997). Predicting burnout with a hassle-based measure of role demands, *Journal of Organizational Behaviour, 18,* 101-115.

Weaver, J.L., Morgan, B.B., Adkins-Holmes, C. and Hall, J.K. (1992). A review of potential moderating factors in the stress-performance relationship, *Technical Report 92, Naval Training Systems Center.*

ACKNOWLEDGMENT

The paper is based on the project No. F. 5-116/2000 (HRP) sponsored by U.G.C., New Delhi.

30

Perceived Support for Innovation Among Scientists in Relation to Organizational Climate and Leadership

Shabu B. Raj*, K. Ramachandran** and Hempal Punia***

The quality of intellect that a nation possesses and utilizes determines its position in technology ranking in the international scenario. In this competitive global scenario, to be technologically superior, a nation establishes and looks towards to its R&D institutions to deliver products and services that are superior to its competitors. Researches with the mission to develop cutting edge technologies require conducive environment, or organizational climate that encourages constant innovation (Haefele, 1962). Organizations who are in pursuit of excellence in technology development are assumed to have certain characteristics in terms of leadership, organizational climate, and innovativeness. An innovative organization fosters the creative functioning of its members, and its leadership respects all members' capacity to function creatively.

Leadership effectiveness is a group process involving group support to attain group goals with due consideration for the individuals in the group. Leadership of an organization apart from having certain qualities is able to transform their followers into team members with commitment to action towards the predetermined goals. This 'people orientation' of leadership is concerned with building and sustaining appropriate motivational factors into the system or creating an environment likely to motivate the members towards the achievement of the goals (Davar, 1993). Integrating individual and organizational goals is one such measure. In general, leadership depends upon, *(i)* the leaders' skills, personal philosophy/value system etc, *(ii)* the type of followers (team members), and *(iii)* the situations in which the leadership qualities are exercised. The manner and approach of providing direction, implementing plans,

*Sc 'B', Defence Institute of Psychological Research, Delhi.
**Sc 'E', Defence Institute of Psychological Research, Delhi.
***STA 'B' Defence Institute of Psychological Research, Delhi.

and motivating people are different from one leader to another due to one or more of the above reasons. This leadership variation has been put into different styles based on some aspect of leadership emphasized. Two contrasting styles are defined by emphasis on task to be done (task oriented style), and persons doing the task (people-oriented style). This dichotomy if seen as a continuum has another style : *(i)* high task orientation (telling), *(ii)* leadership through convincing people about what should be done (selling), *(iii)* discussing with them the task and its strategy (consulting), and *(iv)* giving responsibility to them to plan and achieve results, with enough support (delegating). Blake and Mouton's (1964) managerial grid treats task-orientation and people orientation as two independent dimensions with each dimension ranging from low (1) to high (9), giving rise to a combination of five leadership styles; low-low (style 1, 1), high task with low people-orientation (style 9, 1), low task with high people-orientation (style 1, 9), compromise between two orientations (style 5, 5), and high emphasis on both (style 9, 9). In this grid, style 9,9 is suggested as ideal that managers should aspire.

Fielder's contingency theory indicates that the effectiveness of task-orientation and people-orientation depended (was contingent) on the situation. Hersey and Blanchard (1976) combined the grid approach, and contingency theory to propose the situational theory of leadership, and developed an instrument (LEAD- Leadership Effectiveness and Adaptability Description) to identify, *(i)* leadership styles (dominant and secondary styles), *(ii)* style range or flexibility (how easily a leader is capable of using the various four styles), and *(iii)* adaptability or relevance (how appropriately a leader uses the various styles). Another way of looking at leadership style is on the merit of where the power lies; *(i)* authoritarian (also known as autocratic), *(ii)* participative (democratic), and *(iii)* delegative (free-reign). Although most leaders use all three styles, one of them usually becomes the dominant one.

Authoritarian style is used when the leader tells the team members what has to be done, how it has to be done, without getting their advice/ideas/suggestions. This style is autocratic in nature and is appropriate in conditions where the leader has all the information to solve the problem, is in short of time, and the team members are highly motivated. Shouting at subordinates, using threats and abuse of power is not authoritarian leadership style but an abusive and unprofessional way of leadership.

If the leader has time and wants to gain more commitment and motivation from the team members, participative style has been found suitable. This style involves the leader including some of the team members involved in the decision making process (to determine what to do and how to do it), but the leader maintains the final decision making authority. This leadership style is applicable when the leader has some of the information and the other team members have some of the information. This style improves the team spirit and provides room to make better decisions, and is more applicable in government owned research organizations operating within a different set of rules and regulations.

If the team members are able to analyze the situation and determine what needs to be done and how to do it, and the leader has to set priorities and delegate certain tasks, then delegative leadership style is found to be more suitable. Though the leader allows the team members to make decisions, the responsibility of the decisions lies with the leader. Depending on the dynamics of leadership, influenced by followers, leadership skills, and the context in which leadership is exercised, appropriate style(s) has to be used. In spite of the leadership style that may be used, the organization has to welcome, stimulate/encourage innovation to remain technologically excellent (Khandwalla, 1988).

Every organization has a set of characteristics specific to it that can be ascertained in the way, the organization relates to its members and to its environment. Apart from leadership, the organizational structure, systems, culture, and psychological needs of employees interact with one another to create organizational climate. Organizational climate is a psychological state caused by organizational structures, systems, and managerial behaviour, and it directly affects job satisfaction and performance. Organizational climate is developed by the organizational process, and is perceived or felt by the members of the organization. It is reflected in the attitudes and expectancies held by the members toward the organization. Twelve such processes as dimensions of organizational climate (Pareek, 1988) are : *(i)* Orientation, *(ii)* Interpersonal relations, *(iii)* Supervision, *(iv)* Managing problems, *(v)* Managing mistakes, *(vi)* Managing conflicts, *(vii)* Communication, *(viii)* Decision making, *(ix)* Trust, *(x)* Reward management, *(xi)* Risk taking, and *(xii)* Management of change. The organizational climate arouses various motives in varying degrees, and the members in the organization behave in relation to these motives. This psychological climate of an organization is called as motivational climate. The six motives are achievement, affiliation, influence, control, extension, and dependence. The way the dimensions of organizational climate operate in an organization may indicate the underlying motive of the leadership. Thus there is a matrix or a grid with 12 dimensions and 6 motives with the overall score giving a profile of the organizational climate on the six motives.

As the scientists have to be innovative for developing better technologies, the leadership of such institution is supposed to support the initiation and development of new ideas throughout the system, as well as respect all members' capacity to function creatively. Such an organization needs to be a highly effective work group that attaches high value to creative approaches and solutions to its problems. Therefore, an innovative organization continuously experiments with alternative solutions to its problems, and at the same time its members successfully cope with the frustration inherent in dealing with new approaches, problems, or tasks. The members of an organization may perceive the organization as supportive to their attempts and the results as worth taking pains or making efforts. Siegal and Kaemmerer (1978) have identified three factors in perceived support for innovation : *(i)* support for creativity, *(ii)* tolerance of differences, and *(iii)* personal commitment. The leadership style, and the organizational climate as perceived by research scientists involved in technology development may influence their perception as to how supportive are they for being innovative.

The present study tries to study the nature of relationship between support for innovation, leadership styles (authoritarian, democratic, and delegative), and motivational climates (achievement, affiliation, influence, control, extension, and dependence).

METHOD

Design

A single group correlational study was conducted.

Sample

Total of 35 research scientists were selected to conduct the study from defence institutes. An incidental sampling technique was used.

Tools

(1) Siegal scale of support for innovation (Siegel & Kaemmerer, 1978). This scale consists of three factors, *(i)* support for creativity, *(ii)* tolerance of differences, and *(iii)* personal commitment, which were identified by Siegel & Kaemmerer through factor analysis.

(2) Organizational Climate: MAO-C (Pareek, 1989). This scale consists of six motives; achievement, expert power, extension, control, dependency, and affiliation.

(3) Leadership style survey (Donclark, 2002). This scale has three leadership styles namely, autocratic/authoritarian, participative/democratic, and free-reign/delegative.

(4) Leadership effectiveness scale (Raj, Ramachandran, and Punia, 2004). This five-point scale rates the leadership effectiveness of an individual as perceived by his/her subordinate.

Procedure

The Ss were selected from various Research Institutes of Defence. Assuring confidentiality these subjects were given the questionnaires individually. After getting the filled tools back, the scoring was done as given in the manuals and obtained scores were put to analyses. The scores obtained on the various questionnaires were analysed by using Pearson's Product method of correlation.

RESULTS AND DISCUSSION

Table 30.1 indicates that there is *(i)* significant correlation between achievement motive and extension motive ($p<0.01$, $n=35$), *(ii)* significant negative correlation between achievement motive and control motive ($p<0.01$, $n=35$), *(iii)* significant negative correlation between achievement motive and dependency motive ($p<0.05$, $n=35$), *(iv)* significant correlation between delegative/free-reign leadership style and participative/democratic leadership style ($p<0.01$, $n=35$), *(v)* significant negative correlation between expert influence motive and control motive ($p<0.05$, $n=35$), *(vi)* significant negative correlation between expert influence motive and affiliation motive ($p<0.01$, $n=35$), *(vii)* significant negative correlation between extension motive and control motive ($p<0.01$, $n=35$), and *(viii)* significant negative correlation between extension motive and dependency motive ($p<0.01$, $n=35$).

Achievement motivational climate (Pareek, 1989) is characterized by a concern for excellence, competition in terms of the standards set by others or by oneself, the setting of challenging goals by oneself, awareness of the obstacles that might be encountered in attempting to achieve these goals, and persistence in trying alternative paths to one's goals. Extension motive is characterized by concern for others, interest in super ordinate goals, and an urge to be relevant and useful to large groups, including society. Table 30.1 shows that there is significant correlation between achievement motive and extension motive ($p<0.01$, $n=35$). This implies that the scientists are working on challenging tasks and they devote equal attention to the social relevance of these tasks. The organization in which they perform has a highly developed sense of social responsibility as well as strong sense of its responsibility to fulfill the scientists' needs.

Organizational climates dominated by achievement, expert power, and extension motives are conducive to the achievement of goals, whereas climates dominated by control, dependency, and affiliation motives retard the achievement of goals. Control motive is characterized by a

Table 30.1 : Karl Pearson Coefficient of Correlation Between Scores of Support for Innovation, Six Motivational Climates, Three Leadership Styles, and Leadership Effectiveness

	Achievement Motive	*Support for Innovation*	*Authoritarian/ Authocratic Style*	*Delegative/ Free-regin Style*	*Participative/ Democratic Style*	*Leadership Effective-ness*	*Expert Influence Motive*	*Extension Motive*	*Control Motive*	*Dependency Motive*
Achievement	1.000									
Support for innovation	.106									
Authoritarian/ autocratic	.071	.231								
Delegative/ free-reign	–.020	.224	.325							
Participative/ democratic	–.176	.321	.126	.757**						
Leadership effectiveness	.207	.201	–.223	.309	.330					
Expert influence	.104	.208	.035	–.061	–.112	–.043				
Extension	.481**	.104	.088	–.022	–.227	.285	.058			
Control	–.729**	–.183	–.129	–.062	.149	–.254	–.340*	–.760**		
Dependency	–.403*	–.279	–.016	.051	.210	–.278	–.068	–.475**	.234	
Affiliation	.004	.076	.033	.212	.081	.133	–.513**	.088	–.141	–.163

*P ≤ 0.05 (2 tailed).

**P ≤ 0.01 (2 tailed).

concern for orderliness, a desire to be and stay informed, an urge to monitor events and to take corrective action when needed, and a need to display personal power. Table 30.1 shows that there is significant negative correlation between achievement motive and control motive ($p<0.01$, $n=35$). It implies that the organizational climate characterized by control motive may not be conducive for attaining innovative achievements in science and technology.

Dependency motive is characterized by a desire for the assistance of others in developing oneself. A need to check with significant others (those who are more knowledgeable or have higher status, experts, close associates, and so on), a tendency to submit ideas or proposals for approval, and an urge to maintain a relationship based on the other person's approval (Pareek, 1988). Result table shows that achievement motive and dependency motive are negatively correlated ($p<0.05$, $n=35$). This shows that the scientists set standards as well challenging goals by themselves, and instead of seeking approval and assistance from others, persist in trying to achieve these goals independently, and use their own innovativeness.

Expert influence motive is characterized by a concern for making an impact on others, a desire to make people do what one thinks is right, and an urge to change situations and develop people. Results indicate a significant negative correlation between expert influence and control motives ($p<0.05$, $n=35$). High value on specialization of knowledge, influence of specialists in decisions, and emphasis of unique contributions may be difficult in a bureaucratic set up where procedures are rigid. Research organizations need to have flexible procedures and should give priority to experts' opinion during decision-making.

Results Table also shows significant negative correlation between expert influence motive and affiliation motive ($p<0.01$, $n=35$). A concern for establishing and maintaining close, personal relationships, an emphasis on friendship, and a tendency to express one's emotions are characteristics of affiliation motive. Research scientists are specialists in their knowledge domain, and work in an interdependence mode, than in an affiliation-motivated manner, for the achievement of research goals. Since the results indicate clearly the nature of government research and development set up, teamwork is emphasized for the attainment of common goals. Here, unless good interpersonal relations (an aspect of affiliation) are there, it will be difficult to attain the set goals in time.

There exists significant negative correlation between extension motive and control motive ($p<0.01$, $n=35$) as shown in Table 30.1, which implies that concern for others, and urge for the research activity to be socially relevant, may be difficult in an organizational climate having control motive where events are monitored to take corrective action and to display personal power is prevalent.

A desire for the assistance of others in developing oneself, depending too much on approval, and maintenance of relationship based on other person's approval, is evident in dependency motive. This is very much different from independence as well as interdependence. The extension motive has social relevance as its main characteristic. There is significant negative correlation ($p<0.01$, $n=35$) between extension motive and dependency motive. Extension motive is conducive for achievement of results whereas dependency motive retards the achievement in research and development organizations. The above finding of significant negative correlation supports that the two opposite motives don't exist together.

There exists a significant correlation ($p<0.01$, $n=35$) between delegative/free-reign leadership style and participative/democratic leadership style. Leaders, who want their team members to grow, use a participative style of leadership. As they 'grow' into their jobs, they are given more authority (delegative) over their jobs (Donclark, 2002). The degree of free-reign and integration (participative style aspect) need balance in an ideal research organization. The research scientists deserve freedom and flexibility provided by a free-reign style and the 'we' feeling provided by a participative leadership style.

As it is evident from Table 30.1 that the leadership styles, leadership effectiveness, and the motivational climates were not significantly correlated to perceived support for innovation among the scientists. The inherent limitations of the present study like small sample size may have contributed to the insignificant correlations. These findings may be due to the particular nature of organizational climate prevalent in firms involved in scientific research and technology development. Research organizations can encourage achievement, extension, and expert influence motives for providing a better organizational climate. Autonomy as well as participation in leadership, in a balanced manner, is beneficial for innovation and for producing research output of good quality, in these organizations. The correlates, and determinants of perceived support for innovation need to be identified in a broader study involving more variables related to support as well as motivational organizational climate, and leadership.

From the present findings, it can be concluded that the scientists in research and development organizations have high achievement motive and extension motive, which helps them in pursuing their goals. When the control and dependency motives operate in an R & D organization, it will retard the achievement of goals in time. Therefore, in order to facilitate the scientists to be innovative, control and dependency has to be limited. An R&D organization having a pleasant working climate with delegative-cum-participative/democratic style of leadership encourages the scientists to be innovative and self contented in achieving their goals.

REFERENCES

Blake, R.R., & Mouton, J.S. (1964). *The Managerial Grid*, Houston : Texas.

Davar, R.S. (1993). *Creative Leadership : The People-Oriented Task Approach*, New Delhi : UBS.

Donclark (2002). Leadership Style Survey. http://www.nwlink.com/~donclark/leader/survstyl.html

Haefele, J.W. (1962). *Creativity and Innovation*, New York : Reinhold.

Hersey, P. & Blanchard, K.H. (1976) : *The Annual Handbook For Group Facilitators*, California : University Associates Inc.

Khandwalla, P.N. (1988). *Fourth Eye : Excellence Through Creativity*, New Delhi : Wheeler.

Pareek, U. (1988). *Organizational Behaviour Processes*, Jaipur : Rawat.

Pareek, U. (1989). Motivational Analysis of Organisations climate (MAO-C). In J.W. Pfeiffer (Ed.), The 1989 *Annual Developing Human Resources*, California : University Associates.

Raj, S.B., Ramachandran, K., & Punia, H. (2004). *Leadership Effectiveness Scale*, Unpublished. Delhi : Defence Institute of Psychological Research.

Siegel, S. M. & Kaemmerer, W. F. (1978). Measuring Perceived Support for Innovation in Organizations, *Journal of Applied Psychology*, *63*, 553-562.

31

Positive Work Climate Dimensions and Hardiness in Private Sector Organizations

Sudeepa Bose & Manisha Agrawal**

Individuals react differently under stressful and changing environmental conditions. Kobasa (1979) proposed that hardiness is a constellation of personality dispositions that function as a resistance source in the encounter with stressful life events. These personality dispositions are commitment, control and challenge. The commitment disposition is expressed as a tendency to involve oneself in whatever one is doing or encounters (as opposed to alienation). Thus, committed persons have a generalized sense of purpose that allows them to identify with and find meaningful the events, things and persons in their environment. They invest enough in themselves and in their relationships so that they do not easily give up under pressure.

The control disposition is expressed as a tendency to feel and act as if one is influential in the face of contingencies (as opposed to alienation). Thus, committed persons have a generalized sense of purpose that allows them to identify with and find meaningful the events, things and persons in their environment. They invest enough in themselves and in their relationships so that they do not easily give up under pressure.

The control disposition is expressed as a tendency to feel and act as if one is influential in the face of contingencies (as opposed to helplessness) of life. This implies the perception of oneself as having a definite influence through the exercise of imagination, knowledge, skill and choice. Control enhances stress resistance perpetually by increasing the likelihood that events will be experienced as natural outgrowth of one's actions and therefore, not as foreign, unexpected and overwhelming experiences.

The challenge disposition is expressed as the belief that change rather than stability is normal life and that the anticipation of changes are interesting incentives to growth rather than threats to security.

Kobassa and Puccetti (1983) have suggested that the personality characteristic 'hardiness'—a combination of commitment, control, and challenge—decreases or buffers the

*Department of Psychology, B.H.U., Varanasi.

illness—related effects of stressful life events. Hardy individuals suffer from fewer illnesses because they are able to transform stressful life events cognitively to make them less stressful.

Hardiness is known as stress-resistance-enhancing agent of personality. Kobasa (1979) reported that highly stressed subjects who experienced little illness also reported feeling more committed, internally controlled, and challenged than did highly stressed subjects with high illness levels. Hall, Treuren and Virnelli (1987) have suggested that individual differences in the personality variable of hardiness are related to health and illness.

Researches relating these dispositions with work climate dimensions indicate that regarding participation in decision-making, employees have reported more satisfaction, more interpersonal trust, less role tension, and more organizational commitment when the discrepancies between desired and actual participation were low (Alutto & Acito, 1974). In addition, subordinates who successfully negotiated high-quality relationships with their supervisors were likely to perceive their organization as providing greater autonomy, decision-making latitude, and supportiveness. Scott and Bruce (1994) have reported that an innovation-supportive climate affects individual innovative behaviour. They reported that subordinates who had relationships with their supervisors characterized by high levels of support, trust and autonomy also reported the organization to be supportive of innovation and judged the resource supply to be high. In addition, an innovation-supportive climate accompanied by a participative decision-making process can be further expected to foster interpersonal trust among members of work groups. Trust refers to a mutual understanding between the management and employee. According to Porter, Lawlwer and Hackman (1975) where there is trust there is the feeling that others will not take advantage of me. Trust is likely to have an important influence on the willingness of participants to encourage risky behaviours, such as proposing creative alternatives in a decision-making group.

The present study focuses on examining those dimensions of the work climate in the organization that may be related to the three dispositions of hardy personality among the employees. Modern organizations function in uncertain environments while facing the challenges of competitiveness. These changes take place in the external and internal environment of the individual. It is argued that certain positive dimensions of the work climate in the organizations such as innovative climate, interpersonal trust and participation in decision-making processes can assist the individual in developing the characteristics of a 'hardy' personality. Member's participation in the decision-making process, the level of interpersonal trust between them and their innovative climate can be hypothesized to develop the components of hardiness.

It was hypothesized that : Participative climate would be positively related with hardy personality of the employees, innovative climate will be positively related with hardy personality of the employees. Interpersonal trust for boss, subordinate and colleague will be positively related with hardy personality.

METHOD

Sample

The sample for the study consisted of 100 managerial and supervisory personnel belonging to two manufacturing organizations, of the private sector.

Tools

Measures consisted of four scales, which were related to (1) hardy personality, (2) climate for innovation, (3) participation in decision-making, and (4) interpersonal trust.

The hardy personality scale was developed by Kobasa (1979). This scale consisted of 50 items that measured three components of hardy personality, that is challenge, commitment and control, 17 items measured the element of challenge and control and 16 items measures the element of commitment. The respondent indicated their responses on a four point scale ranging from "not at all true" (0) to "completely true" (3). The reliability coefficient of the scale was. 85.

Among the antecedent variables, innovative *climate* was measured by a scale consisting of 16 items which were to be rated on a five point scales which were adapted from the 'climate for innovation' scale developed by Scott and Bruce (1994). Factor analysis of the scale by means of principal components method with varimax rotations revealed four factors in perceived climate for innovation namely, System support (24.71% Variance), Rigidity (19.80% variance), Encouragement to creativity (7.57% variance), and Conformity (6.67% variance).

Participation in decision-making was measured by 10 items adapted from the scale developed by Agarwal and Agarwal (1994). The reliability coefficient of the scale was .75. Factor analysis by the principal components method with varimax rotations yielded three factors, namely decision-making (21.51% variance), Work related problems (19.34% variance), and Member welfare (19.07% variance). Responses of the participants were measured on five point scales, ranging from (5) 'very great extent' to (1) 'not at all'.

Following McAllister (1995), affect-based and cognition-based interpersonal trust was measured at three levels, that is, at the supervisory, peer and subordinate levels. The scale contained 11 items which measured participants' trust for a boss, a colleague and a subordinate. The reliability of the scale was. 85.

Table 31.1 : Mean Scores and SD on Personality and Positive Work Climate

Variables	*Dimensions*	*Mean*	*SD*
Hardy personality	Challenge	18.59	5.65
	Commitment	17.92	5.90
	Control	21.69	5.49
Positive work climate trust	Subordinate	37.10	7.06
	Boss	38.12	7.62
	Colleague	40.13	6.18
Innovative climate	System support	16.88	3.89
	Rigidity	13.54	3.12
	Creativity	6.84	1.59
	Conformity	14.35	2.609
Participative climate	Decision making	14.02	2.66
	Work related problem	11.41	1.98
	Member welfare	9.75	2.32

Procedure

The study was conducted on the premises of the organizations understudy. The HRM Department in each organization were approached for its cooperation in data collection.

RESULTS AND DISCUSSION

Data were analyzed for measuring the effect of positive work climate dimensions, namely, participation in decision-making processes, factors of innovative climate and interpersonal trust on the perception of hardy personality. The hypothesized relationships between the work climate and hardy personality were analyzed through coorelation analysis and step-wise regression analysis.

Table 31.2 : Correlation Coefficient Analysis of Positive Work Climate Variables with Challenge, Commitment and Control

Variables	*Hardy Personality Dimensions*	*Challenge*	*Commitment*	*Control*
Trust	Subordinate	–.04	–.08	.04
	Boss	–.28**	–.18	–.27**
	Colleague	–.13	–.05	–.06
Innovative climate	System support	–.35**	–.31**	–.41
	Rigidity	–.21*	–.25**	–.22**
	Creativity	–.21*	–.10	–.10
	Conformity	–.20*	–.28**	–.20*
Participative climate	Decision making	–.22*	–.07	–.10
	Work related problems	.04	.15	.09
	Member welfare	.09	.15	.12

*>.05, **>.01.

Table 31.3 : Stepwise Regression Analysis of Positive Work Climate with Challenge of Hardy Personality (N=100)

Independent Variables	*R*	*Rsq.*	*Rsq. Change*	*% Variance*	*Beta Coefficients*	*t*
System support	.35	.12	.12	12	–.34	3.37**
Work-related problems	.39	.15	.03	3	.35	2.98**
Boss	.46	.15	.06	6	–.29	2.71**

*>.05, **>.01.

Table 31.4 : Stepwise Regression Analysis of Positive Work Climate with Commitment (N=100)

Independent Variables	*R*	*Rsq.*	*Rsq. Change*	*% Variance*	*Beta Coefficients*	*t*
System support	.31	.09	.09	9	–.29	2.84**
Work-related problems	.43	.18	.08	8	.19	1.69
Boss	.47	.22	.03	3	–.31	2.95**
Conformity	.54	.29	.04	4	–.35	3.21**
Subordinate	.58	.33	.04	4	.45	3.29**

*>.05, **>.01.

Table 31.5 : Stepwise Regression Analysis of Positive Work Climate with Control of Hardy Personality (N=100)

Independent Variables	*R*	*Rsq.*	*Rsq. Change*	*% Variance*	*Beta Coefficients*	*t*
System support	.41	.16	.16	16	–.51	5.20**
Work-related problems	.49	.24	.07	7	.34	3.44**
Boss	.54	.29	.05	5	–.41	3.63**
Colleague	.58	.33	.04	4	.29	2.48**

*>.05, **>.01.

Table 31.1 shows means and correlations between the all variables. Table 31.2 shows correlation chart of all the variables and Table 31.3, 31.4, 31.5 show stepwise regression analysis of the effects of work climate dimensions on the hardy personality.

Analysis revealed that among the interpersonal trust dimensions, mean score of trust for colleague was higher than the mean score of trust for boss and subordinate. Correlation analysis showed that interpersonal trust for the boss was negatively correlated with challenge and control but interpersonal trust for subordinate and colleague were not significantly correlated with the challenge commitment and control. In the stepwise regression analysis, trust for boss emerged as a significantly negative predictor of challenge, commitment and control but trust for the subordinate was a positive predictor of commitment and trust for the colleague was a significantly positive predictor of control. Earlier, Rempel, Holmes, and Zanna (1985) have proposed three components of interpersonal trust that is predictability, dependability and faith. It can be suggested here that in organizations where employees can trust their subordinates and can depend upon them to perform their functions in a reliable manner, they are likely to feel that the organization has fulfilled its promises to them and hence can cope better with stress in the organization.

Among the factors of participation in decision-making process, decision-making processes showed high mean score and member welfare activities showed lower mean score. Correlation analysis showed that the among the participative climate only decision-making process was negatively correlated with challenge, other factors of participation in decision-making process were not significantly correlated with components of hardy personality. In the stepwise regression analysis, work related problems of participative climate emerged as positively significant predictor of challenge and control. These findings indicate that when employees face problems related to their work then their stress level will be increased and due to this stress, hardiness will increase. Thus factor of hardiness enables the persons to face the changing situation of the organization.

Among the four factors of innovative climate, system support and creativity were positive dimensions of climate for innovation and rigidity and conformity were negative dimensions of climate for innovation. System support had a high mean score and creativity had a low mean score. Correlation analysis showed that system support, rigidity and conformity were negatively correlated with challenge, commitment and control but creativity was negatively correlated with challenge. In the stepwise regression analysis, system support of innovative climate emerged as negatively significant predictor of challenge, commitment and control. These findings indicate that when employees get system support by the organization then their stress level will decrease and hardiness will also decrease. Conformity emerged as negatively significant predictor of commitment. These findings indicate that, if employees get opportunities for creative work and these creative work were supported by the organization then they perform better and then they do not require the hardiness needed for coping with stress in the organization. These findings show that support for innovation and resource supply are functions of the organizational system, which can strengthen innovative behaviour (Scott & Bruce, 1994).

On the basis of present findings it can be suggested that organizational support is most effective in preserving health when hardiness is high because hardiness influences the extent of and manner in which organizational support is being utilized in the management of stressful events. When confronted with such events, hardy persons may seek out contact with others and with social institutions that could decrease the stressfulness of the events.

REFERENCES

Alutto, J.A. & Acito, F. (1974). Decisional participation and sources of job satisfaction : A study of manufacturing personnel, *Academy of Management Journal, 17,* 160-167.

Hull, J.G.; Van Treuren, R.R. & Virneli, S. (1987). Hardiness and health : A critique and alternative approach, *Journal of Personality and Social Psychology, 53,* 518-530.

Kobasa, S.C. (1979). Stressful life events, personality, and health : An inquiry into hardiness, *Journal of Personality and Social Psychology, 37,* 1-11.

Kobasa, S.C., & Pucetti, M.C. (1983). Personality and social resources in stress resistance, *Journal of Personality and Social Psychology, 45,* 839-850.

Porter, L.W., Lawler, E.E. & Hackman, J.R. (1975). Behaviour in organizations, New York : McGraw-Hill.

Rempel, J.K., Homes, J.G. & Zanna, M.P. (1985). Trust in close relationships, *Journal of Personality and Social Psychology, 49,* 95-112.

Scott, S.G. & Bruce, R.A. (1994). Determinants of innovative behaviour : A path model of individual innovation in the workplace, *Academy of Management Journal, 32,* 580-607.

32

Perception of Work, Stress and Coping Among Street Children

Veena Tucker & Poonam Phogat***

"Street children" are those who work and live on the street day and night. Many of them do not have contact with their families and almost all of them use many kinds of drugs. The Street children sleep, play, eat, dress and treat themselves when they are sick. Many of them practice illegal activities such as stealing, gambling etc. (Ferrari, 2003). The needs of street children differ from other community children, as in addition to the usual socio-economic and health problems, they also have to deal with lack of emotional support, insecurity, exploitation and working in unhygienic conditions. Such unhealthy and hazardous environment adversely affect their physical and mental health. Street children are exploited, if they are not handled with care, they can drift into anti-social activities, such as pick pocketing, stealing, smuggling, drug-peddling, gambling etc. Street children come into the world of adults unprepared, with an unrealistic view of life. The community in which the child grows up is a significant influence on his or her development as emphasized in the ecological model of human development. Socialization involves bi-directional interactions between the child and significant others like family, peer, school and community (Berns, 2004). Psychosocial stress may adversely influence individual's psychological growth. Stressful life events are determined by psychological characteristics of the individual and the situations in the environment. For many street children negative psychological characteristics may lead to psychopathology and improper psychological growth in the absence of supportive psychosocial mediators and ineffective coping defenses.

Various stress models describe how street children face deprivations, which are further compounded by poverty and economic constraints. Some of these deprivations are : Diminished social support for children within the family and community; decreased opportunities for socialization; lack of opportunities to consolidate one's self-worth in broader societal sphere;

*Sr. Reader, Gargi College, Delhi.
**Ph.D Scholar, Department of Psychology, University of Delhi.

experience of marginalization and uncertainty of future and poorly planned urban environment.

Various life stressors that street children face in different countries have been examined (Greenblatt & Robertson,1993; Janus *et al.*, 1987 and Rothman & Davis,1985). The most common stressor found in the lives of street children were the lack of proper homes and education, unemployment among parents, violence and hunger. Home rearing patterns can influence children to runaway from home. Highly positive relationship was found between home rearing patterns and the children found on the street. There was equally positive but low relationships between the level of family income and children running away from home (Matchinda, 1999). Ennett, Bailey and Federman (1999) found that the youth without a social network were significantly more likely to report illicit drug use, multiple sex partners and survival sex than youth with a supportive social network indicating that network characteristics were associated in both positive and negative directions with risky behaviours.

Street children cope with their problems either by cognitive restructuring of their circumstances, adopting practical solutions to their problems and by maladaptive approach of avoidance. Street children live with few protective or mediating supports, and many risk factors, facing psychosocial trauma which generates profound problems in personality development (Le-Roux, 1996). Street children describe a broad spectrum of home and work experiences that had led to their living on the streets.They made significant use of various resources found within their social network of peers local communities and NGOs (Baker *et al.*, 1997; Hagan & McCarthy, 1997; Whitebeck & Hoyt, 1999)

Further it is found that among these children, the typical adaptation techniques such as time orientation, self concept, success-failure orientation, reinforcement system, sense of control over environment and coping strategies generally become adversely affected by the conditions of poverty. More professional intervention strategies would help these children learn positive coping skills.

Poverty and Street Children : Poverty exerts an impact by increasing a child's vulnerability to cumulative risk of health hazards. The health hazards on the child also impede the development of cognition and learning. Street children have low levels of education and come from families with five or more siblings. Parents of street children commonly had low education and were mainly found in unskilled occupations, were in contract polygamous marriages, which are also often characterized by marital disruption. Street children also left home because of parental/familial reasons. (Adernito, 2000; Clatts & Davis; 1999; Mustafa & Sharma, 1996; Sampa, 1998 and Segal & Ashtekar, 1999).

Perception of Work : Poverty forces all the street children to work and earn. It becomes an activity that is a must for daily survival. Many of these children were forced earlier to work by their families because of poverty. The concept of work is a social and cultural construction. The expression "child worker" puts together two categories of a different type : the first belonging to a generational and cultural and the second to an economical and social one. The concept of work is a social and cultural construction. There are four main components of work : game, means of subsistence, relationing identity. Work also has a double function of subsisting and socialization (Invernizzi, 2001).

The ideal picture of work and childhood do influence the way the child builds his perception and definition of subsistence activities (Myers, 1989). Also, the studies concerned with the children's point of view are also of the fact that the ideal work as a waged and steady worker is out of reach (Tellez & Abramo, 1985). They do not fully understand the ideal model of work and/or rather tend to redefine it from their own experience. They sometimes tend to valorize the work they are doing for some reason still to be determined. The link between a child and his survival activity comprises three dimensions. The material or socio-economic one deals with material subsistence. The socio-cultural one refers to the child's links with other individuals (customer, employer, other children, policeman etc). At last the identity dimension regards the link built by the child with himself through his work. Through his work the child is looking for a positive personal recognition and self-valuation. Working gives the child a feeling of belonging since it enables him to be recognized as an active member of a family group or any other group. (Tellez & Abramo, 1985)

Health of Street Children : There is an adverse effect of child labour on the health of the child. Hazardous working conditions and impoverished unhealthy environment and starvation are associated with ill heath among street children. Health problems of street children ranged from common health problems like fever, cold eye/ear infections occurring very often. The serious health problems were stomachache, general weakness, animal bites TB and Sexually Transmitted Diseases (Baker, Panter-Brick & Todd, 1997; Butterflies, 2004; Tucker *et al.*, 2001 & UNICEF, 2004)

Coping in Street Children : Street children being 'at risk' face more challenges in their lives. Lack of vocational skills and low social competence make them face hazards and harassment from employers, police and public. WHO (1999) studied of the lives of street children relating to programmes on substance abuse, in seven developing countries and one developed country. Children reported that 'taking to the street is a way of searching for identity, earning a living out of it, and contributing to the family's income. Further most children felt that 'with positive support of the street educators and other elders in the family/community coping with the present stressful situation would become less problematic'. Some of the coping strategies and skills found in street children were prosocial example supporting each other emotionally and materially, playing sports, dancing, performing music, joining a gang for support and protection, being able to fight etc., attending groups, drop-in shelter, clinics run for street children. While others demonstrate skills and strategies utilized within anti-social activities such as drug use, cheating, begging, and commercial/survival sex etc. However, the skills themselves and the planning capacities used in the antisocial activities may be transformed to pro-social activities with proper-interventions and skill training.

The objective of the present study was to explore the lives of street children referring to their perception of work. Further various problems and fears faced by the street children were also assessed. How these children coped with these stresses was also analyzed. The present study used the participatory methods for exploring the lives of the street children. Thus, the purpose of this action research was to take into account the multi-dimensional view of street children where their work was related to their family, education, health and overall psychosocial development.

METHOD

Design

The objective of the present study was to study the perception of work, stress and coping among street children. This action research focused on understanding and analyzing their feelings, thoughts about living and working on the streets, their problems, fears and anxieties and how they cope with this.

Method

The lives of the street children were investigated with the participatory methods.

The various phases in the Participatory Action Research are as follows :

1. Understand and analyze the street children through participatory methods initiated by listening and auto diagnosis.
2. Identification and prioritization of problems—the concept of stress as viewed by the street educators and psychological theories has to be dropped to facilitate learning from the experiences of the street children. Their feeling, memories and coping mechanisms have reflected what is social reality for them. Their illusions and reality may be adaptive from the adult's viewpoint. However, probing into their reality without any assumptions and theories has lead to better understanding. Thus concrete action for helping the street children emerged from this process of understanding of the lives of street children through auto-diagnosis and other PRA methods.
3. In the final phase, street children reflected and analyzed their lives. This would help them in planning, taking action and developing new skills or building on their existing skills and knowledge and increasing their confidence. This process of empowerment may lead to potential change with the help of facilitator.

As the present study is a PAR paradigm, the variables and hypotheses were not explicitly stated.

Sample

The study being a participatory action research, PAR, with both cross-sectional and longitudinal approach. For understanding and analyzing the lives and social reality of street children, a few children were interacted for a longer period of time. The total sample constituted of thirty (n=30) male street children working in and around New Delhi Railway Station. These children were in the age range of 8-18 yrs with mean age of 13.1 and SD of 2.04 working as shoe-shine boys, rag-pickers, tea stall workers, porters etc. earning on an average Rs. 25-40 per day. The sample was purposive and incidental. The sample was constituted of young children (8-12 yrs, n_1= 11, Mean-10 yrs 9 months, SD-1.1) with short duration on the street (0-3 yrs) and older children (13-18 yrs, n_2= 19, Mean-14 yrs 3 months, SD- 1.23) with long duration on the street (above 3 yrs), who were studied through PRA. Most of the children studied were assisted by the NGOs.

Methods Used

Participatory methods like PRA methods of daily activity, problem ranking, focus group discussion, in-depth interviews, case studies, and observation were used. These PRA methods can only be used once the facilitator listens and builds a trust among street children. Use of participatory methods along with case studies elicited qualitative information that helped in understanding and analyzing street children's lives in their social context. Children's emotions, experiences, decisions and needs/wishes were revealed through interaction with them and these collectively described every street child as a unique individual.

Procedure

The procedure began with the selection of site and the NGOs working with street children in those areas. It was found that the NGO Salaam Balak Trust has a drop-in shelter for children at the New Delhi Railway Station. The NGOs were the primary source for contacting the street children for the present study. The investigator started visiting these contact places for familiarization and rapport formation with the street children. In the initial phase of the research observation method was used for studying the lives of street children. Investigator was trained to observe the children regarding their interpersonal interaction, their communication, daily activities *etc.* Detailed day-to-day dairy was maintained wherein the information was recorded. After the investigator felt that the street children had accepted her, the next phase of research was started. In this phase, the various methods as mentioned in the design were used for various objectives.

RESULTS AND DISCUSSION

The results for the various objectives are described below :

Demographic Profile of Street Children

The age of the sample *i.e.* the street children ranged from 8-18 years. Majority (61%) of them were school dropouts who had not gone beyond the primary level. Majority of the children were Hindu (60%) and a few Muslims (40%) and most of them belonged to neighbouring states like Uttar Pradesh (UP), Bihar etc. The average family size was five members. Besides the demographic and socio-economic information of the family (*e.g.* profession and financial status of the parents/family, structure of family number of siblings, education facilities), child's relation with the family members (*e.g.* parental behaviour, sibling relations), child's relation with peers and reasons for leaving home were also assessed through the detailed interviews with the street children.

Analysis of this information pertained to finding the causes for leaving home. Various reasons for leaving home were elicited by the street children. Maltreatment, physical abuse/neglect/rejection by the extended family or stepparent were found to be the most pervasive reason followed by poverty. However most street children faced multiple stresses that compelled them to runaway or leave homes. For example, physical abuse/rejection often combined with poverty and as well as facing the trauma of death of a parent, forced work, ill treatment by step parent etc. In most street children cases the causes of leaving is complex stressful situation marked by poverty, large family & trauma of some kind (losing a family member). Specifically in young children the cause of leaving is ill treatment & neglect by parents/stepparent/family members which is rebelled against by the child. Many of these children were the eldest or youngest or belonged to a family of many daughters with only son.

Table 32.1 : Reasons for Leaving and Frequencies for a Sample of N= 30, Street Children

S.No.	*Reasons for Leaving*	*Frequency (Percentage)*
1.	Physical Abuse	13 (45.23%)
2.	Poverty	9 (28.57%)
3.	Illness/injury/death of parent	4 (11.90%)
4.	Ill-treatment by step-parent	3 (9.23%)
5.	Forced work	7 (23.80%)
6.	Family conflicts	2 (4.76%)
7.	Peer pressure/family influence (for *e.g.* brothers, father etc.)	1 (2.38%)
8.	Discontinuation of education	2 (4.76%)
9.	Lost from home	1 (2.38%)
10.	Others (for *e.g.* no interest in studies, fight at school, delinquent etc)	4 (9.23%)

Assessment of Wishes/Desires of Street Children

The Table 32.2 shows the various wishes/desires elicited by the street children. The results indicate that most of the children, *i.e.* 76.67% wished for happiness and protected with their family & loved ones. They also wished for the welfare of their siblings. 60% of the children wished for basic needs like clothes, food and shelter to be met.

Table 32.2 : Wishes/needs of Street Children and Related Frequencies, N=30

S.No.	*Wishes / Needs*	*Frequency*	*Percentage*
1.	Basic security & fulfilling basic needs	18	60%
2.	Buying things to fulfill desire	4	13.33%
3.	Emotional needs (Being with family)	23	76.67%
4.	Education/Vocational Needs	13	43.33%
5.	Health Related Well Being Needs	8	26.67%
6.	Higher Aspirations /Better jobs & money needs	13	43.33%
7.	Self improvement & overcoming helplessness	3	10.0%
8.	Other Needs (for community, country, religion etc)	2	6.67%

*Total 82 wishes elicited from a sample children where each child stated more than 2 wishes.

Also the next preferred needs found in the wishes of the children were related to education and vocational needs and aspirations of a better jobs and money with both desired by 43% of children. Next 27% of children wanted better quality of life and wellbeing. They also wished that they be healthy and not get sick. The three kinds of wishes that were least desired were different things (like toys, cycle, bat etc.) to fulfill childhood desires of play, improvement in self and personality and some general wishes like progress of country or peace.

Assessment of Fears of Street Children

The fears elicited were either threat because of the particular harsh life situations of these children or to some of their desires and problems arising due to stresses and homelessness. As shown in the results, the most frequent fear, 93.33% was of police harassment and social discrimination by other people. The next frequent fear was the various abstract fears (73.33%) like that of spirits ('Bhoot' and 'Chudael'), nightmares, death, God and natural calamities like earthquake and fire. The third most frequent fears were situational, which reflected the harsh life conditions (40%) in which these children live. The fears were those of accidents and being run over by various vehicles like car, trains etc. and also traveling alone in night. Health related to getting AIDS, cancer or addicted to substances. Next, were the peer related fears (20%) like those of fights between them & also being bullied by older children. Lastly were the fears of losing self-control and committing wrong (6.67 %) whereas family related fears were least frequent 3.33%) fear.

Table 32.3 : Types of Fears and Their Frequencies Elicited from the Street Children (N=30)

S.No	*Fear Category**	*Frequency*	*Percentage*
1.	Abstract/Unnatural fears	22	73.33%
2.	Situational Fears (being alone in night, accident by vehicles etc.)	12	40%
3.	Fear of Harassment (police, social discrimination etc.)	28	93.33%
4.	Health Related Fears (AIDS, Cancer, Addiction etc.)	7	23.33%
5.	Peer Related Fears (fights, bullying by older boys etc.)	6	20%
6.	Family Related Fears (concerning mother's health etc.)	1	3.33%
7.	Fear of Losing self Control (*e.g.* doing wrong)	2	6.67%

Assessment of Future Aspirations/Planning

The responses to future plans were categorized into different groups as shown in Table 32.4. Most of the children (36.67%) reported that they don't know what they will do in future, or had no aspiration at all. They also said that they would continue in the same manner.

Table 32.4 : Future Aspirations of Street Children (N=30)

S.No.	*Future Aspirations**	*Frequency*	*Percentage*
1.	Uncertain/No Planning (Don't know/No Aspiration/ Continue like this)	11	36.67%
2.	Unskilled Work (Domestic servant, pan/tea, stall owner, fruit/ peanut vendor, waiter)	6	20%
3.	Skilled Work (Driver, mechanic, shoemaker, tailor, candle making)	5	16.67%
4.	Fauji/Policeman	5	16.67%
5.	Miscellaneous (Cricketer, Teacher, Dancer etc.)	4	13.33%

*Total 31 future aspirations elicited from a sample of 30 street children.

Next were those children who said that they would start doing an unskilled job (20%) like a domestic servant, pan/tea stall owner, fruit seller, 'chowkidar' or a waiter. About 16.67% of children said that they would get into a semi skilled job with training like driver, mechanic, shoemaker, tailoring or candle making. Another 16.67 % of the children said that they would like to become an army man/policeman. Lastly there were about 13.33% who aspired to become cricketer or dancer or teacher.

Purposes of Saving

All the children were also asked what do they do with the money they earn and that which is saved. Most of the children said that they tried to collect/save some money and send it home. Some said that they used the money for their own purposes. There were others who said that they would use it to go on a tour and visit other places or would use it to start their own shop.

Problem Analysis

Problem Analysis was used to understand the street children's problems and the stress that they experienced as a consequence. These children using cards indicated problems scored out in the severity rating on a 5-point scale. These problems were perceived on the various indices elicited from the children that included disability, frequency, pain and overall severity. The problem analysis (Table 32.5) showed that the problems experienced by the street children varied from food & emotional insecurity to work related problems, police interference and physical & sexual abuse.

Table 32.5 : Problem Analysis by Facilitator and Street Children

S. No.	Problems	*Frequency*		*Disability at Work*		*Pain*		*Overall Severity*	
		F	*SC*	*F*	*SC*	*F*	*SC*	*F*	*SC*
1.	Food Insecurity	1	2	2	1	3	1	3	1
2.	Emotional Insecurity	4	4	3	3	2	3	3	4
3.	Physical Abuse	5	5	2	4	5	3	3	4
4.	Sexual Abuse	3	-	3	-	3	-	3	-
5.	Drug Addiction	4	5	2	3	5	2	4	3
6.	Police Interference	4	5	5	5	4	5	4	5
7.	Social Discrimination	5	4	2	5	3	3	2	3
8.	Depression (well-being)	3	3	2	4	3	4	2	4
9.	General Sickness	4	3	3	5	4	3	3	4
10.	Work relate stress (older boys)	4	4	3	4	3	4	3	3

*5-point rating scale [less (1)- more (5)]; n=30, age= 8-18 yrs and F= facilitator & SC= street children; Work= rag picker, bottles seller, tea-stall workers.

The problems that were perceived to be the most frequent by the facilitator were police interference, social discrimination, drug addiction, work related stress and physical and sexual abuse. The problems perceived to be least frequent was food security only. Police interference, social discrimination and physical abuse were found to be most disabling at work in comparison of facilitator and children's ratings, street children viewed social discrimination whereas facilitator didn't view discrimination as causing high disability.

On the pain index, police interference, depression and work related stresses were rate high by the street children, and food insecurity and drug addiction caused least pain to them. On the other hand physical abuse, drug addiction and police interference was rated high on pain by the facilitator. When all the problems were judged on the index of overall severity police interference, physical abuse, emotional insecurity and depression were found to be highly rated by the street children whereas food insecurity and drug addiction were rated low. The facilitator rated drug addiction and police interference, high on the overall severity whereas problem of social discrimination and depression were rated low. These problems are linked to the work they do.

Assessment of Coping Strategies and Resources

The coping strategies and resources of street children were inferred from the detailed interviews, case studies and observation. The results are described below.

Coping Strategies : A variety of strategies and activities for coping with street life emerged from the stories included :

- Support from peers, both emotionally and materially. They also join gang for support and protection. It was widely evident in their interviews, *e.g.* taking help from mend when sick, helping another child in trouble with employer.
- Fighting and being aggressive shown in behaviour as well as language. This is also a survival strategy. They fight for money also, using it as a means of coping both in happy as well as sad states. This also elicits the theme of searching for one's identity.
- Knowing how to effectively lie and manipulate the authorities and to get away with it. It was seen in the many children being registered at almost all NGO's and taking their benefits and facilities and not being attached to a single NGO. The children also lie to police, act novice when caught or lie about their state. They also keep in mind the weekdays on which police conducts raids on stations and they avoid roaming on those days.
- Engaging in high risk behaviours like fighting, jumping off and onto trains, playing games of dare and chance where physical harm may result. They also use substances like tobacco, gutka, bidi solution on which a major part of their earnings are spent.
- An ability to elicit alms by begging as it requires stamina, intelligence and imagination. Children easily resort to begging as shown in story where for a desire such as an ice cream, they would consider begging.
- Becoming "numb" psychologically, so that they felt nothing. Being in a harsh life and reality, they keep themselves in a shell or behind a wall and do not come up with emotions/feelings. They also try to suppress their experiences of maltreatment.
- Fantasy is one of the most commonly used coping mechanisms. It was evident in the interview where when asked what they would do on their birthday, all children fantasized elaborately how they would go about celebrating their birthday.
- Learning, educational aspirations and acquiring vocational skill.

Some of the coping strategies shown in the children being assisted by NGOs. These included :

- Playing sports-cricket being one of the most liked games in the country; children spent most of their idle time in cricket. There are also matches help from different groups of children.

- Dancing, performing music and plays with NGO. This serves three purposes–one as a coping strategy, second reaching to community and thirdly to the donors for the projects for street children.

Some of these strategies are skills–prosocial, while others demonstrate skills and strategies utilized within antisocial activities. However, the skills themselves and the planning capacities used in the antisocial activities may be transferable to prosocial ends, if such ends are perceived as valid and rewarding alternatives.

Some negative aspects of the children indicated by statements were :

- Low self-esteem—"was thrown out of play because of dirty clothes" or "was thrown out of job".
- Escapism—"will run away from job, if there is a fight with employer. Showing no alternative thinking or problem solving".
- Stealing to have ice cream. Easy acceptance of the desire to commit crime.

Resources

The resources were also identified from the stories and detailed interviews. These resources were categorized in three, namely, self-resources, economic resources and social resources. Self-resources were those qualities that the children possessed and acquired on the street.

Personality characteristics and adaptive coping style that are capacity to work and earn a living; capacity to relate to others; sensitivity to perceive their own as well as others emotions; insight into their lives and situation, not being happy with their lives and in particular drug use, and wanting change in their lives; tolerance of pain; awareness of being discriminated; close attachment to parents, particularly mothers as in stories where the children wanted to spend their earnings with parents, celebrating birthday with parents or mother taking care when the child is sick; sense of responsibility as an earning member of family; and saving capacity.

Economic resources are the money that they earn through working and the availability of cooperative banks for saving their money. Social resources include peer support and gang membership; family contact and support; NGO support (participation in projects; support and care from facilitator; shelter homes; centers for education and vocational training; 'Time out' programmes *e.g.* outings and camps in Delhi as well as outside Delhi and providing bank and money saving facility.) and Other community support such as Police becoming more sensitive to children, donating items like clothes, shoes etc. and some even taking charge of education of some children. Police support to street children is available minimally; visiting doctors, teachers, social work trainees and help from religious places of worship church (night shelter), temples, gurudwara etc. shelter, education, food etc.

Case Studies

Two case studies are given to highlight the problems faced by the street children and referring to each child's strengths and weaknesses.

Case No. 1—Mahendra was a 11yrs old Hindu boy from Fatehpur, Uttar Pradesh. He had studied till the second class. His family constituted of mother, father and a younger brother. He did not like going to school and hence used to roam around. His father was a labourer at farm and was addicted to alcohol. He used to beat him for not studying. Some of his friends worked at marble mines in Gujarat, so he left home with friends to work. Unable to get work he left Gujarat and went to Kanpur. Failing to get any work there also he came to Delhi one year back and picks rag around New Delhi Railway Station area. He had been using Salaam Balak Trust's (SBT) drop-in shelter for basic facilities like food, clothes and sleeping. He attended non-formal educational classes. He said that SBT's staff would help street children on being caught by the police. For recreation they also go for trips in Delhi every month.

He feared being police, as he was once caught in suspicion of theft in the train and was put in the jail. Then his parents came to rescue him but was left on the street by parents and he continued surviving by rag picking. He also feared fighting with other boys at the station as they use blades, razors etc. to harm him. Since he picked rags in dumps he also feared of getting hurt by broken glass pieces and stones.

When given problem situations, he showed resignation and feelings of helplessness in the adverse situations. It was also inferred that adults were viewed as more powerful and that he resigned easily to the authority of adults. In the exercises on perception of emotions, he showed high awareness of feelings and perception of bodily changes during intense emotions. Mahendra showed realistic perception of positive emotions. However lacked social support and facilities to channel such positive emotions as on being happy unable to play and enjoy. Similarly he showed acute sense of experiencing negative emotions of sadness and anger and reactions to such intense emotions. For *e.g.* he said that when he gets angry," I get terrible headaches" ("Sar me dard hota hai") and when he feels sad, "It hurts me deeply" ("Aatma roti hai").

Strengths

(a) He had future orientation: he said that he will save the money safely in a bank so that he can use it later for his own grocery shop. He also said that he would make his children study so that they would stand on their feet.

(b) He has family contact and misses his home. He wants to serve his parents and do something for his younger brother.

Weakness

Inspite of using SBT's facilities he appears dirty and faces the problem of being caught by police. In conclusion, he belongs to a poor family where there were no restrictions and no motivation to study. Hence the suggestions for intervention are counseling him to stay at the shelter home and continue his education, as he is still young. He should also be taught how to mange money and save it rather than wasting it.

Case no. 2—Mohd.Rafiq was 17yrs old illiterate Muslim male from Banaras. His family included an elder sister, two elder brothers and a younger brother. His father had left home and started living with another woman in Ajmer when he was very young. After his mother's death he had left home 6yrs back in anger to search for his father. He wanted to confront his father on this issue. He said, "My father is dead for me as he left us alone to survive" ("mein apne papa ko papa nai manta. Mere liye vo mar gaye hai, nai to vo hamara khayal karte"). His family was engaged into the traditional art of making Banarasi Sarees. His brother and maternal aunt ill treated and forced him to work. Since then he had been with the NGO, Salaam Balak Trust and worked as a volunteer. He was also taking vocational training for tailoring. He said that he wanted to study and stand on his own feet. He also said that he liked to dance when he was happy and wanted to become a dancer. He said that he feared falling into addiction as he earlier used to take drugs and solution but now has stopped after the NGO's intervention. He said that he also feared police and death. In the perception of emotions exercises he said that he was unable to control his anger and when he got angry he felt like hurting himself as well as hurting the other. Once in anger he hit his fist in the wall and broke his finger. When he felt sad, he thought of why it happened to him? ("Ye mere sath kyun hua").

Rafiq had a tendency towards addictive substances and lacked of self-control as earlier he had been addicted but had left after the NGOs interventions, and said that he was tempted to take addictive substances. In the problem situation of employer not giving salary he indicated delinquent tendency when he replied the child would run away with the shop owner's money and will not get caught.

Strength & Weaknesses

He has now stopped consuming addictive substances and was working as a volunteer. He was also showing capability to take on responsibility and fulfilling it. For recreation he watched movies and danced. However his weakness was that he had been addicted once and was still not very strong willed that he would not go back into addiction. Another weak point was that he had no contact with his family. Also his aggression was uncontrollable and also sometimes resulted in self-harm.

The investigator visited the contact point again after a year and it was learnt that he had got job at an export company in Gurgaon and was earning Rs. 3000/- per month. In conclusion, he should maintain constant contact with the NGO and the facilitators supporting him so that he doesn't engage in addiction again. He should also be taught to manage his money and save it for future.

The presence of street children in urban areas is not a new phenomenon. They have been a part of the urban scene mainly due to unabated migration from the villages to cities in search of a livelihood. Acute poverty of their families has denied them a proper shelter, forcing them to squat on public land on pavements, below flyovers, at or near railway stations, bus stations and other public places. Street children are, thus, a living and sordid symbol of urban malaise, their growing numbers giving the problem a high degree of visibility in cities where squatter settlements as well as the numbers of such children are mushrooming. The lives of street children have been explored from their perspective in the present study.

The causes of street children phenomenon have been found to be associated with various psychosocial variables. The main reasons for leaving home or running away from home were found to be poverty, physical abuse or neglect by family, illness/injury/death of parent and forced work besides other reasons of peer influence and delinquent tendencies etc. The factors were not exclusive of each other and in most cases there was a combination of factors like poverty, death of parent, along with forced work or ill treatment by step-parent, or poverty, discontinuation of education and forced work etc. (Whitebeck & Hoyt, 1999). Sometimes physical abuse at home and undesirable peer influence were the reasons for child running away from home. Similar findings have been reported from some of the studies on street children. Aptekar (1988) found that physical violence and abuse at home by parents was the primary reason for running away from home. Also many studies have shown that street children have high experiences of maltreatment, sexual abuse, and discrimination and faced traumatic events (Lalor, 1999; Manihara, 1997; Panter-Brick, Todd, & Baker, 1996; Sampa, 1998 & Suda, 1997).

Most of the children belonged to lower socioeconomic class, which are poor, large families with extreme parental rejection, neglect and maltreatment of the child. These families showed strained parental relations and parents were not nurturing, unconcerned and distant from the child. The families were very poor, resulting in neglect or discontinuation of education of the child. Many children were forced to work and share the financial responsibility towards family. Hence, most street children faced extreme deprivations, neglect, and maltreatment for a long period of time. These children lacked family and peer support. (Gelles, 1998; Kotch, Muller & Blakely, 1999 & Sampa, 1998).

Perception of Work

Interacting with the street children and the observation of their daily activities showed the way children perceived their work. Children were also asked about their future plans/ aspirations. Most of the children had no future aspirations regarding the type of work they would like to do and many wished of getting an unskilled job like being a domestic servant/ worker; owning a tea/pan shop, fruit seller, 'chowkidar' or waiter. Some of the children desired to become an army men/policeman etc. and rest of them (13%) desired to become cricketer, teacher, dancer etc. The aspiration to become a policeman was present in the children as they see that police has a lot of power over others. The children also faced harassment and discrimination from the police; hence they wanted to attain a status of authority where others would not be able to harm them.

These children were aware of the harsh working conditions of their work. Their work was not ideal work as a waged and steady work was out of reach. It has been reported by Tellez and Abramo (1985) that working children do not fully understand the ideal model of work and/or rather tend to redefine it from their own experiences. They sometimes valorize the work they are doing for some reason still to be determined. It could be to increase their self-esteem and have a more substantial identity. Children were also asked about the way they spent/used and saved money. Work for street children is survival and subsistence of many of their families. The amount of earned money and subsequent savings are small. Street children are young and not supposed to work. Their circumstances forced them to work. Invernizzi (2001) described the socialization of working children through four activities namely work as survival, playing, relationship and building one's identity. Family background of the street children reflected that the street children have not been exposed to the ideal middle class protected family and School environment. Majority of these children have experienced the consequences of poverty both at home and on the street. The street child is exposed to work as a necessity for subsistence, which is combined with socialization. Street children working as rag picker, shoe shiners, in tea stall and even as beggars, have not learned the work skills, social competencies, value of work and money management. Many a times these children play a role of victim to gain sympathy of adults to make more money, for example, while begging, rag picking or working at tea stalls. Though the children did not show clear definition/meaning of work, for them working meant long hours involving efforts and subsequent malnutrition and health problems. Activities of many street/working children contribute to material survival of the family and have the same function as that of a waged worker. Moreover older children may see work in terms of competence as seen in their future plans and desire to learn a vocational skill. These children had a desire to learn a vocation with the help of NGO and then start their own work in future like candle making, tailoring, driving vehicle etc. Street children wished for a 'happy future' along with their family and also desired for the well being of their sibling. Some of these were supporting their families financially and showed concern for the well-being of their siblings. Children even faced parental neglect and rejection showed strength and positive attitude of responsibility and this may be resilient factor for their survival and adjustment on the street without a family.

Through work, the child is trying to survive and looking for a positive personal recognition and self-evaluation, especially where this working child is also supporting family members. Wherever the work involves competencies as seen in the skilled work the child is motivated to excel and it would improve the self-valuation and identity of the street child. It is reflected in their desires for a better job and money and self-improvement. They wished for general well-being and better health. Many of them were aware of their unhygienic working conditions and desired for better life.

Problem Analysis

Problems were also rated on the indices of frequency, disability, and pain. It was found that police harassment was perceived to be most frequent, painful and disabling both by the street children and facilitator. Physical abuse was perceived to be most frequent, disabling, but not painful as compared to the facilitator who perceived it to be more painful Emotional insecurity was perceived to be more frequent, however moderately painful by street children but the facilitator did not consider it painful. Similarly depression was found to be moderate in frequency, high in disability and high on pain and overall severity by the street children. On the other hand facilitator perceived it to be moderate on frequency, low in disability at work and moderate. The facilitator did not consider it to be severe. Hence the street children perceived emotional insecurity and depression as more painful and severe as compared to the facilitator, as the facilitator lacked an internal frame of reference. It must also be remembered that not all young children who have experienced familial maltreatment and societal discrimination end up in trouble. Many survive and do well, their stories are very important for in them, we may be able to see resilience to work in the face of adversity, and be able to identify effective strategies for better assisting those who appear to be as vulnerable but not as resilient. Case studies of street children in the present study show that despite adversities in life, they enjoyed gaining pleasure from traditional Indian games like 'gulli-danda', choker, and cricket etc. It was also reflected in the wishes that children elicited, where 76.66% wished for "being with family and loved ones" and having a happy family in future.

Perception of work is also related to other problems faced by the street children. Problem analysis comparisons of street children and facilitator showed that as compared to facilitator who also judged the problems of street children, police harassment and drug addiction were perceived to be more severe whereas social discrimination and depression as less severe. Hence both facilitator and street children perceived police interference and social discrimination as major obstacles in street child's life. D'lima and Gosalia (1982) and Paniker and Nangia (1992) reported that street children were arrested because the police considered them vagrants or suspected they might have committed crimes. Even the NGOs Salaam Balak Trust having the support of Delhi Police have not been able to solve the problem of police interference and insensitivity towards these children. It was also reflected in the fears of children where police harassment was perceived to be the major threat.

Coping Strategies

Coping strategies of the street children relating to their problems of basic needs fulfillment, work situations, peer relations have been explored through qualitative methods like case studies, daily activities and observation. Forming close peer bonds, seeking support from peers, joining street gangs helped the child adjust to the harsh environment and may be compensated for the lack of home and family. Using drop-in shelter, seeking support of sympathetic facilitators and counselors could built up the resilience of the deprived child and promote well-being. Emotional coping strategies of being aggressive, tendency to show high risk behaviour of using drugs, gambling, watching porn movies, stealing, begging and other anti-social activities were the survival strategies. These coping styles were seen in the children who were influenced by the street 'gangs'. Lacking self-confidence and social skills, these children fail to engage in satisfying peer relationships and drift into increasingly deviant peer groups which provide them some kind of corrective environmental experience that might buffer earlier neglect from the parents. Street children want to be accepted and seek identity. As Jackson and McBride (1985) reported that gang members identify themselves with names, clothes, tattoos, slang, sign language etc., in the present study also there were evidences of such gangs functioning. Younger children are compelled to join a 'gang' to save themselves from being exploited and bullied by older boys.

Street children's erratic working hours and work (rag picking, sweeping in trains, working in tea-stalls etc) make them prone to intense physical strain and harassment. They try to cope by using drugs like chewing tobacco ('gutka') drinking 'whitener' solution, ganja etc. Case studies showed that children reported "smoking makes them alert", "drinking solution make them forget their fatigue and get refreshed". They missed their homes and families, remembering those with whom they were attached to like their mothers, sisters. These thoughts were depressing and made them cry and withdrawn.

Police harassment and abuse by older street boys was painful. However, they tried to forget these incidences and moved from one place to another. Peer support was found to be very essential, which gives a street child support and protection. Sharing and talking with each other they are able to survive in the harsh conditions. Those children assisted by the NGOs started sharing their problems with the facilitator. A child's own attitude toward him and positive psychosocial characteristics were related to self-related resources resulting in resilience. Some of these are sense of responsibility toward the family, warm feelings towards some family members like mother, hope for future, saving money, learning vocational skills etc. It is emphasized in the ecological model (Berns, 2004) that competence and skills of the street child in coping with the stress would affect his/her adjustment and may pose high risk for drug use and impede the psycho-social development.

Many researches explaining the street child phenomenon in detail highlighting the possible causes and the negative outcomes of street life. However little empirical work has been done on the social networks of street children which helps them to survive the harsh realities of street (Kipke *et al.,* 1997). These street children often congregate in groups which are differentiated by degrees of involvement in deviant activities and amplify the pressure on child to use alcohol and drugs or to engage in unprotected sex (Ennett, Bailey & Federman, 1999; Kipke *et al.,* 1997). It's however important to acknowledge that peers on the street often play dual roles in the life of a homeless adolescent. They are sources of nurturance and support as well as of risk. These "street families" provide both physical and emotional association as well as protection from the many dangers of street life (Hagan & McCarthy, 1997; Whitebeck & Hoyt, 1999).

Addressing the problem of street children would emphasize the development of close, guardian-like relationship between resource persons (of govt. & non-govt. organizations) and the homeless youth (Cauce *et al.*, 1994). Such trusting relationships with adults on the street appear to serve a protective function and afford to potential to break the cycle of victimization and re-victimization. It is critical to recognize, that adolescent homelessness represents a failure of our society on multiple levels : social, political and economic. These structures of the society should address this issue and embark upon a change, however to have a desired attack on the problem, we need to learn to intervene effectively. Programmes that focus on acquiring effective social skills, making positive attachments and access to health, welfare, educational, vocational and recreational services have potential to ameliorate some stress that street children may experience.

REFERENCES

Aderinto, A.A. (2002). *Social Correlates and Coping Measures of Street Chidlren : A Comparative Study of Street and Non-street Children in South-western Nigeria,* Child Abuse and Neglect *24*, 199-213.

Aptekar, L. (1988). Street Children of Cale, Durham, NC : Duke University Press.

Baker, R., Panter, B. C. & Todd, A. (1997). Homeless street boys in Nepal : Their demography and life-style, *Journal of Comparative Family Studies,* University of Calgary, Alberta, Canada.

Berns, M. (2004). *Child, Family, School, Community : Socialization and Support,* Wadsworth : USA.

Butterflies (1997). *History of Butter Flies Programmes of Street Working Children.* Report by Butterflies, NOG, New Delhi.

Clatts, M.C. & Davis, W.R. (1999). A demographic & behavioural profile of homeless youth in New York City : Implications for AIDS outreach prevention, Medline Anthropological Q., *13*, 365-74.

Cauce, A.M., Morgan, C.J., Lohr, Y., Wagner, V., Moore, E., Wurzbacher, K., Weeden, K., Tomlin, S. & Blamchard, T. (1994). Effectiveness of intensive case management for homeless adolescents : Results of a 3-month follow-up, *Journal of Emotional and Behavioural Disorders*, 2, 219-227.

D'Lima, H. & Oosalia, R. (1992). Street children of Bombay, A situational analysis, National Labour Institute, Noida, India.

Dohrenwend, B.S. (1978). Social stress and community psychology, *American Journal of Community Psychology,* 6, 1-14.

Ennett, S.T., Bailey, S.L. & Fedennan, E.B. (1999). Social network characteristics associated with risky behaviours among runaways and homeless youth, *Journal of Health and Social Behaviour, 40*, 63-78.

Ferrari, A. (2003). Rehabilitation of street children in Africa : An experience in Nairobi, Kenya. In J. Gerald Young *et al.* (Eds.), *Brain, Culture and Development* (pp. 160-167). Macmillan India Ltd.

Gelles, R. J. (1998). The youngest victims : Violence toward children. In R. Bergen & Kennedy (Eds.), *Issues in Intimate Violence* (pp. 5-24). Thousands Oaks, CA : Sage.

Greenblatt, M. & Robertson, M. (1993). Life-styles, adaptive strategies, and sexual behaviours of homeless adolescents, *Hospital and Community Psychiatry, 44* , 1177-1180.

Hagan, J. & McCarthy, B. (1997). Mean streets : Youth crime and homelessness, New York : Cambridge University Press.

Invernizzi, A. (2001). The work of children is not only work. In Manfted, L., Overwien. B. & Recknage, A. (Eds.) *Working Children's Protagonism : Social Movements and Empowerment in Latin America, Africa and India,* (c) IKO, London.

Jackson, R.K. & McBride, W.D. (1985). *Understanding Street Gangs,* Sacramento : Custom.

Janus, M., McCormack, A. Burgess, A., & Hartman, C. (1987). *Adolescent runaways : Causes and consequences,* Lexington, MA : Lexington.

Kipke, M.D., Montgomery, S.B., Simon, T.R. & Unger, J.B. (1997). Homeless youth : Drug use patterns and HIV risk profiles according to peer group affiliation, *AIDS and behaviour, 1*, 247-259.

Kotch, J.B., Muller, Gi. O. & Blakely, C.H. (1999). Understanding the origins and incidence of spousal violence in North America. In T.P. Gullotta & S.J. McElhaney (Eds.), *Violence in homes and communities* (pp.1-38). Thousands Oaks CA : Sage.

Lalor, K.J. (1999). Street children : A comparative perspective, *Child Abuse and Neglect, 23*, 759-770.

Le Roux, J. (1996). *Adolescence; 31,* 965-971.

Manihara, S. (1997). Street children : An international problem. In R. Bama (Ed.), *My Name is Today, Childin news,* (v), 1.

Matchinda, P. (1991). *Child Abuse and Neglect,* Mar. *23,* 245-255.

Mustafa, M. & Sharma, O. (1996). *Child Labour in India : A Bitter Truth,* Deep and Deep Publication, India.

Panicker, R. & Nangia, P. (1992). *Working and Street Children Delhi*, National Labour Institute, Noida, India.

Panter-Brick, C., Todd, A. & Baker, R. (1996). Growth status of homeless Nepali boys : Do they differ from rural and controls? *Social Sciences and Medicine,* 42, Pergamon Press, Oxford, UK.

Rothman, J. & Davis, T. (1985). *Status Offenders in Los Angeles Country : Focus on Runaway and Homeless Youth,* School of Social Welfare, Los Angeles, CA : University of California.

Salaam Balak Trust (1998). SBT-Annual Report, NGO, New Delhi.

Sampa, A. (1998). *Journal of Psychology in Africa, South of Sahara, the Caribbean and Afro Latin America, 2*, 1-23.

Segal, U.A. & Ashtekar, A. (1994). Child *Abuse and Neglect, 18*, 957-967.

Suda, C. (1997). *Child Abuse Review, 6*, 199-217.

Tellez,V.S. & Abramo, H. (1985). "Experiencia urbana trabajo e identidad. Apuntes a una investigation sobre menores proletario en Sao Paulo", in Carrion, D. Vainstoc, A. (eds.) La ciudad y los ninos. Quito.

Tucker, V., Tucker, S., Phogat P. & Pandey A. (2002). Effectiveness of participatory techniques with street children for planning intervention programmes. In V. Veeraraghavan., S. Singh & K.

Khandelwal (Eds.), *The Child in the New Millennium* (pp. 136-141). Mosaic Books : New Delhi, India.

UNICEF (2004). The State of the World's Children, 2004, UNICEF, New York.

Whitebeck, L.B., Hoyt, D.R. & Yoder, K.A., Cauce, A.M., & Pradise, M. (1999). *Deviant Behaviour and Victimization among Homeless and Runaway Adolescents,* Technical Report, Ames, IA : University of Iowa.

World Health Organization (1999). Report of the Consultation on Child Labour Prevention, WHO, Geneva.

SECTION—V

Illness : Pathology and Coping Strategies

33

Personality Behaviour Patterns and Cardiovascular Diseases

*Akbar Husain**

The theme underlying in this article is the role played by personality and behaviour patterns in vulnerability to illness. The idea that personality is relevant to disease etiology has a long history in psychosomatic medicine, beginning with psychodynamic conceptualizations in which psychic conflicts or specific attitudes were thought to increase risk for particular disorders (Alexander, 1950; Grace and Graham, 1952). More recently, Friedman and Booth-Kenley (1987) have suggested a hypothesis linked with 'disease-prone personality', a constellation of negative affective trait such as anxiety, depression, and hostility that increase disease risk in a general fashion across different medical problems.

The present paper emphasizes the role of some personality variables and behaviour pattern in disease risk, including Type A behaviour, unpleasant emotions (anger, hostility, depression etc.), pessimism/explanatory style, irrational thinking and stress.

Type A Behaviour

The Type A Behaviour Pattern (TABP) has been one of the most influential constructs in studies of psychosocial factors in disease etiology. Type A Behaviour Pattern is that behaviour which takes place when characterologically predisposed persons are challenged or blocked by an environmental condition (either social or physical environment). The characteristics tend to be associated with Type A personality are : competitiveness, high levels of anger and hostility, quick actions, punctuality and rigidity, impatience, energetic gestures, self-centered concentration, extreme desire for recognition and competitive drives, feelings of time urgency and time pressures.

In a series of longitudinal studies, Friedman and Rosenman (1974), Jenkins, Zyzanski and Rosenman (1978); Matthews and Haynes (1986) have found that people (both men and

* Professor, and Chief Editor, Journal of Indian Academy of Applied Psychology, Department of Psychology, Aligarh Muslim University, Aligarh.

women) who have Type A personality styles are more likely to develop coronary artery and heart diseases. Stress and Type A personality seem to go hand in hand. Psychologists, cardiologists, and epidemiologists have found the positive association between TABP and high levels of catecholamines and cortico-steroids specially when under stress (Krantz, Contrada, Hill & Friedler, 1988; Pope & Smith, 1991; Smith, 1992). Moreover, a number of studies have found the positive relationship between TABP and coronary atherosclerosis and angina pectoris (Eaker, Abbot & Kannel, 1989; Stevens, Turner, Rhodewatt & Taibot, 1984).

A number of studies failing to support any relationship between coronary heart disease and Type A Behaviour have been reported (Appels, & Muller, 1987; Shekelle *et al.*, 1985). Eaker and others (1989) found no association between Type A Behaviour and myocardial infarction or fatal cardiac events. Miller *et al.*, (1991) have put forth several explanations for these discrepancies. First, questionnaire measures are less sensitive than the structured interview. That is, Type A questionnaire did predi t coronary heart disease in the western collaborative group and Framingham studies, but not in other studies. Second, the cultural context of Type A Behaviour has changed. Third, the global Type A construct is too broad, and that only specific components may be pathogenic.

The Type A people have difficulty in coping with chronic day-to-day stressors (*i.e.*, tends toward anxiety, frustration and worry). Altering and modifying TABP enables us to overcome the problem as a risk factor in cardiovascular disease among aged patients in particular and others in general. The new learned behaviour (*i.e.*, content and tranquil) increases the chance for creating TABP and decreases TABP within patients, since anger is an element in Type A personalities. In sum Type A people can be viewed as stressing themselves because of their own attitudes toward their position in the world.

Unpleasant Emotions

Psychological stress is accompanied by negative emotions and associated behaviours including depression, frustration, aggression, hostility, fear and anger. These emotions are found to be associated with the development of cardiovascular disease, especially angina pectoris (Jenkins, 1983). The negative emotions appear to be related to immune system function and health outcomes. Most patients especially at the time of leaving hospitals found to be depressed, anxious, neurotic, and frustrated. All these factors have negative effects and are harmful to the health of the patients unless they are controlled and managed. Negative emotions increase irritability as well as emotional liability.

Anger

It is considered to be a negative emotion. Anger may be defined as an emotion characterized by strong feeling of displeasure, which are triggered by real or imagined wrong (Davidoff, 1987). Berkowitz (1962) considers that anger refers to an emotional state presumably resulting from frustration, which even congruent with a suitable cue instigates aggressive responses. There are two dimensions of anger, anger-in and anger-out. Anger-in refers to how often anger feelings are experienced but not expressed, whereas anger-out refers to the extent that an individual engages in aggressive behaviours when motivated by angry feelings. In addition to anger—in and anger-out, two other dimensions of anger are identified, *i.e.*, anger control and anger total. Anger control may be defined as a tendency not to become angry even in anger provoking situations. Anger—total reflects a configuration of all the anger dimensions.

Anger is found to be one of the most crucial elements in coronary problems (Smith & Pope, 1990). A number of researches have identified direct relationship between suppressed anger or inhibited aggression and high blood pressure (Gentry *et al.*, 1982; Gold & Johnston, 1990, Johnson, Gontry & Julins, 1982; Spielberger *et al.*, 1985). Expressed anger is linked to coronary heart problems (Feshback, 1986; Hecker, Chesney, Black & Frantsch, 1988; Wood, 1986). Anger should be avoided at any cost. Rubin (1969) believes that the cost is very high—that in order to avoid this essentially natural, normal and essential feeling, we are obliged to engage in what he calls "perversions". We "put off" our angry feelings, transferring our anger from the original situation or person to a safer object (expressed on the kids and spouse). We dilute our feelings by rationalizing the thoughts why we should not be angry, and we "put down" anger, pushing the feelings almost instantaneously from consciousness. The net effect of our attempts to be nice, non angry people is to create a "slush fund" of feelings that result in anxiety, depression, overeating, insomnia, and overall self-sabotage. In sum, playing the role as a nice person is stressful because that role requires us to deny significant parts of ourselves—we must pretend that a portion of reality is not there. The expression of anger can prevent heart disease patients to break away from the nice guy role and to work hard at being more honest with ourselves and others.

Hostility

According to Buss (1981), hostility consists "of the mulling over of past attack on oneself, rejection and deprivation". This suggests that hostility is the result of punishment, repeated punishment and suffering at the hands of others may lead to a generalized dislike of humanity, and a tendency to perceive the pain and discomfort of people as reinforcing. Buss suggests that hostility involves negative evaluation of people and events .... and may be inferred when the attack is reinforced more by injury than by attaining the "extrinsic reinforcer". Kaufman (1970) writes of the hostile person, "we think of him as one who has a habit or propensity for disliking others, wishing harm or aggregating against them". Thus, hostility is a more ensuring condition of enmity, involving angry feelings and a tendency to inflict them.

In recent years, attention has been focused particularly on hostility, since this is the element that has been found to predict coronary heart disease most strongly (Dembroski, MacDougall, Costa & Grandits, 1989). In a longitudinal study, hostility predicted increased risk of coronary artery disease and mortality due to all causes. Weekes and Waterhouse (1991) have found that hostile attitudes may have a subordinate corrective role in the development of CHD and may contribute to coronary risk because of an association with more fundamental components of the coronary-prone personality. Dembroski and Costa (1987) found the relationship between potential for hostility and coronary heart disease. Results of Helmers and others (1993) study indicated that in patients with coronary artery disease, hostility traits are significantly correlated with extent of daily life ischemia with severity of exercise—induced myocardial ischemia. Fukunishi, Hattori, Nakamura & Nakagama, (1995) found that Myocardial Infarction (MI) patients had stronger cynical hostility and lower social desirability than college students, and hostility was related to narcissism before and after controlling for social desirability in both MI patients and college students.

Depression

Depression appears to be the one most important unpleasant emotion related to cardiovascular diseases. Sword (1977) defines depression-prone personality, he states : "It is a person who works hard, is ambitious, has a high sense of integrity, tells the truth, never gets mad, is very responsible and conscientious, pays bills on time (or at least tries to), is pleasant to everyone, smiles outwardly even when feeling like hell inside, has a strong sense of duty, and sets very high standards of performance for others but even more so for himself". A large number of studies found an increased mortality from cardiovascular disease among depressed patients (Norton & Whalley, 1984; Rabins, Harvis & Koven, 1985; Sharma & Marker, 1994; Tsuang, Woolson, & Fleming, 1980; Weeke, 1979; Weeke, Juel, & Vaith, 1987). The findings of Anda *et al.* (1993). Study indicated existence of relation between depression and the development of ischemic disease. Booth-Kewley and Friedman (1997) analyzed 55 studies that had examined the relation between personality and cardiovascular disease. They found that the strongest effect size in the 55 studies they analyzed was not for Type A personality or anger but for depression. They commented that "depression appears to be reliably associated with cardiovascular heart disease ... but has generally been overlooked".

Frasure-Smith and colleagues obtained structured psychiatric examinations of 22 patients 5-15 days after they suffered myocardial infarction. The patients were contacted again 6, 12 and 18 months after discharge from the hospital. Sixteen percent of these patients showed evidence of major depression while hospitalized for their index myocardial infarction. This is consistent with the other surveys that regularly show 15%-20% of postinfarction patients developing major depression (Hance *et al.*, 1996; Schiefer *et al.*, 1989). After 6 months (app.) 17% of the depressed patients in the study by Frasure-Smith, Lesperance and Talagic (1993) had died, compared with 3% of the nondepressed patients. With control for other independent predictors of risk, the relative hazard for the depressed patients was almost 3.5 times greater than for the non-depressed patients. The strongest medical predictor of mortality after myocardial infarction is generally heart failure, and it is associated with just about the same 3.5 fold increase in mortality.

It is amply clear that depression is strongly associated with more frequent and more malignant cardiovascular disease. In fact, it is likely that depression's effect is not limited to cardiovascular disease but involves all vascular diseases including stroke (Morris, Robinson & Sammuels, 1993).

Irrational Thinking

Irrational thinking is a key element in the development of cardiovascular diseases. Ellis's rational emotive therapy (RET) states "that sustained emotional reactions are caused by internal sentences that people repeat to themselves, and these self-statements reflect sometimes unspoken assumptions—irrational beliefs—about what is necessary to lead a meaningful life," (Davison & Neale, 1994, p. 563). The basic tenet of RET is that we cause ourselves unnecessary anxiety, guilt, and so on, by irrational "self-talk". The aim of therapy is to eliminate self-defeating beliefs through a rational examination of them. Ellis (1962) believes that most of us suffer needlessly because we do not respond on a rational level. In a series of studies, researchers have found that people who have Type A personality, expressed anger, suppressed hostility, depression, anxiety behaviour patterns and so on are likely to develop coronary artery and heart diseases, and hypertension. What we believe that a number of irrational beliefs can cause emotional turmoil and thus consequently may develop or suffer from cardiovascular diseases.

There are some preliminary evidences which show that RET is useful in reducing the Type A behaviour pattern (Haaga, 1987) and may be useful in treating excessive anger, depression, etc. (Haaga & Davison, 1989). People can effectively and satisfactorily deal with life's problems if they can reject impossible ideas or accept the rational process at work. Rational thinking can promote psychological health. An old epigram emphasizes "Think and you won't sink".

Stress

It refers to a bodily (physical) or mental (psychological) tension resulting from factors that tend to alter an existent *equilibrium* (Webster, 1988). The term stress has been defined in numerous ways. Stress has been defined in at least four different ways : *(a)* stimulus-based definitions, *(b)* response-based definitions, *(c)* intervening process definitions, and (4) the more comprehensive definitions, combination of the three. In medicine, the result is produced when a *structure, system,* or *organism* is acted upon by forces that disrupt equilibrium or produce strain. In health care, the term denotes the physical (gravity, mechanical force, pathogen, injury) and psychological (fear, anxiety, crisis, joy) forces that are experienced by individuals (Tyber, 1989). For example, cold, heat, infection, haemohorrage, toxic substances, and the like are considered to be as physical stressors (Selye, 1936). Challenges that affect the functions of the body and its balance are called psychological stressors. The most common are : the loss of loved one, failures, frustrations, helplessness, hopelessness, and loneliness. Such stressful events are harmful and injurious to health due to their meanings and values as perceived as well as evaluated by the concerned individual. The thing which may challenge our integrity and equilibrium is stressor, and the caused reaction (the result) by that stressor is stress. It is mainly of two types : physical stress, and psychological stress, and each type is created and determined by its specific stressor.

Stress has been accepted as one of the major factors in the aetio-pathogenesis of Coronary Artery Disease (CAD) and its manifestations. It is well known for its effect on human body as a whole and particularly on the neurophysiological, autonomic, endocrine, and immune system (Folklow, 1993; Glazer & Kiecott-Glazer, 1984; Smith & Davito, 1984). As being a mental state, stress is responsible about altering our neurophysiological function either for good or bad (health or disease). No doubt, the matter depends on our perceptions, and judgements for the environmental stressors which first of all stimulate and evoke our central nervous system (CNS). Physical stress responses produce a healthy heart, while the emotional state (*i.e.*, the fight-flight situations) is associated with the chance of being more prone to suffer from the heart diseases (Hedman *et al.*, 1990; Linden, 1991; Lovallo *et al.*, 1985; Lovallo, Pincomb & Wilson, 1986).

A large number of studies were conducted to examine the effect of stress and stressors on health, particularly on the cardiovascular system. Freeman, Nixon and Reavelay (1987) studied incidence of silent myocardial ischemia (MF) in 30 patients during a short-period of intense spontaneous stress and uncertainty (the waiting period for outcomes of coronary angiography). They found a significant relationship between silent myocardial ischemic events and the intense stress periods. Fredrickson, Lundberg & Tusmisto (1991) found that elevated cardiovascular reactivity is not only due to mental stress and stressors but due to the *elevations* of low-density Lipoprotein Cholesterol (LDL) which may cause stress and as an outcome leads to coronary heart disease.

In long-term perspective studies the "vital exhaustion" syndrome is found to be associated with an "increased relative risk of initial infarction (Appels & Mulder, 1988). They also found that "vital Exhaustion" was positively associated with stable and unstable angina pectoris. Moreover, it was associated with an increase in a diverse cardiac episodes in the year and a half following angioplasty (Appels & Mulder, 1989).

Epidemiological evidence from the Northridge earthquake in Los Angeles in the year of 1994, showed that more than half of all immediate death cases were due to sudden death, and not due to injuries: there was a significant high number of sudden cardiac deaths on the day of the quake, comparatively with the following days of the traumatic events. Death records show that sudden cardiac deaths were five times greater than those expected on the day of the quake (Mitterman *et al.*, 1995). Emotional distress and its outcome mainly psychophysical stress were found to be a cause behind their sudden coronary troubles deaths.

Pessimism/Explanatory Style

Peterson, Seligman and Valliant (1988) showed the relevance of pessimism to general physical health. These investigators construed pessimism as an explanatory or attributional style, a way of accounting for negative events in one's life, and pessimists as people who explain negative events as being due to stable, enduring and global factors in themselves rather than as incidents resulting from chance or external causes. To put it more briefly, there are three dimensions of explanatory style: stability versus instability, globality versus specificity, and internality versus externality.

Explanatory style emerged from the reformulation of the learned helplessness model as a way of accounting for the diversity of people's responses to uncontrollable bad events (Abramson *et al.*, 1978). Explanatory style is a prime candidate as a psychological precursor of good or bad health because it affects the severity of deficits following uncontrollable aversive events (Peterson & Seligman, 1984a).

Research with human subjects suggests that individuals who explain bad events pessimistically have poor immune function, depression, poor problem solving, low self-esteem and higher morbidity (Kamen, Rodin & Seligman, 1987; Maier & Seligman, 1976; Peterson, 1988; Seligman, 1975), and over a one year span, make more doctors visits than do individuals who explain bad events optimistically (Peterson, 1988). Peterson *et al.* (1988) found that a pessimistic explanatory style predicted poor health at ages 45 through 60, even when physical and mental health at age 25 were controlled. Pessimism in early adulthood appears to be a risk factor for poor health in middle and late adulthood. Pessimists may fail to seek medical advice at the appropriate time, may experience more negative life events due to relative inability to maintain relationships, or may display poorer health-related behaviours (Lin & Peterson, 1990). Kamen-Siegel, Rodin, Saligman & Doyer (1991) have shown that a pessimistic explanatory style is associated with poor immune function in elderly men and women, suggesting that resistance to infection may be compromised.

Conclusions

From this literature, it can be concluded that personality and behaviour patterns are resources which do have an impact on physical health. Influence of cardiovascular disease was significantly associated with personality and behaviour patterns (Type A behaviour, unpleasant emotions—anger, depression, hostility – stress, irrational thinking, and pessimism/ explanatory style). It remains to be resolved whether particular personality or behaviour patterns have specific relationships with specific disorders (*e.g.*, coronary artery disease, hypertension etc.) or whether the associations relate to general vulnerability.

REFERENCES

Abramson, L.Y., Seligman, M.E.P. & Teasdale, J.D. (1978). Learned helplessness in people : Critique and reformulation, *Journal of Abnormal Psychology, 87,* 49-74.

Alexander, F. (1950). *Psychosomatic Medicine,* New York, Norton.

Anda, R.F., Williamson, D.F., Jones, D., Macera, C., Eaker, E., Glassman, A.H. & Marks, J. (1993). Depressed affect, hopelessness, and the risk of ischemic heart-disease to cohort of US adults, *Epidemiology, 4,* 285-294.

Appels, A. & Mulder, P. (1988). Excess fatigue as a precursor of myocardial infarction, *European Heart Journal, 9,* 758-764.

Appels, A. & Mulder, P. (1989). Fatigue and heart disease. The association between "vital exhaustion" and past, present and future coronary heart disease, *Journal of Psychosomatic Research, 33,* 727-738.

Appels, A., Mulder, P., Van't Hop, M., Jenkins, C.D., Van Houten, J. & Tan, F. (1987). A prospective study of the Jenkins Activity Survey as a risk indicator for Coronary heart disease in the Netherlands, *Journal of Chronic Disease, 40,* 959-965.

Berkowitz, L. (1962). *Aggression : A Social Psychological Analysis,* McGraw Hill.

Booth-Kewley, S. & Friedman, H.S. (1997). Psychological predictors of heart disease : A quantitative review, *Psychological Bulletin, 101,* 343-362.

Buss, A.H. (1961). *The Psychology of Aggression,* John Wiley.

Davidoff, L.L. (1987). *Introduction to Psychology,* McGraw Hill Book Company.

Davison, G.C., & Neale, J.M. (1994). *Abnormal Psychology,* New York : John Wiley & Sons., Inc.

Dembroski, T.M., & Costa, P.T. (1987). Coronary-prone behaviour : Components of the Type—A pattern and hostility, *Journal of Personality, 55,* 211-235.

Dembroski, T.M., MacDougall, J.M., Costa, P.F., & Grandits, G.A. (1989). Components of hostility as predictors of sudden death and myocardial infarction in the Multiple Risk Factor Intervention Trial, *Psychosomatic Medicine, 51,* 514-522.

Eaker, E.D., Abbott, R.D., & Kannel, W.B. (1989). Frequency of uncomplicated angina pectoris in Type A compared with Type B persons, *American Journal of Cardiology, 63,* 1042-1045.

Ellis, A. (1962). *Reason and Emotion in Psychotherapy,* New York : Lyle Stuart.

Feshback, S. (1986). Reconceptualizations of anger : some research perspectives, *Journal of Social and Clinical Psychology, 4,* 123-132.

Folklow, B. (1993). Physiological organization of neurohormonal responses to psychological stimuli : Implications for health and disease, *Annals of Behavioural Medicine, 15,* 236-244.

Frasure-Smith, N., Lesperance, F. & Talajic, M. (1993). Depression following myocardial infarction: Impact-onto-month survival, *JAMA, 270,* 1819-1825.

Fredrikson, M., Lundberg, U. & Tusmisto, M. (1991). Serum Lipid Levels and cardiovascular reactivity, *Journal of Psychophysiology, 5,* 89-95.

Freeman, L.J., Nixon, P. & Reavelay, D. (1987). Psychological stress and silent-myocardial ischemia. *American Heart Journal, 114,* 4477-4482.

Friedman, H.S. & Booth-Kewley, S. (1987). The 'disease-prone personality' : A meta-analytic view of the construct, *American Psychologist, 42*, 539-555.

Friedman, M. & Rosenman, R.M. (1974). *Type A Behaviour and Your Heart*, New York : Knoff.

Fukunishi, I., Hattori, M., Nakamura, H. & Nakagama, T. (1995). Hostility is related to narcissism controlling for social desirability : Studies of college students and patients with myocardial infarction, *Journal of Psychosomatic Research, 39,* 215-220.

Gentry, W.D., Chesney, A.P., Gary, H.G., Hall, R.P. & Harburg, E. (1982). Habitual anger-coping style : Effect of mean blood pressure and risk for essential hypertension, *Psychosomatic Medicine, 44,* 195-202.

Glaser, R. & Kiecott-Glaser, J.K. (Eds.) (1994). *Handbook of Human Stress and Immunity,* San Diego : Academic.

Gold, A. & Johnston, D.W., (1990). Does anger relate to hypertension and heart disease. In P. Bennett, D. Spurgesn and J. Weinman (Eds.), *Current Developments in Health Psychology,* London : Harmsod.

Grace, W.J. & Graham, D.T. (1952). Relationship of specific attitudes and emotions to certain bodily disease, *Psychosomatic Medicine, 14,* 243-251.

Haaga, D.A. (1987). Treatment of the Type A behaviour pattern, *Clinical Psychology Review, 7,* 557-574.

Haaga, D.A. & Davison, G.C. (1989). Outcome studies of rational-emotive therapy. In M.E., Bernard, and R. DiGiuseppe (Eds.), *Inside rational-emotive therapy,* New York : Academic Press.

Hance, M., Carney, R.M., Freedlamd, K.E. & Skala, J. (1996). Depression in patients with coronary heart-disease : A 12 months follow-up, *Journal of Hospital Psychiatry, 18,* 61-65.

Hecker, M.H.L., Chesney, M., Black, G.W. & Frautsch, N. (1988). Coronary-prone behaviour in the western collaborative group study, *Psychosomatic Medicine, 50,* 153-164.

Hedman, A., Hjemdahl, P., Nordlander, R. & Astrom, H. (1990). Effects of mental and physical stress on central haemodynamics and cardiac sympathetic nerve activity during QT internal-sensing rate-responsive and fixed rate ventricular inhibited pacing, *European Heart Journal, 11,* 903-915.

Helmers, K.F., Krantz, D.S., Howell, R.H., Klein, J., *et al.*, (1993). Hostility and myocardial ischemia in coronary artery disease patients : Evaluation by gender and ischemic index, *Psychosomatic Medicine, 55,* 29-36.

Jenkins, C.D. (1983). Psychosocial and behavioural factors. In N.M. Kaplan, and J. Stamler, (Eds.), *Prevention of Coronary Heart Disease : Practical Management of the Risk Factors,* Philadelphia, PA : Sanders.

Jenkins, C.D., Zyzanski, S.J., Rosenman, R.H., *et al.* (1976). Risk of new myocardial infarction in middle aged men with manifest coronary heart disease, *Circulation, 53,* 342-347.

Johnson, E.H., Gentry, W.D. & Julius, S. (Eds.) (1992). *Personality, Elevated Blood Pressure and Essential Hypertension,* Washington : Hemisphere.

Kamen, L.P., Rodin, J. & Seligman, M.E.P. (1987). Explanatory style and immune functioning. Unpublished Manuscript, Philadelphia : University of Pennsylvania.

Kamen-Siegel, L., Rodin, J., Seligaman, M.E.P. & Doyer, J. (1991). Explanatory style and cell-mediated immunity in elderly men and women, *Health Psychology, 10,* 229-235.

Kaufman, M. (1970). Underground exciting to gold, *New York Times, March 23.*

Krantz, D.S., Contrada, R.J., Hill, D.R. & Friedler, E. (1988). Environmental stress and behavioural antecedents of coronary heart disease, *Journal of Consulting and Clinical Psychology, 56,* 333-341.

Lin, E.H. & Peterson, C. (1990). Pessimistic explanatory style and response to illness, *Behaviour Research and Therapy, 28,* 243-248.

Linden, W. (1991). What do arithmetic stress tests measure? Protocol variations and cardiovascular responses, *Psychopathology, 28,* 91-102.

Lovallo, W.R., Pincomb, G.A. & Wilson, M.F. (1986). Predicting response to a reaction time task : Heart rate reactivity compared with Type A behaviour, *Psychophysiology, 23,* 648-656.

Lovallo, W.R., Wilson, M.F., Pincomb, G.A., Edwards, G.L., Tompkins, P. & Brackett, D. (1985). Activation patterns to aversive stimulation in man : Passive exposure versus effort to control, *Psychophysiology, 22,* 283-291.

Maier, S.F. & Seligman, M.E.P., (1976). Learned helplessness : Theory and evidence, *Journal of Experimental Psychology, 105,* 3-45.

Matthews, K.A., Haynes, S.G. (1986). Type A behaviour pattern and coronary disease risk : update and critical evaluation, *American Journal of Epidemiology, 123,* 923-960.

Miller, T.Q., Turner, C.W., Tindale, R.S., Posavac, E.J. & Dugoni, B.L. (1991). Reasons for the trend towards null findings in research on Type A behaviour, *Psychological Bulletin, 110,* 469-485.

Mitterman, M.A., Maclure, M., Sherwood, J.B., Murray, R.P., Tofler, G.H., Jacobs, S.C., Friedman, R., Bemson, H. & Muller, J.E. (1995). Triggering of acute myocardial infarction onset by episodes of anger, *Circulation, 92,* 1720-1725.

Morris, P.L.P., Robinson, R.G., Andrzejenski, P., Samuels, J., & Price, T.R. (1993). Association of depression with 10 year post-stroke mortality, *American Journal of Psychiatry, 150,* 124-129.

Morris, P.L.P., Robinson, R.G., & Samuels, J. (1993). Depression, introversion and mortality following stroke, *Australian-Newzealand Journal of Psychiatry, 27,* 443-449.

Norton, B. & Whalley, L.J. (1984). Mortality of lithium-treated population, *British Journal of Psychiatry, 195,* 277-282.

Peterson, C. (1988). Explanatory style as a risk factor for illness, *Cognitive Therapy and Research, 12,* 119-132.

Peterson, C. & Seligman, M.E.P. (1984). Causal explanations as a risk factor for depression: Theory and evidence, *Psychological Review, 91,* 347 = 374.

Peterson, C., Seligman, M.E.P. & Vaillant, G.E. (1988). Pessimistic explanatory style is a risk factor for physical illness : A thirty-five year longitudinal study, *Journal of Personality and Social Psychology, 55,* 23-27.

Pope, M.K. & Smith, T.W., (1991). Corticosecretion in high and low cynically hostile men, *Psychosomatic Medicine. 53,* 386-392.

Rabins, P.V., Harris, K. & Koven, S. (1985). High fatality rates of lute-life depression associated with cardiovascular disease, *Journal of Affective Disorders, 9,* 165-167.

Rubin, T.I. (1969). *The Angry Book,* New York : Macmillan.

Schleifer, S.J., Macari-Hinson, M.M., Coyle, D.A., Slater, W.R., Kahn, M., Gorlin, R. & Zucker, H.D. (1989). The nature and course of depression following myocardial infarction, *Archives International Medicine, 149,* 1785-1789.

Seligman, M.E.P. (1975). *Helplessness : On Depression, Development, and Death,* San Francisco : freeman.

Selye, H. (1936). Thymus and adrenals in the responses of the organism to injuries and intoxicants, *British Journal of Experimental Psychology, 17,* 234-248.

Sharma, R. & Marker, H.R., (1994). Mortality in affective disorder, *Journal of Affective Disorders, 31,* 91-96.

Shekelle, R.B. Hulley, S.B., Neaton, J.D., Billings, J.H., Borhani, N.O., Gerace, T.A., Jacobs, D.R., Lasser, N.L., Mittlemark, M.B., Stamler, J. (1985). The MRFIT behaviour pattern study II, Type A behaviour and incidence of coronary heart disease, *American Journal of Epidemiology, 122,* 559-570.

Smith, O.A. & Devitto, J.L. (1984). Central neural integration for the control of autonomic responses associated with emotion, *Annual Review of Neurosciences, 7,* 43-65.

Smith, T.W. (1992). Hostility and health : Current status of a psychosomatic hypothesis, *Health Psychology, 11,* 139-150.

Smith, T.W. & Pope, M.K. (1990). Cynical hostility as a health risk : Current status and future directions, *Journal of Social Behaviour and Personality, 5,* 77-88.

Spielberger, C.D., Johnson, E.H., Rissel, S.F., Crane, R.J. & Wordon, T.J. (1985). The experience and expression of anger. In M.A. Chesney. & R.H. Rosenman (Eds.), *Anger and Hostility in Cardiovascular and Behavioural Disorders,* New York, Hemisphere.

Stevens, J.A., Turner, C.W., Rhodewatt, F. & Talbot, S. (1984). The Type A behaviour pattern and carotid artery atherosclerosis, *Psychosomatic Medicine, 46,* 105-113.

Sword, R.O. (1977). The depression prone personality : Almost "too good" to be true, *Dental Survey, 53,* 12.

Tyber's *Cyclopedic Medical Dictionary* (16th Edition) (1989). Philadelphia : F.A. Davis Company.

Tsuang, M.T., Woolson, R.F., & Fleming, J.A. (1980). Premature deaths in schizophrenia and affective disorders : An analysis of survival curves and variables affecting the shortened survival, *Archives General Psychiatry, 37,* 979-983.

Webster's *Ninth New Collegiate Dictionary (Next Digital Edition),* (1988), Springfield, MA : Merriam-Webster.

Weeke, A. (1979). Causes of deaths in manic-depressive. In M. Schsu. & E. Stromgren, E. (Eds.), *Origin, Prevention and Treatment of Affective Disorders,* London : Academic Press.

Weekes, B.S. & Waterhouse, I.K. (1991). Hostile attitudes and the coronary prone personality, *Australian Psychologists, 26,* 33-36.

Weeke, A., Juel, K., & Vaeth, M. (1987). Cardiovascular death and manic-depressive psychosis, *Journal of Affective Disorders,* 287-292.

Wood, C. (1986). The hostile heart, *Psychology Today, 20,* 10-12.

34

Slackening Memory in Elderly : Alarming Signal of Alzheimer's Disease

I.S. Muhar & N.R. Sharma***

India is one of those developing countries where the average life span used to be markedly less than the Western world. During the post independent era, the country made significant improvements particularly in her per capita income, literacy rate, healthcare services apart from an overall prosperity. The better medical care led to the eradication of certain diseases like small pox and the control of many other fatal diseases leading to reduced mortality rate and enhancement in the average span of life. The percentage of 60+ population has gone up although it is still lower than the Western figure. We now have a sizeable number of people above 60 years of age as revealed by the latest census report. The Government of India recognizes all people of 65 years and above as Senior Citizens who are entitled for marginal special benefits but nothing compared to the Social Security cover provided to them by the developed countries. Currently there are about 76 million senior citizens in the country and the figure is likely to jump to 100 million by 2013. The country is not adequately equipped to look after their special health needs. Some of the age related diseases are new to our health caring agencies. In fact, Gerontology is still in its infancy in this country. It is thus not surprising that the overall awareness of old age diseases like Alzheimer's Disease(AD) is extremely low.

Alzheimer's Disease named after the German Psychiatrist who first described it in 1906 is a progressive brain disorder that causes a gradual and irreversible decline in memory, language skills, perception of time and space and ultimately to care for oneself. The onset of the disease is usually so gradual that even the immediate family members fail to notice it. The early symptoms consist of forgetting of recent events like placing of keys, forgetting names, failing to remember as to how many chapatties he/she has already taken. The most

*Formerly Professor of Psychology and Director, Distance Education, M.D. University, Rohtak. Present address: #518, Sector: 10-D, Chandigarh 160011.
E-mail: "inderjitm@yahoo.com"
**Reader Department of Psychology, M.D. University, Rohtak.

recent thing done by a patient is usually forgotten. Sometimes the patient after taking an afternoon nap fails to decide whether it is night or morning, the day and date also start troubling him. The most common routine activities which were of least concern become difficult, confusing and demanding. The workmanship in ordinary household activities like pressing of clothes, cutting vegetables, making chappaties show decline.

It is not unusual of the person to keep on asking the same question again and again or repeating the same story word by word, appearing to be in a confused, restless and bewildered state. Getting lost even in familiar surroundings is also seen in some patients. There is emotional blunting and loss of intelligence. The usual initiative or zeal in doing things in time is gone. In other words AD is not simply forgetfulness although it may start that way. It seriously impairs a person's ability to carry out daily activities like dressing, feeding oneself or recognizing one's close loved ones as happened with the late former President Reagon who could not recognize even his wife Nancy in the later stage of his Alzheimer's.

The fall in the overall efficiency, sociability, degree of involvement in work and hobbies, difficulty in finding appropriate words while communicating could be noticed by an aware and alert family member but is generally missed in view of the age of the patient as these indicators start appearing from 65 years onwards and then get intensified with the passage of time. In the meantime the Long Term Memory remains relatively unaffected leading to an innocent acceptance of the critical but subtle changes and decline as normal ageing process thus missing a golden opportunity of an early diagnosis of the disease. It has been most appropriately labeled as a memory robbing disease or incurable brain wasting disease.

Raburn, a geriatric neurologist at the Texas Tech School of Pharmacy said that "Alzheimer's is a graceful failure of the (brain) system and it takes a long time for it to occur. The disease can be in the brain up to 30 years before it becomes apparent." With Alzheimer's neurons are damaged and lose their ability to send signals. The temporal lobe, which is responsible for memory, language and regulating emotions, is heavily affected by the disease. The three phases of the disease, go from the initial stage, which often can't be detected, to mild cognitive impairment and, finally to full-blown Alzheimer's.

Incidence

Age is the major risk factor for Alzheimer's disease. It is the most common cause of dementia in people over 65 years. About 10% of Americans over 65 are affected with AD; of that age 85 or older, the incidence increases to 50%. The Indian Alzheimer's Society on the other hand, detected only 1 AD case out of 1000 in below 65 years age. This number increased to 4-5 in 65+ age group. By 80, the incidence increased to 1 out of every 5. Although the statistics don't tally but the trend is the same – with advancing age the rate of AD also increases.

Symptoms

As mentioned above, AD patients have two distinct set of symptoms: Cognitive (memory loss, disorientation, confusion, difficulty with reasoned thought) and Behavioural (agitation/anxiety, delusions/hallucinations, depression, insomnia and wandering). The severity of symptoms increases with time.

Etiology

The short answer is we do not know. It may be combination of factors : some we are born with, some in our environment and some which happen to us. Things that more likely lead to AD are known as risk factors and age is definitely one of the important ones.

AD is characterized by progressive destruction and death of nerve cells in the brain. Most Alzheimer's researchers believe that the cause of the disease is the accumulation of sticky plaques made of "amyloid beta" proteins in the brain. This is what has been known as amyloid hypothesis. Alzheimer's research during the past two decades had almost taken for granted the existence of this hypothesis since there was no challenge to it although conclusive evidence is still lacking. The defenders argued that these sticky plaques lead to shrinkage or atrophy in certain regions of the brain and a decrease in chemicals called neurotransmitters that ferry important messages between nerve cells. The result of these cell and chemical losses is a steady decline in mental functioning.

For the first time neurobiologists—Bishop and Robinson (2003) of Australia's Monash University found that when they injected the notorious protein called beta-amyloid into the brains of adult rats, the results were not exactly what the dominant theory had predicted. They suffered no more cell death than brains injected with innocuous salt water. Bishop concludes "amyloid is not likely to be directly responsible for the neuro degeneration" that causes Alzheimer's. Instead, according to evidence she and others have collected, "amyloid is either an innocent bystander in Alzheimer's or is a protector of brain under assault from toxic compounds". Kelleher (2004) remarks that when you compare one Alzheimer's brain with another, for example, there is only a weak correlation between amyloid plaques and loss of neurons, degree of dementia or synaptic loss. In his opinion amyloid "is the poorest correlate of the pattern and severity of Alzheimer's". Removing it won't help an Alzheimer's brain.

Kelly and his research colleagues at the Scripps Research Institute (2004) have proposed a new theory about the cause of Alzheimer's disease. According to their hypothesis, the disease arises as a consequence of inflammation, which creates abnormal metabolites out of normal brain molecules. These abnormal metabolites then modify "amyloid beta" proteins in the brain and cause them to misfold. Misfolded amyloid beta proteins are thought to be a major player in Alzheimer's disease. The inflammation process that creates these metabolites can be triggered by numerous stimuli, including infections that precede the onset of Alzheimer's disease by a significant amount of time – perhaps years. The findings are being published in the forthcoming issue of the Journal—Proceedings of the National Academy of Sciences.

In view of the disease's devastating effect, its high incidence in elderly population and the manifold increase in American research grants as a result of its President's AD, a large number of researcher's got involved in attempts to strike at a breakthrough in its etiology. Twenty years back hardly 250 research papers were published on Alzheimer's disease and dementia throughout the world. As per the figures quoted by the Alzheimer's Association (2003), 3700 delegates from 78 countries attended the Dementia Research Conference in Sweden and more than 3000 research articles have been already published. The 9th International Conference on Alzheimer's Disease and Related Disorders in July 2004 was attended by above 5000 researchers. Special mention may be made of two research findings which are likely to be published in 2004.

Researchers led by Balln working at the Philadelphia College of Osteopathic Medicine's Center for the Study of Chronic diseases of Ageing had discovered in 1998 the presence of Chlamydia pneuomoniae in 90 percent of brains taken from individuals who had suffered from Alzheimer's Disease. Their latest work published in the April 2004 issue of Neurobiology of Aging shows that when this bacteria is sprayed into the noses of mice not predisposed to amyloid plaques can cause progressive deposition of amyloid plaques, thus creating a partial model of Alzheimer's Disease.

Klein and his team working at the Northwestern University (2004) found that patients with Alzheimer's disease have up to 70 times more a toxic protein ("amyloid b-derived diffusible ligands" (ADDLs). Klein said "if we can develop drugs that target and neutralize these neurotoxins, it might be possible to not only slow down memory loss, but to actually reverse it, to bring memory function back to normal"

There is still no scientific evidence of risk from cooking in aluminum utensils or from drinking tea which has traces of aluminum or use of mobile phones.

Diagnostic Process

Rahimi (2004) said that "we don't want to have mass hysteria of everyone who forgets their keys wanting to get tested for Alzheimer's. But if it starts causing a problem, obstructing their daily living then that person needs to be evaluated."

The Alzheimer's Association based at Chicago (1996) has discussed the various steps involved in the process. Some of the main components of the procedure are summarized below :

Compilation of the Case History

Relevant information is gathered from the patient and a close member of the family individually. It includes known medical history, the various symptoms which brought the patient to the doctor. In order to have a rough evaluation of the mental status the person's sense of time and place, ability to understand, remember, talk and do simple calculations is assessed. The patient may be asked questions like : what is your name? Where do you live and its address? What did you eat in the dinner last night? Who is the present Prime Minister of the country? What year is it? Which day of the week it is? The person is also asked to do simple mental exercises, such as spelling a word backwards, writing a sentence or copying a drawing. The information given by the person may be later on cross checked separately from the family member. If necessary the person is referred to a Psychologist for Psychometric evaluation.

Psychometric Testing

In the process he is administered tests of memory, span of attention, intelligence, personality, cognitive functioning, emotional maturity, speed and dexterity etc. The testing is time consuming and is spread over different sessions and days so as to eliminate the effect of fatigue and boredom. The obtained scores are interpreted in terms of the standardized norms for the particular age and sex and a report prepared highlighting problem areas if any.

Physical and Neurological Examinations

They are useful in ruling out other contributory factors to the problem.

Pathology Laboratory Tests and Scans

Apart from routine blood tests special attention need to be given to test vitamin B-12 and thyroid hormone levels in the blood. Deficiency of vitamin B-12, hyper and hypo thyroid functioning are well recognized for causing dementia like symptoms. Fortunately their effect is reversible if recognized in time. The doctor may also advise some of the following scans to see structural changes in the brain : CT(computerized tomography), MRI (magnetic resonance imaging), PET (positron emission tomography) or SPECT (single proton emission computed tomography). PET shows how different areas of the brain respond when the patient is asked to perform different activities while SPECT shows the circulation of blood in certain regions of the brain and is useful in evaluating brain functions. It might indicate abnormalities that are signs of AD.

A natural question which comes to one's mind at this stage is whether we can arrive at the diagnosis on the basis of such sophisticated scans alone. A good answer has been provided by Jagust (2003) of the University of California, Davis. He elaborates that the utility of these scans may be best understood if we think of a scan as a piece of puzzle. If a person with memory problems gets a brain scan but receives no other assessment, a doctor cannot state accurately whether this person has Alzheimer's. When images of the brain are combined with other diagnostic information, or other pieces of the puzzle, the doctor may then be able to put together a more comprehensive picture of what's happening in the brain. It is thus unlikely that any imaging method would entirely replace a thorough diagnostic assessment. Raburn strongly feels that "the heart and soul of the evaluation is the history." The person may not notice any changes but a family member sees behaviour changes and knows what the patient no longer can do.

In spite of the above mentioned exhaustive diagnostic procedure, it may be clarified that the diagnosis arrived at would at best be only tentative which may be 80 to 90% accurate in life. A conclusive diagnosis of AD can only be made by direct examination of the patient's brain for characteristic plaques and tangles after death in an autopsy.

Treatment

There is no cure, no known way to prevent the illness and the benefits of current treatments are modest at best. Discovering it early may give the patient a better quality of life. Research workers throughout the world are actively engaged in unraveling the mystery of this fatal disease. Once the etiology is understood, it may be possible to come out with effective drugs which either prevent or cure the disease. The recent finding of Balln (2004) linking a common bacteria (Chlamydia pneumoniae) with Alzheimer's disease has been already referred to earlier in this paper. At present there is no option but to rely on the limited number of drugs like Donepezil and Rivastigmine which have been in use for less than a decade. These drugs supposedly attempt to slow the progression of the disease by maintaining levels of critical message sending neurotransmitters in the brain. They at best help in a better management of the patients. Relatively recent agent-Galantamine which is an extract from the snowdrop and daffodil plants is regarded as the best agent for restoring memory. It is superior to Donepezil and Rivastigmine as it has the unique ability to increase the receptiveness of nicotinic receptors to acetylcholine. Galantamine is still not available in India. Another drug-Namenda, which works on different neurotransmitter, was approved by US Health Authorities last year to be used for moderate to severe patients. Grady (2004) feels that these drugs are designed to aid thinking and memory, but they do not change the underlying course of the illness. Moreover they do not help every one, and when they do help, even their strongest fans agree, the effect is usually modest. In a research meeting on Alzheimer's drugs at John Hopkins University held recently one of the experts commented that there was just one chance in 10 that the drugs would have an effect, and that patients should try them for six to eight weeks and then quit if there was no improvement. There is, however, a word of caution in this connection from researchers like Raburn. In her opinion no drug can completely halt the progression of the disease. The mistake some caretakers make is stopping the use of a drug when it no longer seems to be working. "When the drugs are stopped and out of the system, that person's functioning will deteriorate, she said "They crash." She further comments that drugs to treat Alzheimer's work best when the disease is diagnosed early. The worldwide helplessness with respect to the treatment part, however, is apparent from the fact that a former President of the United States—Ronald Reagan died of the disease in less than a decade after he announced the diagnosis in spite of the best medical aid in the World. When Reagan was first diagnosed, there were no drugs to treat the disease. Now we have a handful of approved drugs which claim modest help and dozens of drugs in the research pipeline. The World has to be indebted to Reagan for speeding up Alzheimer's research.

Kolata (2004) feels that researchers have now started looking towards a new direction. Several studies have suggested a link between Alzheimer's and cholesterol which is produced by the brain and liver. As such the administration of anti-cholesterol drugs is likely to protect one from AD. Similarly other researchers predicted that medications that reduce inflammation, a hallmark of Alzheimer's in areas of the brain where cells are dying, might prove useful. A high blood pressure could also act as a predisposing factor. Wolozin—a pharmacologist at the Loyola University Medical School in Maywood in fact examined the records of 56,790 patients at three American hospitals. It was found that those patients who were on Statins (cholesterol reducing drugs) for quite sometime had 70% less prevalence of Alzheimer's. Research on the effects of anti inflammatory and blood pressure reducing drugs on Alzheimer's Disease is in progress in many laboratories. Allen (2004) has reported two studies which claim that diabetes is linked to increased risk of Alzheimer's. It was calculated that diabetics had 65% higher risk of developing AD than nondiabetics. However, further work is needed to determine whether treating diabetes could lower the risks of Alzheimer's and cognitive decline. Lister's (2004) recent study has lent further support to the medicinal antiseptic effect of curcumin (a chemical compound extracted from turmeric) on many diseases. He has also hinted at its prophylactic property against neurodegenerative conditions such as Alzheimer's and its possible benefit for slowing down the progression of the disease. He further points out that India, which produces and consumes most of the world's turmeric, has much lower rates of Alzheimer's among the elderly than the Western countries. Lister's this corollary, however, should be accepted with a pinch of salt since the longevity in India has gone up recently and its elderly population is much smaller than the West and the statistics could be confounding and misleading.

It was known that AD shortens patient's lives but there have been few longitudinal studies lending a scientific backing. Larson (2004) of Group Health Cooperative's Center for Health Studies and the University of Washington have published a study which states that people newly diagnosed with AD survived about half as long as those of similar age. Not only this but Taylor's (2004) research shows that older caregivers have a 63 percent chance of dying prematurely—before their counterparts who don't provide care—precisely because of the stress, depression, physical strain and unrelenting responsibilities of care giving. Reagan knew that this disease puts heavy burden on the family. In fact he was so upset about it that he wrote "I only wish there was some way I could spare Nancy from painful experience."

REFERENCES

Allen, J.E. (2004). Diabetes linked to increased risk of Alzheimer's, *Los Angeles Times* (The details of the study conducted by Zoe Arvanitakis, David Bennett and their colleagues at the Rush University Medical Center, Chicago could be seen in the May 2004 issue of the *Archives of Neurology)*.

Alzheimer's and Related Disorders Society of India. (n.d.) Alzheimer's Disease, Retrieved, April 27, 2004, from http://www.alzheimerindia.org/ardsi_disel.html.

Alzheimer's Association (1996). Steps to Getting A Diagnosis : Finding out if it's Alzheimer's Disease, Retrieved, August 19, 2003, from www.alz.org.

Balln, B., *et al.* (2004). Common bacteria linked to Alzheimer's, Neurolobiology of Aging (To be published April, 2004).

Bishop, G. and Robinson, S. (2003). In Begley, S. Scientists fight a narrow view of Alzheimer's cause, *The Wall Street Journal, Retrieved April 16, 2004, from* http://www.mlive.com.

Grady, D. (2004). Alzheimer's drugs frustrate doctors (in print).

Jagust, W. (2003). Advances—Progress in Alzheimer's Research and Care, Newsletter, 22(4), Alzheimer's Association, Chicago.

Kelleher, R. (n.d). In Begley, S. (2004). Scientists fight a narrow view of Alzheimer's cause, *Associated Press.*

Kelly, J.W. *et al.* (2004). New Theory About Alzheimer's Disease, *Proceedings of the National Academy of Sciences.*

Klien, W.L. (2004). Memory Loss During Alzheimer's Reversible, *Proceedings of the National Academy of Sciences.*

Kolata, G. (2004). A Glimmer of Hope for Fading Minds, *New York Times,* Retrieved, April 14, 2004 from http://www.nytimes/2004/04/13/health/13PREV.html.

Larson, E.B., *et al.* (2004). Life expectancy after Alzheimer's diagnosis demystified, Annals of Internal Medicine.

Lister, S. (2004). Curry keeps Alzheimer's at bay, Retrieved, April 20, 2004 from *http://www.timesonline.co.uk.*

Raburn, L. (April 12, 2004). In Swan, OLP. Alzheimer's treatment works best early on, *Billing Gazette,* Retrieved, April 14, 2004 from *http://www.billingsgazette.com.*

Rahimi, A.(n.d) In Hart, A. (2004). Forgetful? How to tell if it is Alzheimer's, *Savannah Morning News,* Retrieved, April 15, 2004.

Taylor, L. (2004, April 19). Home care for Alzheimer's patients is a major health risk for caregiver spouse. *The Seattle Times,* Retrieved, April 20, 2004 from *http://seattletimes.nwsource.com/cgi-bin/PrintStory.*

35

Informative Counselling and Awareness Level of HIV/AIDS Amongst Drug Dependents

*Jitender Dahiya** & *Dinesh Kataria***

HIV is the name of a newly recognized retrovirus that causes AIDS, a body condition that slowly destroys the body's immune system. Without these important defences, a person with AIDS cannot fight off germs and cancers (Michael, Mahesh and Ravinderan, 2003).

AIDS is a worldwide epidemic. Reports say that about one-third infected are between ages of 15-24 years. Ninety-five percent of new infections are occurring in developing countries and almost 50% are women (Report on the global HIV/AIDS epidemic WHO, Geneva, 2003).

The projections of the WHO indicate that by A.D. 2010, half of the AIDS cases in the world will be from India. The total annual economic loss due to HIV/AIDS in India is estimated to be Rs. 3447 billion. The figure emphasizes the societal burden posed by HIV infection in India (Pandav, Anand, Shamanna, Chawdhury & Nath, 1997).

Although no perfect cure of AIDS have been discovered yet, some anti-HIV drugs keep HIV in check. However, unfortunately, the infected has to die. In addition, unfortunately 95% of the world's HIV infected people cannot afford these medicines (Pavri, 2000).

Behaviour associated with drug dependence is an important factor in the spread of HIV infection. Using or sharing unsterilized needles, etc., while injecting heroin, cocaine, or other drugs, leaves a drug dependent vulnerable for contracting HIV.

It has been shown that drug and alcohol use interfere with judgment about sexual and other related behaviours, making it more likely that users have unprotected sex. This places them at increased risk for contracting HIV from infected sex partners (Holmberg, 1996).

In India, drugs are often used in open public places such as the roadside, parks, playgrounds and market complexes. Generally, syringes and needles are purchased from pharmacies without any prescriptions. In fact, buying of new syringes is too expensive for many drug dependents.

*Counsellor, Distt. Red Cross Society, Rohtak.
**Assistant Professor & Head, Department of Psychiatry, Lady Harding Medical College, New Delhi.

Therefore, they tend to focus on buying the drugs rather than purchasing new injecting equipment. That's why; the sharing of equipment among India's injecting drug users (IDUs) is widespread (Reid & Costigan, 2002). Injecting drug use is also a major problem in metro cities such as Mumbai, Kolkata, Delhi and Chennai (Panda, 2001). However, the life style of drug dependents leads them to the high risk behaviour of getting HIV infection through various ways.

In relation to HIV/AIDS, counselling plays its important role in three ways, *i.e.* Preventive-counselling (awareness & information, alerting for high risk behaviour etc.), Pre-counselling (providing information to suspected persons, before bringing him/her for blood test-elisa test for HIV) and Post-counselling for sero-positives and their family members (D'Souza, 2002).

Preventive counselling is very important for all types of clients in the following way *(a)* for those seeking help because of past or current risk behaviour and planning their future, *(b)* for those not seeking help but who practise high-risk behaviour, *(c)* for those not involved in any risk behaviour currently so that they may be aware of HIV/AIDS. The goal of such counselling is to maintain low-risk behaviour where change has been practiced. Preventive counselling would include risk assessment, risk reduction counselling and information on HIV/AIDS. Counsellors function more as health educators who provide clear and simple information, clarify misinformation and assist in decision-making and implementation of behavioural changes (D'Souza, 2002).

Since, one of the authors is working in drug deaddiction centre, during his dealing with the drug dependents, it was realised that most of the incumbents were ignorant about the causes, prevention or the risk behaviours. Therefore, a need was felt to impart the informative counselling and to check if the informative counselling about HIV/AIDS could enhance the level of awareness amongst such incumbents. However, the design of the study was finalized with the following objectives.

Objectives

1. To study the effect of informative counselling on drug dependents by comparing the awareness level at the time of admission and discharge.
2. To analyze the impact of informative counselling on drug dependents on the basis of their socio-demographic profile.
3. To know whether the awareness/educative programmes/informative counselling are helpful in behaviour change in their real life.

METHOD

Design

A single group, before-after design was employed.

Sample

The study was conducted at Red Cross Drug Deaddiction Centre; Rohtak (Haryana), from August to November 2004, with the drug dependents who arrived there for seeking treatment. Initially, the study was started with 82 dependents, but 12 dependents were dropped out due to certain limitations. However, the study was completed with 70 subjects. The selection of the sample was totally restricted to the availability basis in one centre only. However, it covered the people from various places like all over Haryana, Delhi, and some from U.P. & Rajasthan. No homogeneity was considered in the sample as per their type of drug dependence, age, education and socio-economic status (SES) background.

Tools

Personal Data sheet form

"HIV/AIDS Awareness Questionnaire" by Asthana (1999) was administrated on all respondents. The questionnaire measures three major areas of the HIV/AIDS awareness.

1. Modes of HIV transmission and location of HIV in the body (24 questions).
2. Symptoms of HIV infection (12 questions).
3. Tests and protection (16 questions).

Procedure

First of all the personal data sheet form was filled up.

In the first phase of the study, the questionnaire of HIV/AIDS awareness was filled by the subjects on the first day of their indoor admission, after establishment of a proper rapport and narrating them all necessary instructions. Some of them were illiterate or were not able to understand the language so they were helped by the investigator in tick marking their answers. The subjects facing severe withdrawals were asked later to fill up their questionnaire. This process was labelled as Pre-Testing.

After this, the usual treatment was given to all the subjects. Nothing was told specifically about the questions mentioned in the questionnaire, but were regularly counselled about their drug dependent life style. Regarding the information on HIV/AIDS, relationship of drug abuse with the infection of HIV and other STDs was informed about along with the counselling. The indoor stay of the respondents varied between 3 to 4 weeks.

Then in the third phase, the respondents were tested again on the same questionnaire on the last day of their treatment. The data generated after gathering the required information, was analyzed by applying the t-test.

RESULTS AND DISCUSSION

The results of whole group of 70 drug dependents, without considering their age, education, type of drug used etc. have been shown in the result table 35.1.

Table 35.1 : Showing the Scores of Pre and Post Testing, with Their Mean, S.D., t Value & Level of Significance, of the Total Group of Drug Dependents

Scores	*Pre-testing*	*Post-testing*	*SD*	*SDe*	*t- Value*
Total	1527	2407	8.028	.96	13.10*
Mean	21.81	34.39			

* $P < 0.01$.

The above result table reveals that informative counselling given on HIV/AIDS had a significant positive impact upon their existing knowledge, and they learned a lot about HIV/AIDS from the process, because the t-value is significant at .01 level. Similar results have been obtained by various earlier studies like Wells, Hoppe, Simpson & Gillmore (1995) and

Surender, Guruswami & Verma (1997). It was found that IEC programmes increased the knowledge of subjects at all levels. Subjects who had much misconception about the mechanism involved in acquiring HIV through various routes could know about correct routes of transmission through the IEC programmes.

Lindsey (1989) and A-Owaishi; Rashed, Mohammad, Anwar & Hind (1999) found that the training was too effective for increasing the knowledge of subjects, when they analysed the pre-and post testing for HIV/AIDS awareness training. However, in the present study similar results have been obtained, that respondent's knowledge was increased through the informative counselling.

Further the whole group was divided on the basis of their socio-demographic profile *i.e.* their socio-economic status level, education, domicile, age and their type and duration of drug dependence. The first subgroup was formatted on the basis of their socio-economic status level, *i.e.* low, middle, and upper middle groups. The obtained results have been shown in result table 35.2.

Table 35.2 : Showing the Mean Scores of Pre & Post-test of Subjects along with SDe, t Values and Level of Significance of Three Groups Based on Their Socio-Economic Status Level

SES Level	*Pre-Test*	*Post-Test*	*SDe*	*t Value*
Low SES Level N=29	17.72	30.23	1.4	9.0*
Middle SES Level N=29	22.55	35.38	1.6	7.82*
Upper Middle SES Level N=12	29.92	41.92	2.27	5.92*

* $P < 0.01$.

The results reveal that all three types of SES groups benefited significantly from the process of information counselling, because the obtained t-values for low, middle, & upper middle groups are significant at .01 level. Allman (1997) found that different societies had different views on the issue of HIV/AIDS. Some of them had low awareness level while other societies showed better awareness level, but IEC programmes worked positively for all types of societies. In this study also, although at the time of pre-testing the low SES group had lesser knowledge than high SES group but as a result of Informative Counselling, knowledge level equally increased in this group.

Another classification was as per the education level. The results have been shown in the following table :

Table 35.3 : Showing the Mean Scores of Pre & Post Test of Subjects along with the SDe, t-Values and Level of Significance of the Three Sub Groups as per Their Education Level

Education Level	*Pre-Test*	*Post-Test*	*SDe*	*t Value*
Low Education Level N=37	18.14	30.08	1.4	8.37*
Middle Education Level N=20	19.75	35.60	1.55	10.21*
High Education Level N=13	35.46	44.77	1.69	5.49*

*$P \leq 0.01$.

The result table 35.3 tells about the educational distribution of the group and their learning of the subject matter as a consequence of informative counselling. Though a large proportion of respondents belonged to a low education level N= 37, but some of them were educated up to the post-graduate level or even B.A.M.S. doctors, or graduates + Diploma in pharmacy etc. (N=13). The Result table indicates that higher level of education means higher level of awareness. However, all the subgroups independent on their education level learned significantly from the informative counselling, hence the process may be helpful to all irrespective of their education level.

Result table 35.4 indicates the difference in rural and urban population.

Table 35.4 : Showing the Mean Scores of Pre & Post Test of Subjects along with the SDe, t Values and Level of Significance of the Two Sub Groups Based as per their Domicile *i.e.* Urban or Rural Background

Domicile	*Pre-Test*	*Post-Test*	*SDe*	*t Value*
Urban based N=29	23.86	37.07	1.36	9.69*
Rural based N=41	20.37	32.49	1.3	9.1*

* P ≤ 0.01.

The result table reveals that both groups belonging to urban and rural areas were benefited significantly form the process, because both t-values *i.e.* 9.69 for urban, and 9.1 for rural are significant at .01 level.

The next distribution of the group was based on their type of drug use. The statistics is described in the following result table 35.5.

Table 35.5 : Showing the Mean Scores of Pre & Post Test of Subjects along with the SDe, t-Values and Level of Significance of the Three Sub Group Based on their Type of Drug Use

Type of Drug Use	*Pre-Test*	*Post-Test*	*SDe*	*t Value*
Opium +Smack N = 36	17.58	30	1.19	10.39*
I.V. Use + Cough syp etc. N = 17	25.24	39.41	1.96	7.23*
Alcoholics N = 17	27.35	38.65	2.37	4.76*

* P < .0.1.

Though there is a large range of substances used by drug dependents but in the present study the respondents were divided into three categories as per their most preferred brand they used. These categories were as : those who used opiates *i.e.* opium or smack or both (N=36), Alcoholics, (N=17), & I.V. Users + cough syrup or others drugs like sulpha, bhang, sedative tablets etc. (N=17). The result table shows that all the obtained t-values are highly significant at .01 level. Thus all groups were benefited from the informative counselling given to them during their treatment while staying in the centre.

Duration of use could be another factor affecting the influence of counselling. Longer duration could hinder changing the attitude. The results regarding this variable have been depicted in table 35.6.

Table 35.6 : Showing the Mean Scores of Pre & Post Test of Subjects Along with the SDe, t-Values and Level of Significance of the Three Sub Groups as per their Duration of Use

Duration of Use	*Pre-Test*	*Post-Test*	*SDe*	*t Value*
In use more than 16 yrs N=13	17.85	29.77	2.01	5.93*
In use between 8 to 16 yrs N=18	23.61	35.06	2.14	5.1*
In use less than 8 yrs N=39	22.31	35.62	1.26	10.52*

* P < 0.01.

In the present table the respondents were distributed in to three groups on the bases of their involvement in drug use in terms of years. Some of them were using drugs even more than 37 years. On the other hand some patients were comparatively beginners and were using drugs just from 11-12 months. The table shows that the impact of informative counselling was significant on each group and they enhanced their knowledge of HIV/AIDS, because the obtained t-values were significant at .01 level.

The last result table, *i.e.* table 35.7 is based on the results of the group when divided age wise.

Table 35.7 : Showing the Mean Scores of Pre & Post Test of Subjects Along with the SDe, t-Values and Level of Significance of Three Sub Groups as per their Age Level

Age Level	*Pre-Test*	*Post-Test*	*SDe*	*t Value*
Younger Age Group, *i.e.* 18-24 N=14	29.21	40.36	1.59	7.01*
Middle Age group, *i.e.* 29-40 N=31	22.16	35	1.65	7.78*
Elder Age group, *i.e.* 41-64 N=25	17.24	30.28	1.42	9.17*

* P < 0.01.

The first glance of the result table tells that younger age group already had better awareness but the elder age group had lesser awareness of the subject matter because the obtained mean value of pre-testing of younger group was the highest and the mean value of pre-testing of the elder group was the lowest. But the informative counselling worked equally for all the groups because all the t-values, *i.e.*, 7.01, 7.78, & 9.17 respectively for younger, middle and elder age groups were significant at .01 level, which means each group irrespective of their age level was benefited from the process.

Some earlier studies indicate that having knowledge is not the guarantee of behaviour change in practical life. Gupta, Mathur, Singh, Saxena & Saxena, (2004) in their study found a low correlation between actual knowledge and its implication for health. However, it is important to understand that information & awareness is the minimal necessary condition & requirement for bringing any change in the attitudes. Therefore, authors felt a need for evolving information, education, and communication strategies to focus on raising awareness on HIV/AIDS.

Although, it is clear that education/awareness programmes are essential to control the spread of HIV. Studies have proved that early, large-scale and focused prevention programmes can reduce infection rates in high-risk groups and the risk of spread of HIV among the wider population. An excellent example is Thailand, where prevention efforts have probably averted millions of HIV infections. Cambodia is another example where preventive measures have been effective. Strategies to prevent HIV transmission should remain a priority in combating HIV/AIDS (Michael, *et al.* 2003). This study is also an attempt in the same direction, *i.e.* to bring an improvement in the awareness of the people about HIV/AIDS so as to prevent the Indian population from this deadly disease. And the most positive conclusion is that the information counselling enhanced the knowledge of every type of group taken as a diverse population for the study. This means that informative counselling can prove to be a highly relevant tool to prevent the HIV/AIDS in India.

REFERENCES

Allman, D. (1997). *Concepts, Definitions and Models for Community Based HIV Prevention Research in Canada, and a Planning Guide for the Development of Community-Based Prevention Research,* HIV Social, Behavioural and Epidemiological Studies Unit, Faculty of Medicine, University of Toronto.

A-Owaishi, Rashed, M., Mohammad, A.A, Anwar, S., & Hind, S. H. (1999). Knowledge, attitude beliefs and practices about HIV/AIDS in Kuwait, *AIDS Education & Prevention, 11,* 163-173.

Asthana, M. (1999). *Manual for AIDS Awareness Questionnaire,* Rupa Psychological Centre, Varanasi.

D'Souza, B. (2002). *STD and HIV/AIDS Counselling,* chapter 1st in Thomas, G. (Ed.) Counselling on HIV and Family Matter-AFE-06, IGNOU : N. Delhi.

Gupta, N., Mathur.; Singh, A.K.; Saxena, M.P. & Saxena, N.C. (2004). Reproductive Health Awareness of school-going, unmarried, rural adolescents, *The Indian Journal of Paediatric, 71,* 797-801.

Holmberg, S.D. (1996). The estimated prevalence and incidence of HIV in 96 large U.S. Metropolitan areas, *American Journal of Public Health, 86,* 642-654.

Lindsey (1989). Knowledge and Beliefs about AIDS and AIDS Prevention, *International Dissertation Abstract, 10,* 235-239.

Michael, P.J., Mahesh, G., Ravinderan, G.D. (2003). *Global and National Scenario of HIV/AIDS,* chapter 1st. In Ravinderan, G.D. (Ed.) Basics of HIV/AIDS – AFE-01: IGNOU, N. Delhi.

Panda (2001). Interference between Drug use and Sex work in Manipur, *National Medical Journal of India, 14,* 209-211.

Pandav, C.S., Anand, K., Shamanna, B.R., Chawdhury, S., & Nath, L.M. (1997). Economic consequences of HIV/AIDS in India, *National Medical Journal of India, 10,* 27-30.

Pavri, K.M. (2002). *Challenges of AIDS,* National Book Trust India, Delhi.

Reid G. & Costigan G. (2002). *Revisiting the Hidden Epidemic : A Situation Assessment of Drug Use in Asia in the Context of HIV/AIDS,* The Centre for Harm reduction, The Burnet Institute, Australia.

Surender, S., Guruswami, M. & Verma, R.K. (1997). Knowledge and attitudes of school children about HIV/AIDS : Evidence from rural Maharashtra, *The Indian Journal of Social Work, 58,* 599-615.

Wells, E.A., Hoppe, M.J., Simpson, E.E. & Gillmore, M.R. (1995). Misconceptions about AIDS among children, who can identify the major routes of HIV transmission, *Journal of Paediatric Psychology, 20,* 671-676.

36

Neurotic Tendency in Women Sexually Abused in Childhood

Nazirul Hasnain* & Divya Kumar**

The term "neurotic" is used to define the behaviour of an individual who cannot manage effectively with stressful circumstances. "Neurotic" would define the individual who would have serious difficulty in coping with many normal "everyday" pressures. But, behaviours defined as neurotic would not necessarily reflect pathological constructions in the personality. Neuroticism implies neurotic tendency in individuals rather than a disorder in itself. It may differ from individual to individual in quantity. People who show emotional instability, anxiety, apprehensions, immaturity, submissiveness, and tender-mindedness-like characteristics are said to be possessing neuroticism. These people may or may not be suffering from any classified neurotic disorder, say, phobia, hysteria, obsessive – compulsive behaviour etc., but essentially have a tendency towards being neurotic.

Just as everyone is at times anxious, so everyone at times uses defenses, and the use of one or other of these defenses can only be regarded as neurotic if it becomes habitual and is resorted to under circumstances in which there is no need to use defenses at all, or in which it would be more appropriate or more efficient to use some other defense. The person who always tries to master situations obsessionally, who always avoids dangers, or who always submits to others, is behaving neurotically since his behaviour ceased to be spontaneous and becomes subject to restrictions which limit his enjoyment and self development. Wolpe (1958) defines neurotic behaviour as the behaviour acquired in anxiety generating situation and suggesting that the core of neurotic behaviour lies not in any particular behaviour or motor activity, but in anxiety itself, which is usually the central constituent of neuroses and is always present in the causal situations. Neurotic behaviour according to Eysenck (1957), is learned and not due to injury or lesions, is maladaptive and involves strong emotions, particularly anxiety. According to Freud, all neurotic symptoms are secondary and superficial.

*Professor, Dept. of Psychology, Jamia Millia Islamia, New Delhi, 110025.
**Department of Psychology, Jamia Millia Islamia, New Delhi, 110025.

Neurotic behaviours develop due to psychological and interpersonal causal factors. They predispose an individual to develop specific maladaptive behaviours. The factors of anxiety—defence, faulty—learning, blocked personal growth, pathogenic interpersonal relationships, and socio-cultural environment determine the development of neurotic patterns in behaviour (Carson and Butcher, 1992).

A number of theories of personality identify dimensions or traits of personality in terms of emotions. Eysenck (1961) has proposed three fundamental dimensions of personality : extroversion-introversion, neuroticism, and psychoticism. Extroversion- introversion includes the traits of sociability which can also be related to emotion (*e.g.*, interest as expressed toward people vs. shyness). Neuroticism includes emotionally defined non-specific negative emotional responsiveness. Psychoticism may represent emotions gone awry or the absence of emotions appropriate to circumstances. Neuroticism varies along a continuum and degree, hence everyone has neurotic tendency to a lesser, moderate or a high degree. Eysenck's studies have offered a substantial support for the view that there are two separate and independent dimensions of neuroticism and psychoticism, both of which could be regarded continuous with normality.

Child sexual abuse by nature is threatening and disruptive, hence, the victims of such maltreatment are prone to feelings of anxiety, even well after the abuse has transpired. Based upon childhood experiences of sexual abuse, significant number of adult abuse survivors appears to associate relationships with maltreatment. As a result, they may accept some level of aggression in intimate relationships as normal or appropriate. Women in the latter group may be prone to sexual or physical victimization by others, perhaps especially in sexual or romantic relationships (McCord, 1985; Runtz, 1987; Russel, 1986). When a child is sexually abused, the perpetrator has complete power on the victim and uses it to harm him/her. The victim learns that not having power and control can mean danger and hurt. After being abused, the survivors often feel uncomfortable in situations where they feel that they have no control. They may try to avoid such situations or try to gain control in whatever way they can. The feeling of lack of control of helplessness in control may cause them to fear tendencies to comply or submit. Sexual abuse survivors often report difficulties in forming and sustaining intimate relationships (Courtois, 1988; Elliot & Gabrielson-Cabush, 1990; Finkelhor, Hotaling, Lewis and Smith, 1989). One of the most disruptive and painful aspects of child sexual abuse is its impact on the survivor's ability to trust. The untreated survivor's continued difficulties with trust may lead to considerable isolation from—and rejection by—the social milieu. As a result, true friendships may be rare for such survivors as may be enduring romantic relationships. Similarly, the survivor may have considerable difficulty bonding with the psychotherapist; instead he or she may see the clinician either as a potential enemy or as someone who must be groomed, bribed, or manipulated into providing interpersonal safety.

Literature on sexual abuse and on neuroticism points towards a relationship between the two. Ernst, Angst and Monika (1993) in the course of a 10-year longitudinal investigation of young Swiss adults, assessed childhood sexual abuse (CSA) and found that abuse cases tended to be more depressed and anxious; they reported more suicidal attempts, more sexual problems, and slightly more psychiatric symptoms and neuroticism than did subjects who did not report CSA. Bohan (1997) carried out a study on well-being, anxiety, conflicts, and values of 30 women from an obstetrics/gynecology clinic. Mean scores for anxiety and conflicts in the 15 women who reported CSA were significantly higher than those in the 15 women who had experienced no abuse. Convoy, Weiss and Zverina (1996) assessed 150 female psychiatric patients. Women, particularly those with a neurotic diagnosis were victimized incestuously. The results of an investigation by Zlotnick, Shea, Pearlstein, Begin, Simpson and Costello (1996) on the relationship of childhood incest to dissociation indicated that the incest survivors had higher Dissociative Experience than those with abuse in adulthood. Talbot, Duberstein, King, Cox and Giles (2000) examined the relationships between specific dimensions of CSA and personality traits in adulthood. Personality was measured with the NEO-Five-Factor Inventory, which yields scores on neuroticism, extraversion, openness to experience, agreeableness, and conscientiousness. Findings suggest that there are associations between personality traits and CSA characteristics in psychiatric patients. Specifically, women who experienced intercourse by a parent had low scores on openness to experience and extraversion, and may be more introverted than women whose sexual abuse history does not include parental incest.

None of the studies mentioned above reflect upon the effect of Indian socio-cultural environment on the relationship between childhood sexual abuse and neurotic tendency. In a socio-cultural environment like ours, where the sanctity of womanhood and the respect attached to it is almost dependent upon her sexual purity, an incident like sexual abuse in one's childhood can amount to high levels of anxiety, despair, trauma, confusion, and negativity. However it is disgusting to know that such shameful incidents seem to be prevalent in our country. Thee women survivors may suffer from a host of concomitant initial and long-term repercussions of childhood sexual abuse. This becomes important because it has been found that the negative long-term consequences of childhood sexual abuse differ because of the differences in perception and interpretation of the experience (Dale, 1999) and events and cultural background (Najoff-Bulman, 1985, 1989). Against this backdrop, the present study was conducted to measure and compare the neurotic tendency of adult women with severe childhood sexual abuse, moderate childhood sexual abuse, and no report of childhood sexual abuse.

METHOD

Design

A multigroup design, with three groups was used.

Sample

In order to select the participants, a Biographical Inventory was developed which contained questions that required the participants to indicate whether they had experienced sexual abuse in their childhood, who the perpetrator was, and what was the mode used by the abuser?

A total of 150 female college undergraduates were approached individually by the second author and were requested to answer the questions truthfully. The students were assured of confidentiality and anonymity. Out of 150 students, 57 reported one or the other type or more than one types of CSA and an absence of CSA was reported by the remaining 93. Among 57 students, 24 reported being severely abused and 33 were moderately abused. Those who reported the incidents of touching, stroking or rubbing in a sexual way, hugging and kissing in a sexual way, flashing or exposing of genitals by an adult, performing or making them perform oral sex or having sexual intercourse, were put in the 'severely sexually abused' category. Those who reported incidents of being looked at in a sexual way, making lewd or suggestive comments, being shown pornographic material by an adult were put in the 'moderately abused' category.

As per the availability and willingness of the students for further research, 20 students form each category were taken. A third group of 20 female undergraduates who reported no incident of sexual abuse in their childhood was also included as a control group. This group was called the 'non-abused' group and the participants in this group were taken in a random way out of the 93 participants who reported an absence of CSA.

Tool

Kundu Neurotic Personality Inventory (KNPI) was used to measure neurotic tendency in the participants. The inventory consists of 6 statements. The participants responded on a 5 category response scale ranging from 'always;, 'yes', 'entirely' to 'never', 'no, not at all'. The weightage even to the responses in each item determine the score for that item. Each statement is designed to score for positive or negative response as it represents symptoms of neurotic tendency. For five items (Nos. 41, 51, 55, 56 and 58) negative responses are indicative of neurotic tendency and for other items it is positive response that indicates neuroticism. Scores of 1, 2, 3, 4 and 5 were given to the above mentioned items for respective categories and scores of 5, 4, 3, 2 and 1 were for respective categories on rest of the items. The weights of each response were added up to determine the total score. Theoretically the minimum and maximum possible scores are 66 and 330 respectively. Split-half reliability for males, females, and neurotics has been reported as 0.85, 0.80 and 0.72 respectively and odd-even reliability has been reported as 0.86 and 0.87 for males and females respectively and coefficients of correlation between this scale and scale of neuroticism in Bernreuter Personality Inventory have been reported as 0.65 and 0.80 for males and females respectively.

Procedure

During the collection of initial information through the Biographical Inventory, the participants were asked to give their phone numbers for future contact. The participants were met individually and the second author administered the test. One college was covered at a time.

RESULTS AND DISCUSSION

The mean neurotic tendency scores of the three groups were calculated and t-test was applied to find out the significant difference between the means of the two comparing groups.

Table 36.1 : Mean, SDs, SEds, and t-ratio between the Mean Neurotic Tendency Scores of the Groups

Comparing Group	*N*	*Means*	*SD*	*SEd*	*t*
Severely Abused	20	228.20	19.74	4.476	3.049*
Moderately Abused	20	211.50	14.48		
Severely Abused	20	228.20	19.74	8.054	4.51*
Non-Abused	20	191.85	30.12		
Moderately Abused	20	211.50	14.48	7.47	2.63*
Non-Abused	20	191.85	30.12		

* $p < .05$.

Perusal of Table 36.1 shows that the mean neurotic tendency scores of severely abused and moderately abused participants were 228.20 and 211.50, and their SDs were 19.74 and 14.48 respectively. The SEd and the t-ratio were calculated as 4.476 and 3.049 respectively. The t-ratio was found to be significant at .05 level of confidence. The mean neurotic tendency scores of severely abused and non-abused groups were 228.20 and 191.85, and their SDs were 19.74 and 30.12 respectively. The SEd was found to be 8.054. The t-value between the two means came out to be 4.51, which was found to be significant at .05 level of significance. The mean neurotic tendency scores of moderately abused and the non-abused groups were 211.50 and 191.85, and their SDs were 14.48 and 30.12 respectively. The SEd was 7.47. The t-value between the two means was calculated as 2.63, which was found to be significant at the .05 level of significance. Thus all the comparisons came out to be significant.

The results of the study suggested significantly higher neurotic tendency in 'severely abused' than in 'moderately abused' participants; significantly higher neurotic tendency in women reporting both severe and moderate CSA history as compared to women reporting an absence of CSA history.

The significantly greater neurotic tendency among 'severely abused' as compared to 'moderately abused' indicates that levels of severity may play an important role in the amount of damage done. This finding can be supported by research done by Finkelhor and Browne (1986), which suggests that nature of the abuse, type of sexual act, whether physical contact with victim was made—may also affect the degree of damage done or development of neurotic tendency. Further evidence for this finding comes from a research conducted by Talbot *et al.* (2000) that examined the relationships between specific dimensions of childhood sexual abuse (CSA) and personality traits in adulthood. It was found that women whose abuse history included both parental abuse and intercourse had low scores on openness to experience and extraversion and were more introverted than women whose sexual abuse history did not include parental incest. In a study conducted by Zlotnick *et al.* (1996), incest survivors reported more dissociative symptomatology.

A look at Table 36.1 shows that neurotic tendency was significantly more in both 'severely abused' and 'moderately abused' than in 'non-abused' participants. These results are pointer of the relationship between CSA experiences and neuroticism. Child sexual abuse usually involves intrusion, threat, devaluation and / or pain. As a result, the child or adolescent abused victim may form a classically conditioned association between various social or environmental stimuli and danger, so that a variety of otherwise relatively neutral interpersonal events stimulate fear (Beck, Emery and Greenber, 1985). Ernst *et al.* (1993) assessed CSA in the course of a 10 year longitudinal investigation, and found out that abuse cases tended to be more depressed and anxious, and reported slightly more neuroticism than did subjects who did not report CSA. Convoy *et al.* (1996) in their study on psychiatric patients found that women, particularly those with a neurotic diagnosis, were victimized incestuously. In a study carried out by Bohan (1997) mean scores for anxiety and conflicts in the women who reported CSA were significantly higher than those for the women who had experienced no abuse. Hasnain and Kumar (2004) reported significantly poorer well-being in women who reported severe or moderate sexual abuse than in women who did not report any CSA. However, non-significant difference between well-being of severely abused and moderately abused women was reported.

REFERENCES

Beck, A.T., Emery, G., and Greenberg, M. (1985). *Anxiety Disorders and Phobias : A Cognitive Perspective,* New York : Basic Books.

Bohan, M.J. (1997). Assessing adult women sexually abused in childhood for anxieties, conflicts and values : a biopsychosocial approach to well-being, *Dissertation Abstracts International : Section B: The Sciences and Engineering, 57,* 46-94.

Carson, Robert A. and Butcher, James, N. (1992). *Abnormal Psychology and Modem Life,* New York : Harper Collins Publishers Inc.

Convoy, H., Weiss, P., and Zvervina, J. (1996). Sexual abuse in childhood in different diagnostic groups of psychiatric male and female patients, *Ceska a Slovenska Psychiatrie, 92,* 217-225.

Courtois, C.A. (1988). *Healing the Incest Eound : Adult Survivors in Therapy,* New York : W.W. Norton.

Dale, P. (1999). *Adults Abused as Children,* New Delhi : Sage Publications.

Elliot, D.M. & Gabrielson-Cabush, D.L. (1990). *Impaired Object Relations in Professional Women Molested as Children.* Paper presented at the annual meeting of the American Psychological Association, Los Angeles.

Ernst, C., Angst, J., and Monika, F. (1993). The Zurich Study : XVII. Sexual abuse in childhood : Frequency and relevance for adult morbidity data of a longitudinal epidemiological study, *European Archives of Psychiatry and Clinical Neuroscience) 242,* 293-300.

Eysenck, H.J. (1957). *The Dynamics of Anxiety and Hysteria,* London : Routledge and Kegan Paul.

Eysenck, H.J. (1961). Classification and the problem of diagnosis. In H.J. Eysenck (Ed.), *Handbook of Abnormal Psychology,* New York : Basic Books.

Eysenck, M.W. and Morley, S. (1974). Neuroticism, Extraversion, Locus of control, and work style, *Journal of Indian Academy of Applied Psychology,* Indian Medlars Centre.

Finkelhor, D. & Browne, A. (1986). Initial and long-term effects : A conceptual framework. In D. Finkelhor (Ed.), *A Sourcebook on Child Sexual Abuse,* Beverly Hills, CA : Sage.

J. Finkelhor, D., Hotaling, G., Lewis, I.A., and Smith, C. (1989). Sexual abuse and its relationship to later sexual satisfaction, marital status, religion, and attitudes, *Journal of Interpersonal Violence, 4,* 279-399.

Hasnain, N. and Kumar, D. (2004). Psychological well-being of women reporting sexual abuse in childhood. Paper presented to 8th *International and 39th National Conference of the Indian Academy of Applied Psychology on 'Positive Health and Well-being', July 15-17, 2004 Held at Department of Psychology, M.D. University, Rohtak.*

Janoff-Bulman, R. (1985). The aftermath of victimization : Rebuilding shattered assumptions. In C.R. Fingley (ed.) *Trauma and its wake : The study and treatment of post-traumatic stress,* New York : Brunner.

Janoff - Bulman, R. (1989). Assumptive works and stress of Traumatic events : Application of the schema construct, *Social Cognition, 7,* 113-136.

McCord, J. (1985). Long-term adjustment in female survivors of incest: An exploratory study, *Dissertation Abstracts International, 46,* 650B, Arizona Board of Regents, Arizona State University Libraries.

Runtz, M. (1987). *The Psychological Adjustment of Women who were Sexually and Physically Abused during Childhood and Early Adulthood : A Focus on Revictimization.* Unpublished master's thesis, University of Manitoba, Canada.

Russel, D.E.H. (1986). *The Secret Trauma : Incest in the Lives of Girls and Women,* New York : Basic Books.

Talbot, N.L., Duberstein, P.R., King, D.A., Cox, C., and Giles, D.E. (2000). Personality traits of women with a history of childhood sexual abuse, *Comprehensive Psychiatry, 41,* 130-136.

Wolpe, J. (1958). *Psychotherapy by Reciprocal Inhibition,* Palo Alto : Stanford University Press.

Zlotnick, C., Shea, M.T., Pearlstein, T. Begin, A., Simpson, E., and Costello, E. (1996). Differences in dissociative experiences between survivors of childhood incest and survivors of assault in adulthood, *Journal of Nervous and Mental Disease, 184,* 52-54.

37

Exploring Role of Spirituality in the Psychological Recovery of Cervical Cancer Patients

Neena Kohli & Roli Shukla**

Psychologists and other social scientists have generally kept their distance from religion and spirituality. Few professional training programmes in psychology address religious and spiritual issues (Bergin, 1983; Shafranske & Malony, 1990). Though mental health professionals, seek out referrals from religions groups, they rarely make referrals to clergy or other religious leaders (Koenig, Bearon, Hover, & Travis, 1991). Furthermore, the gap between psychology, religion and spirituality can also be felt in the empirical area. Systematic reviews of the empirical literature indicates that religion and spirituality are understudied variables in health related research in a number of disciplines, including psychology (Weaver, Kline, Samford, Lucas, Larson & Gorsuch, 1998), psychiatry (Larson, Patterson, Blazer, Omran & Kaplan, 1986), family practice (Craige, Liu, Larson, & Lyons, 1988), and gerontology, (Sherrill, Larson, & Greenword, 1993).

Several possible reasons for the neglect of religion and spirituality variables include : *(a)* religion and spirituality are less central and important to psychologists and other health related researchers than to the public as a whole (Bergin, 1991; Shafranske, 1996), *(b)* religion and spirituality are mistakenly assumed by some to fall outside the scope of scientific study (Thomson, 1996) and *(c)* religion and spirituality are believed to necessarily receed during an age that reflects the rise of science and rational enlightenment (Hill, Pargament, Hood, McCullough, Swyers, Larson & Zinnbauer, 2000). When religion and spirituality have been studied, they have often been included only as add-on variables, in the context of other research agendas.

Spirituality and religion represent related rather than independent constructs (Hill *et al.*, 2000). Although any definition of a construct as religious and spiritual is limited and therefore debatable, spirituality can be understood as a search for the sacred, a process through

* Department of Psychology, University of Allahabad, Allahabad.

which people seek to discover, hold on to, and when necessary, transform whatever they hold sacred in their lives (Pargament, 1997, 1999). This search takes place in a larger religious context, one that may be traditional or non-traditional (Hill, *et al.,* 2000). The search is what distinguishes religion and spirituality from other phenomena. The sacred is the common denominator of religious and spiritual life. It represents the most vital destination sought by the religious/spiritual person, and it is interwoven into the pathways many people take in life.

The term spirituality has had a long and diverse history. William James (1902/1961) regarded religion as the "feeling, acts, experiences of individual men (sic) in their solitude... in relation to whatever they may consider the divine". Thus, in essence he equated religion with spirituality and ignored institutional religion (Hauerwas, 2001). Simpson and Weiner (1991), in the Oxford English Dictionary, offer a substantial 10 pages of reference material on the concept of spirituality. Two related themes seem to dominate. First, is the notion of being concerned with life's most animating and vital principle or quality, often described as giving life or energy to the material human elements of the person. Second spirituality includes a broad focus on the immaterial features of life, regarded as not commonly perceptible by the physical senses (*e.g.*, sights, hearing) that are used to understand the material world. In popular usage, that which is spiritual is defined in diverse ways usually in distinction from material reality as experienced by the senses. Some view spirituality as primarily relational, a transcendent relationship with that which is sacred in life or with something divine, beyond the self. The concept itself is multidimensional and defies simple clear-cut boundaries. It often seems easier to point to what spirituality is not (*i.e.*, something material) than to what it is.

Religion is an institutional phenomenon. Though often centrally concerned with spirituality, religions are social entities or institutions, and unlike spirituality, they are defined by their boundaries. Religions are differentiated by particular beliefs and practices, requirements of membership, and needs of social organization. What is spiritual or transcendent may be a central interest or focus, but religions are also characterized by other non-spiritual concerns and goals (*e.g.*, cultural, economic, political, social). Thus, religion can be seen as fundamentally a social phenomenon, whereas spirituality is usually understood at the level of the individual within specific contexts. Viewed in this way, the field of religion is to spirituality, as the field of medicine is to health.

The present study focussed on cervical cancer patients. Cervical cancer is the commonest malignancy among females in India. It accounts for 24 percent of all malignancies. (Biennial Report National Cancer Registry, the Indian Council of Medical Research, 1988). The exact cause of cancer of the cervix is unknown, but certain predisposing factors are multiple sexual partners, poor male sex hygiene, vaginal infection and venereal diseases. The symptoms of cervical cancer are unusual discharge and bleeding. Women from the poor strata are more vulnerable to cervical carcinoma. If diagnosed at an early stage (stages 1 and 2) it is curable. Even if diagnosed late, life can be prolonged considerably. As a chronic disease, cervical cancer creates certain adjustment problems. Patients need enormous social and psychological resources to cope with the problems of treatment, adjustment with reality and rehabilitation.

The major objectives of this study are *(a)* to develop a measure of spiritually and *(b)* to explore the role of spirituality in the psychological recovery of cervical cancer patients.

METHOD

Sample

The sample comprised 40 Hindu female cervical cancer patients undergoing therapy at the cancer unit of Kamla Nehru Hospital, Allahabad. The sample included only stage 3 patients (in such cases the carcinoma extends to the pelvic wall or the lower third section of the vagina). The treatment for all the patients was radiotherapy.

The age of these patients varied from 40 to 70 years. As far as their education was conserved, 90 per cent of the patients were illiterate and 75 per cent of the patients were from similar background. The monthly family income of 90 per cent was less than Rs. 1,000 month.

Tools

An interview schedule was prepared in Hindi which included items from three domains *(a)* information about the history of illness and treatment, perception of severity of illness and extent of recovery, *(b)* measure of spirituality, and *(c)* measure of psychological recovery.

A set of 12 statements about spiritual beliefs was posed. The statements referred to *(a)* sense of completeness during prayers, *(b)* forgiveness etc. Each item was rated on a 5-point rating scale on which I implied "fully agree" and 5 implied "fully disagree".

RESULTS AND DISCUSSION

One of the objectives of the study was the development of a measure of spirituality. To achieve this objective, a 12-item measure of spirituality was developed. Examples of items were : (1) While praying, I have a feeling of completeness, and (2) I experience closeness with God. The mean score on each of the items and item-total correlation are presented in Table 37.1.

Table 37.1. Measure of Spirituality : Means, Variance and Item Total Correlation

Spirituality Items	*Mean*	*Scale Mean if item Deleted*	*Scale Variance if Item Deleted*	*Corrected Item Total Correlation*
S1	3.70	28.7500	19.9359	.2990
S2	3.75	28.8000	20.4718	.2200
S3	3.18	28.2250	22.7942	–.2669
S4	3.08	28.1250	20.1122	.2421
S5	2.88	27.9250	19.6096	.2879
S6	3.20	28.2500	23.3205	–.0955
S7	3.17	28.2250	20.3327	.2691
S8	3.80	28.8500	20.3872	.2716
S9	3.13	28.1750	21.5840	.0536
S10	3.85	28.9000	21.1692	.1647
S11	3.83	28.8750	21.5481	.1476
S12	3.40	28.4500	19.8949	.2722

A look at the Table 37.1 reveals that two items *viz.* S3 (I am capable of forgiving others, who did wrong with me) and S6 (Even during crisis situations, I rely upon my internal strength) correlated negatively with item total correlation. These items were dropped from further analysis. After deletion of these two items, the cronbach alpha α of the scale = .55.

Though cronbach alpha (.55) and the sample size on which the scale was administered was small (N=40), yet it is an important beginning, in the development of a measure of spirituality.

The second major objective of the present study was to explore the role of spirituality in the psychological recovery of cervical cancer patients. For this correlations were computed between spirituality and psychological recovery (r = –.039). Thus study failed to unravel linkages between spirituality and psychological recovery.

There could be several explanations for this finding. The measure of spirituality, as stated above, needs further refinement. A look at Table 37.1 shows that for all the items except item No. S5 (Mean=2.88) the mean score was above 3.00 This points to the fact, that all the patients were not high on spirituality. But spirituality is a complex variable. Studies conducted by Oman, Kurata, Strawbridge and Cohen (2002) and Hummer, Rogers, Nam & Ellison (1999) suggest that any association between religion or spirituality and cancer mortality can be explained by the confounding effects of prior health status. This raises the possibility that the temporal relationship of religion and spirituality and health is reversed in people who are at risk for cancer morality. That is, those who become sick are then more likely to become religious or spiritual. In the present study the focus was on exploring the role of spirituality in recovery of patients, but the fact that patients became less spiritual after the diagnosis of illness or were less spiritual before the onset of illness was not investigated.

Examination of five well-designed studies related to the role of some aspect of religion or spirituality on physical recovery from acute illness showed that in four of these studies, the hypothesized association between religious coping and more favourable physical outcomes in hospitalised patients was not supported (Fitchett, Rybarczyk, DeMarco, & Nicholas, 1999; King, Speck & Thomas, 1999; Koenig, Larson, Hays, McCollough, George & Branch 1998; Pargament, Koeing, Tarakeshwar, & Hahn, 2001).

Only one of these five studies found religion or spirituality to be associated with a recovery advantage. Oxman, Freeman, and Manheimer (1995) studied six-month mortality in patients undergoing elective cardiac surgery A significant association between the single item "strength and comfort from religion" and mortality was observed (OR=0.31, p=0.04) after adjustment for confounders and established risk factors. However, eight different ways to assess religion and spirituality were tested (five single items, a private religiousness scale, a public religiousness scale, and a total religiousness scale) with no persisting hypotheses for these repeated attempts and no adjustments for multiple looks. If for example, the Bonferroni transformation were used to adjust the significance level for the eight attempts to find the association, the cut-point of significance would be 0.006, thus, relegating the observed association of 0.04 to non-significance (Powell, Shahabi, & Thoresen, 2003).

The present study focussed on psychological recovery. Psychological recovery is linked to physical recovery. According to the bio-psychosocial model of health, the mind and the body are interconnected. Thus the findings of the above studies can be generalized to psychological recovery. The present study failed to unravel linkages between spirituality and psychological recovery (r = .036, p<.81).

Another possible reason for a non-significant correlation is the size of the sample (N=40). With an increase in sample size, even a small correlation value would have been significant. However, with patient population, even a small sample size appears reasonable.

To conclude, this study has opened the possibilities of future research in this very important yet controversial area and the intriguing evidence to date warrants continued and careful investigation.

REFERENCES

Bergin, A.E. (1983). Religiosity and mental health : A critical reevaluation and meta-analysis, *Professional Psychology : Research and Practice, 14,* 170-184.

Bergin, A.E. (1991). Values and religious issues in psychotherapy and mental health, *American Psychologist, 46,* 394-403.

Craigie, F.C., Liu, I.Y., Larson, D.B. & Lyons, J.S. (1988). A systematic analysis of religious variables in *The Journal of Family Practice,* 1976-1986, *Journal of Family Practice, 27,* 509-513.

Fitchett, G., Rybarczky, B.D., DeMarco, G.A. & Nicholas, J.J. (1999). The role of religion in medical rehabilitation outcomes : A longitudinal study, *Rehabilitation Psychology, 44,* 333-353.

Hauerwas, S. (2001). *With the Grain of the Universe,* Grand Rapids, MI : Brazos Press.

Hill, P.C., Pargament, K.I., Hood, R.W. Jr., McCullough, M.E., Swyers, J.P., Larson, D.B. & Zinnbauer, B.J. (2000). Conceptualizing religion and spiritually : Points of commonality, points of departure, *Journal for the Theory of Social Behaviour, 30,* 51-77.

Hummer, R.A. Rogers, R.G., Nam, C.B. & Ellison, C.G. (1999). Religious involvement and U.S. adult mortality, *Demography, 36,* 273-285.

James, W. (1961). *The Varieties of Religious Experience : A Study in Human Nature,* Cambridge, MA : Harvard University Press. (Original work published 1902).

Koenig, H.G., Bearon, L.B., Hover, M. & Travis, J.L. (1991). Religious perspectives of doctors, nurses, patients and families, *Journal of Pastoral Care, 45,* 254-267.

Koenig, H.G., Larson, D.B., Hays, J.C., McCullough, M.E., George, L.K. & Branch, P.S. (1998). Religion and survival of 1010 male veterans hospitalised with medical illness, *Journal of Religion and Health, 37,* 15-29. (*et al.*).

Larson, D.B., Pattison, E.M., Blazer, D.G., Omran, A.R. & Kaplan, B.H. (1986). Systematic analysis of research on religious variables in four major psychiatric journals, 1978-1982, *American Journal of Psychiatry, 143,* 329-334.

Oman, D., Kurata, J.H., Strawbridge, W.J., & Cohen, R.D. (2002). Religious attendance and cause of death over 31 years, *International Journal of Psychiatry in Medicine, 32,* 69-89.

Oxman, T.E., Freeman, D.H. & Manheimer, E.D. (1995). Lack of social participation or religious strength and comfort as risk factor for death after cardiac surgery in the elderly, *Psychosomatic Medicine, 57,* 5-15.

Pargament, K.I. (1997). *The Psychology of Religion and Coping : Theory, Research, Practice.* (New York : Guilford Press).

Pargament, K.I. (1999). The psychology of religion and spirituality? Yes and no, *International Journal for the Psychology of Religion, 9,* 3-16.

Pargament, K.I., Koenig, H.G., Tarakeshwar, M.A. & Hahn, J. (2001). Religious struggle as a predictor of mortality among medically ill elderly patients: A 2-year longitudinal study, *Archives of Internal Medicine, 161,* 1881-1885.

Powell, L.H., Shahabi, L. & Thoresen, C.E. (2003). Religion and spirituality : Linkages to Physical Health, *American Psychologist,* 58 (1) 36-52.

Shafranske, E.P. (1996). Religious beliefs, affiliations, and practices of clinical psychologists. (In E.P.

Shafranske (Ed.), *Religion and the Clinical Practice of Psychology* (pp. 149-162), Washington, DC : American Psychological Association.

Shafranske, E.P. & Malony, H.N. (1990). Clinical psychologists' religious and spiritual orientations and their practice of psychotherapy, *Psychotherapy, 27,* 72-78.

Sherrill, K.A., Larson, D.B. & Greenwold, M. (1993). Is religion taboo in gerontology? Systematic review of research on religion in three major gerontology journals, 1985-1991, *American Journal of Geriatric Psychiatry, 1,* 109-117.

Simpson, J.A. & Weiner, E.S.C. (1991). *The Oxford English Dictionary* (2nd ed.). Oxford, England : Oxford University Press.

Thomson, K.S. (1996). The revival of experiments in prayer, *Americal Scientist, 84,* 532-534.

Weaver, A.J., Kline, A.E., Samford, J.A., Lucas, L.A., Larson, D.B. & Gorsuch, R.L. (1998). Is religion taboo in psychology? A systematic analysis of research on religion in seven major American Psychological Association Journals : 1991-1994. *Journal of Psychology and Christianity, 17,* 220-232.

38

Cultural Beliefs : Impact on Mental Health and Treatment in Psychiatric Patients

Priti Singh[*], *Jagtar Singh*[**] & *S.C. Bhargava*[***]

The influence of culture on symptoms, treatment methods and response in illnesses is well known. Physical illnesses like exanthamatous fever are considered as a result of curse by sheetala mata and even highly educated people stick to worshipping in place of treatment. Life threatening conditions like snakebite is treated by chanting mantras.

Psychiatric illnesses because of their behavioural and emotional presentation are always considered as mysterious in Indian society. Their aetiology, symptom and treatment are surrounded by many myths and misconcepts. Patients and caretakers have their own beliefs which directly affect overall management and well being of the patients. Mental illnesses are supposed to be caused by ghosts, spirits, evileye, magic, tona totaka. The origin may be related to drugs, season, worries, sexual malpractices by many persons and dealt accordingly for treatment.

Reddy (1998) in his study—'Cultural beliefs and expectations' found that patients and their relatives have certain presumed causes for the illness like God's ungraciousness, evil spirits alcohol, narcotic substances, sins, sexual preoccupations, lunar cycles etc. 58% of his subjects related mental illness to Gods, ungraciousness, 50% to evil spirits and 58% to alcohol. Studies in west also reflect misconcepts. Wolff (1996) found in a population based study that 80% of population consider environmental factors as causative agents for mental illness.

With the above background the present study aims to—

1. Find out knowledge and beliefs in-patients and caretakers regarding presentation, causes and management of psychiatric disorders.
2. To plan strategies for improving mental health literacy.

[*] Reader, Dept. of Psychiatry, Pt. B.D. Sharma PGIMS, Rohtak-124001.
[**] Ex-Post-Graduate Student.
[***] Associate Professor and Head, Dept. of Psychiatry, Pt. B.D. Sharma PGIMS, Rohtak.

METHOD

Sample

The study was conducted in OPD of Psychiatry Department; of Pt. B.D. Sharma PGIMS, Rohtak. 100 first-degree relatives of patients and 100 neurotic patients attending OPD for first time formed the study group.

Material Used

A specially designed questionnaire was administered to the subjects. Questionnaire was divided into two parts :

First part comprised of 25 commonly considered causes of illness.

Second part has 15 presumed treatment modalities.

Procedure

The subjects were asked to tick yes/no on the basis of their understanding regarding causes and treatment. Information regarding symptoms were obtained during simple interviewing. Socio-demographic profile was also taken for each subject.

RESULTS AND DISCUSSION

Table 38.1 : The Socio Demographic Profile of the Sample

Age		*% of Patients*	*% of Relatives*
	Below 40	64	67
	40 and above	36	33
Sex	Male	55	77
	Female	45	23
Background	Rural	87	70
	Urban	13	30
Marital Status	Married	70	84
	Unmarried	23	14
	Widow/Widower	6	—
	Separated	1	2
Education	Illiterate	46	33
	Literate	54	67

Table 38.2 Reflects features which were perceived as part of psychiatric illness. Biological functions like sleep and appetite. Aggression/violence and oversocialization were considered as important presentation.

Table 38.2 : Perceived Features of Psychiatry Illness

		% of Patients	*% of Relatives*
1.	Disturbance in biological functions	56	60
2.	Persistent mood changes	42	48
3.	Aggressive/violence	88	94
4.	Oversocialization	74	80
5.	Abnormal perception	36	40
6.	Physical symptoms	24	30

Table 38.3 reflects the presumed causes of mental illnesses. Over thinking and poor sleep were most frequently presumed causes of psychiatric illnesses in both groups. Substance abuse, head injury, ghosts and spirits were also given significance. 62% of patients believed that illness was due to Gods ungraciousness.

Table 38.3 : Presumed Causes of Psychiatric Illness

		% of Patients	*% of Attendants*
1.	Change in psychological physical and physiological functioning		
	Excessive thinking	80	84
	Excessive work	35	49
	Poor sleep	86	82
	Excessive study	26	41
	Digestive disturbance	20	32
2.	Alcohol and substance		
	Alcohol	40	50
	Substance other than alcohol	59	60
3.	Organic		
	Head injury	50	51
	Epilepsy	42	42
	Encephalitis and infection	36	44
4.	Sex related concepts sterilization	11	29
	Excessive thinking absent sex	38	41
	Habits	20	26
5.	Concepts related to fate	46	56
	Ghosts/spirits	54	25
	Evil eye	19	26
	Sin	23	29
	Gods ungraciousness	62	32
6.	Miscellaneous	36	45

Considering the treatment modalities, significance was given to drugs by patients as well as relatives. Electro-convulsive therapy was also considered as important treatment modality by both groups. Presumed treatment modalities are reflected in table 38.4.

Current study reveals many factors related to our culture. There are many beliefs, which surround the patients and their relatives understanding about psychiatric illness.

Right from the starting of psychiatric illness the symptoms are not considered as part of an illness and they keep on lingering for a long time. Symptoms like sleep and appetite changes are ignored by many.

Persistant mood change, which is diagnostic of mood disorder was given importance only

Table 38.4 : Presumed Treatment Modalities

Treatment Modality	*% of Patients*	*% of Attendants*
Drugs	77	70
ECT	58	68
Change in place	10	21
Worship	14	31
Sedative/Hypnotics	23	38
Marriage	16	33
Vitamins/Energy providing drugs	20	38
Drip	20	24
Specific diet	9	28
Yoga/Meditation	9	10
Hypnosis	6	10
Psychological treatment	6	8
Consultant with tantriks/black magic	10	10

by 42% of patient and 48% of attendants. Abnormal perception (hallucinations) which is core feature of psychosis is considered a part of illness only by 36% of patients and 40% of attendants.

Somatic/physical symptoms which are important presentation of neurotic disorders and considered as part of psychiatric illness only by 24% patients and 30% of attendants.

Regarding presumed causes majority believed that mental illness are caused by excessive thinking and worries. Similar findings were reflected in Reddy's studies (1988). Next importance was given to sleep deprivation. Alcohol and other psychoactive substance were considered as causative agents by 26 and 20% patients and 41 and 32% of relatives. 21% of subjects in Jorm's study (2000) believed the same.

Even in modern era of science and technology a good percentage of caretakers and patients believed in concept of fate, ghosts/spirits, Gods ungraciousness, similar concepts were reflected in study by Reddy.

77% of patients and 70% of attendants believed in drug treatment. Negative views were because of side effects and concepts of dependence and brain damage. Negative views regarding medication were also found Jorm, Korten, Jacomb, Christensen, Rodgers and Pollett (1997). Only 58% of patients and 68% of attendants believed in Electro Convulsive Therapy (ECT).

Negative views regarding ECT were also found by Jorm (2000). It is considered as harmful. Psychological treatments are viewed more positive in western studies (Jorm 1997, 2000) in contrast to present study where only 6% of patients and 10% of attendants were in favour of psychotherapy. People still believe in treatment like change in place, worship, marriage and black magic.

As far as presentation to psychiatrist are concern, efforts are to be made to improve public knowledge of mental disorders which is less as compared to physical illness. Efforts should be made not only to improve public awareness but also to make health workers more aware of incidence of mental health problems. These two can be done by involvement of broad range of educational material through TV, radio, print media etc. Disease specific subgroups like relatives of patients with specific disorders. Efforts should also be made to improve the quality of information presented in media through expert input.

A step towards improving the mental health literacy is taken through district mental health programme where health workers at various levels are being trained to recognize mental illness. Similarly school teachers are being trained to identify illnesses among their students. Much more is required to improve community awareness.

REFERENCES

Angermeyer, M.D., Bruce, G., Angermeyer, A.M. (1996). Stigma perceived by patients attending modern treatment setting, *The Journal of Nervous and Mental Diseases* 176; 4-11.

Fisher, J.D., Farina, A. (1979). Consequences of beliefs about the nature of mental disorder, *Journal of Abnormal Psychology*, *88*, 320-327.

Jorm, A.F., Korten, A.E., Jocomb, P.A., Christensen, H., Rodgers, B. & Pollett, P. (1997). Public beliefs about causes and risk factors for depression and schizophrenia, *Social Psychiatry and Psychiatric Epidemiology*, *32*, 143-148.

Jorm, A.F. (2000). Mental Health Literacy—Public knowledge and beliefs about mental disorders, *British Journal of Psychiatry*, *177*, 396-401.

Reddy, K.R. (1988). Cultural believes and expectations of the patients – A consideration of the customer's view point, *Indian Journal of Psychology Medicine*, *11*, 93-100.

Wolff, G., Pathare, S., Craig, T. & Julian, L. (1996). Community knowledge of mental illness and reaction to mentally ill people, *British Journal of Psychiatry*, *168*, 191-198.

39

A Challenge to Well-Being—HIV/AIDS and Coping Strategies

Rajesh Nair**, *Sunita Malhotra *and Sapna Sachdeva Nair******

Human Immune Deficiency Virus (HIV)/Acquired Immune Deficiency Syndrome (AIDS) have been considered as a major threat to the sustainable development of the country and has impact beyond national boundaries. It is not just a medical problem but basically a social problem. The most disturbing fact is that the productive age group, *i.e.* 15 to 49 years has been largely infected by the disease. A community as we know is composed of people, therefore, well being of community depends upon that of the members who compose it. A community or for that matter a nation cannot be expected to prosper when underneath it is being hollowed in terms of losing its primary breadwinners in the family, thereby affecting the country's per capita productivity and loss of labour. In the absence of any medicine for cure, relying on behavioural and social change seems to be the only alternative. In the present discussion an attempt has been made to putforth the facts and figures of the AIDS epidemic in India and the challenges posed by this social problem and to uncover some of the coping strategies adopted by people living with HIV infection. Lastly some of the intervention strategies aimed at fostering more adaptive coping efforts have also been proposed.

Acquired Immune Deficiency Syndrome is the final and fatal stage of infection with Human Immuno Deficiency Virus. It is a complex syndrome of diseases which manifest in deterioration of human immune system. The virus enters and destroys the crucial white blood cells known as T4 lymphocytes which are capable of protecting the body from various diseases. With the collapse of immune system, the AIDS patient develops a variety of infections ordinarily checked by a normal system. Two retroviruses that cause immune deficiency are : HIV1 and HIV2. There are 10 genetic subtypes of HIV-1: A to I and O. HIV-1C is most common in Central and South Africa and India. There are significant differences between rates of transmission and

*Consultant (NGOs), National AIDS Control Organisation (NACO), New Delhi.
**Professor, Deptt. of Psychology, M.D. University, Rohtak.
***Consultant, Hindustan Latex Family Planning Promotion Trust (HLFPPT), New Delhi.

disease development for different types of HIV. Infection with subtype E seems to be associated with significantly faster decline in immunity.

HIV/AIDS—Its Magnitude

While a few decades back the most dreaded four letter disease "AIDS" seemed so unfamiliar to most of us, within no time it has wormed its way into all sections of society affecting not only the individuals but also their families, community and nation at large (Figure 39.1). The impact of the epidemic turns out to be far worse than the forecasters had predicted. The epidemic remains extremely dynamic, growing and changing character as the virus exploits new opportunities for transmission.

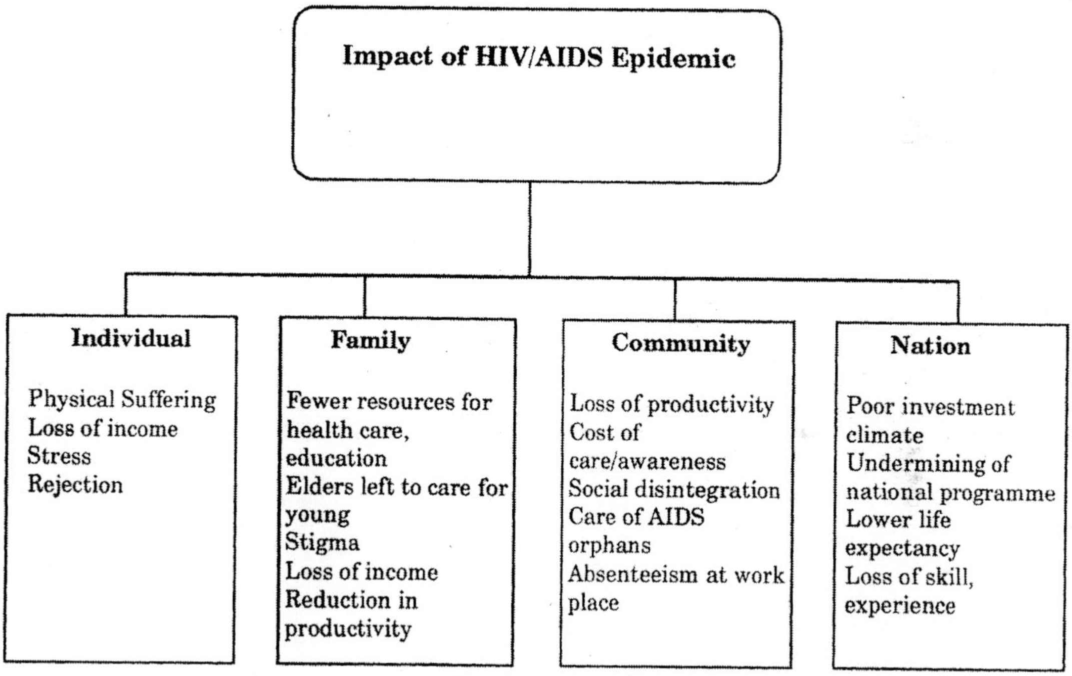

Fig. 39.1. : Impact of HIV/AIDS epidemic.

Rates of infection are high in many countries in Sub-Saharan Africa. In South East Asia, India is estimated to have the largest burden. There also seems to be a change in the distribution of HIV/ AIDS epidemic in this region. At one time it was seen to be transmitted in high risk populations, *i.e.* Commercial Sex Workers (CSWs) and Intravenous Drug Users (IDUs), in some labour migrants and in urban areas whereas today, the epidemic is being seen in the partners of high risk groups, young people and in urban, peri urban and rural areas (Fig. 39.2).

HIV/AIDS in India : Some Disturbing Trends

1. About 5.1 million people are estimated to be infected with HIV.
2. According to HIV/AIDS surveillance report there are 44,275 AIDS cases in India (National AIDS Control Organization, 2003).

3. Nearly 50 percent of infections occur among young people below 25 years.
4. Almost 90% of the cases fall within most economically productive age group and one in four cases of HIV are among women.
5. Everyday estimates indicate that 1500 people in India become newly infected with HIV.
6. Given India's large population a mere 0.1 percent increase in prevalence rate would increase the number of adults living with HIV/AIDS by over half a million persons.

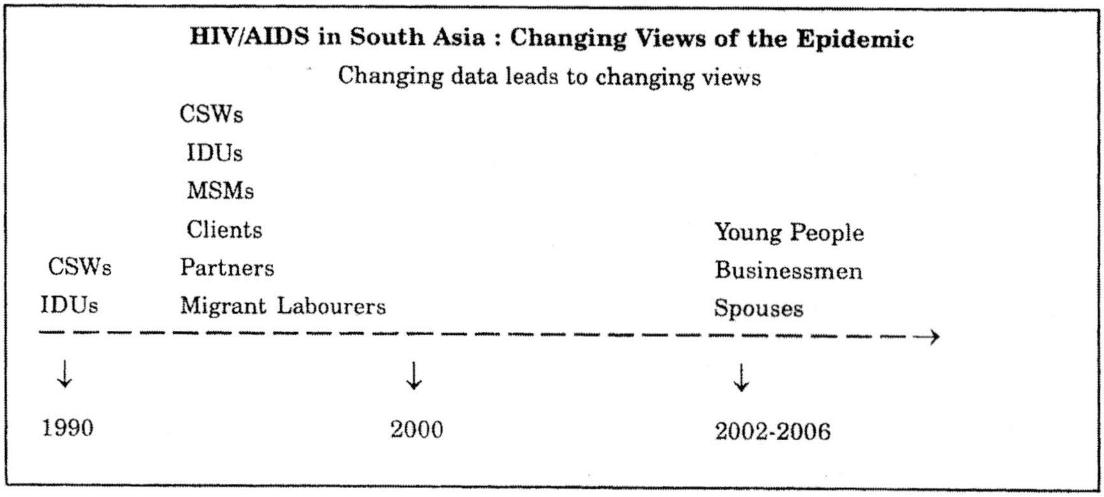

Fig. 39.2 : HIV/AIDS in South Asia.

Source : South Asia Inter Faith Consultation on Children, Young People and HIV/AIDS 4-6 December 2003, Kathmandu, Nepal. (UNICEF)

Looking at the data it can be said with confidence that in today's times AIDS is the most serious public health problem with unprecedented medical, psychological and societal implications. Some of the key challenges that our country is facing right now are :

- Magnitude and diversity—India is a country with variety and diversity of settings and situations. Even one percent of incidence actually translates to millions of cases.
- Risk and vulnerability—Understanding of risk and various dimensions of risks that puts the individual at risk.
- Spread to general population (youth, women)—Surveillance data shows spread of virus from high risk groups to general population and from urban to rural. Women and youth more likely to be affected, calling for different approaches for them.
- Stigma and discrimination—From the beginning the disease has been perceived to spread by sexual transmission and the issue of shame and fear has caused the public to treat people suffering from HIV/AIDS in a discriminatory fashion.
- Denial and Self exemption—Person infected with this virus has also been denied the social status. The other critical problem is the issue of self exemption or the tendency to see oneself outside the domain of the risk.

- Gender and human rights issue—The weaker power of decision-making and the inability of negotiation of safer sex practices puts women at risk. Also depriving services violates the rights of people.

Individuals living with HIV infection live with their condition, in majority of cases well over a decade (Longini, Scott, Byers, Ward, Lemp and Hethcote, 1989). The survival of people infected with HIV is likely to be prolonged even further with the understanding of biological markers of HIV disease and prognosis will increase as advances in antiretroviral therapies and control of common presenting opportunistic infections improves (Cotton, 1989), and early interventions occur. During the progression from the time of infection to full blown AIDS, the infected person may not show any signs of illness. Therefore, the real measure of scope of epidemic is the number of people living with HIV (PLWHIV) hence it is meaningful to talk about people living and coping with HIV. With the understanding that the researches that examine HIV related coping and adaptation could provide valuable information for clinical understanding and management of the psychiatric sequelae of HIV/AIDS, the following section delves into the issues related to the coping of people living with HIV positive status.

Coping with HIV

Living with the diagnosis of HIV can be frightening and anxiety producing experience, including the uncertainty of future, fear of death and disfigurement. Besides these issues, dealing with stigma or the adverse responses of others adds an additional layer of difficulty and may pose severe threats to the individual. A broad range of reactions to AIDS have been noted, encompassing denial, feelings of external control, feelings of alienation and isolation and generally subjective distress (Nichols, 1983). Nichols (1985) observed that the psychological effect of AIDS on patients has been described by others as an adjustment reaction to catastrophic stress (Haussman, 1983). The emotional responses that are elicited are similar to those evoked by any of a variety of catastrophic stresses (Weiss,1976). Situational distress occurs in three phases: crisis, transitional phase and the deficiency state. Reactions to AIDS follows the same pattern with frequent addition of a fourth stage *i.e.,* the preparation of death.

Walker (1991) and McKusick (1992) identified a number of challenges being faced by HIV positive people close to death :

- Find self acceptance.
- Make clear their wishes for final treatment.
- Attempt to deal with and hopefully heal rifts with family and friends.
- Find ways to say goodbye and yield to death.

Depression is one of the most frequently reported psychiatric manifestations of HIV infection (Morris, 1996). As many as one-half of HIV-infected persons report significant levels of depression (Low-Beer, Chan, Yip, Wood, Montaner, O'shaughnessy & Hogg, 2000; Penzak, Reddy & Grimsley, 2000) making depression a particularly important factor in determining health and in HIV-infected women's evaluation of their health. Depression has been linked with poor adherence to antiretroviral therapy (Catz, Kelly, Bogart, Benotsch and Mc Auliffe, 2000) and also contributing to the hastening of HIV disease progression (Mayne, Vittinghoff, Chesney, Barrett and Coates, 1996). As individuals become symptomatic and exhibit an increased number of symptoms, they experience greater depressive symptoms and engage in unhealthy self-care behaviour (Valente & Saunders, 1997) further undermining their health and perceptions of well-being.

Researchers who study coping have described how individuals with HIV/AIDS use various social and psychological strategies to cope with illness related to stressors (Fleshman & Fogel, 1994). The subsequent paragraphs explore specific coping strategies used by HIV-infected individuals.

HIV Positive People and their Coping Strategies : Some Empirical Evidences.

Lazarus and Folkman (1984) described two general strategies that people living with HIV/AIDS may use—problem focused coping and emotion focused coping. Problem focused coping strategies target the source of stress, for example seeking medical care, seeking social support, making healthy changes in life style, etc. whereas emotion focused coping targets how a person feels without addressing the problem. Examples of it include denial of condition, avoidance and escape from stressors etc. Denial, a form of emotional coping can be beneficial at times. However, if it persists for an extended period of time, it can delay the onset of medical intervention and may therefore have deleterious health effects. For example, in a group of men and women living with HIV/AIDS, use of denial as coping stratergy was associated with greater pain (Hart, Gore, Maldonado, Lagana & Blake, 2000). On the other hand information seeking, which is generally considered as positive or adaptive coping may also be associated with adverse outcomes in certain conditions. The study of coping intervention for HIV positive gay men by Chesney, Folkman & Chambers (1996) included a coping skills group, an HIV/AIDS education and information group, and a no-treatment control. The anxiety level of HIV/AIDS education and information group increased, suggesting that the additional knowledge, while possibly helping with respect to strategies of management of their illness, was also anxiety provoking, especially in the absence of training in skills for coping with anxiety. Also important here is to specify that while some researchers consider social support as a form of problem focused coping, there are some who have taken social support as an independent variable or the other form of coping.

Siegel and Krauss (1991) proposed conceptual frameworks that contextualize HIV related changes and noted emergence of 3 major challenges in coping with HIV :

- Dealing with the possibility of curtailed life span.
- Dealing with the reactions to a stigmatizing illness.
- Developing strategies for maintaining physical and emotional health.

Though the influence of gender and race on the use of coping strategies is less established among individual with HIV but in one of the few such studies, Solomon, Gleghorn, Astemborski & Vlahov (1993), looked for the differences in social support and coping strategies among HIV-infected male and female intravenous drug users. The study revealed that HIV-infected women had greater avenues of social support and used more socially based coping strategies whereas HIV-infected men displayed more active coping strategies. Hackl, Somlai, Relly and Kalichman (1996), conducted a study to examine the salient life issues and coping strategies used by HIV-infected women. Five themes of concern were identified: stigma, child concerns and care-taking roles, social support needs, death, dying and despair issues, and HIV/AIDS information needs. The primary coping strategies most often employed by these women were denial, concealment of their health status from others, isolating oneself from others, and crying.

It has been further suggested that the coping strategies used immediately after the diagnosis differed from those used at later stages. For example Reeves, Merriam and Courtenay (1999) on the basis of in-depth interviews with eighteen HIV—infected individuals reported that two types of coping strategies utilized immediately after diagnosis, *i.e. affective* which ranged from complete denial to intense anger and *behavioural*. The period of transition was reported to serve as a launching pad for sucessful coping strategies, characterized by three particularly salient occurences : confronting the challenge, taking control and responsibility, and action.

The literature is also well supplied with anecdotal accounts of individuals who report richer and more meaningful lives as a result of encountering stressful situations including potentially life threatening illness like HIV/AIDS. The way in which HIV infected subjects respond to their condition might also have a role in molding disease parameters. Taylor, Kemeny, Reed, Bower and Gruenewald (2000) in their study of HIV positive men, found that the ability to find meaning and benefit in the experience predicted a slower immune decline over time and longer survival, even after controlling for potential psychosocial and health confounds. Earlier Goodkin, Blaney, Feaster, Fletcher, Baum, Mantero Atienza, Klimas, Million, Szapocznik and Eisendorfer (1992) also observed a significant relationship between active coping and increased natural killer cell cytotoxicity in HIV-infected persons, whereas avoidance coping was found to be related to increased psychological distress (Fleishman & Fogel, 1994). Goal setting therefore is important because living with HIV is characterized by pervasive uncertainty about future and so those infected with HIV need to feel entitled to set goals and focus on quality rather than quantity of life. On similar lines Chidwick and Borrill (1996) discovered that individuals who managed their lives successfully after HIV positive diagnosis shared characteristics of coping more efficiently after two years had elapsed since the diagnosis, having perception of good physical health and feeling that they had appropriate and sufficient social support. In yet another such study of 736 individuals with AIDS it was noted that these individuals practiced a variety of coping behaviours categorized as positive coping, social support seeking, and avoidance coping. Their coping behaviours were associated with health behaviours, affect, and disease progression in both cross-sectional and longitudinal analyses (Fleishman & Fogel, 1994). Moreover, religious behaviours (*e. g.* Service attendance, prayer) have also been found to be associated with medical outcomes and religious coping more generally (placing trust in God, seeking comfort in religion), to lower levels of psychological distress (Woods, Antoni, Ironson & Kling, 1999). On the basis of foregoing overview and evaluation of literature it can be concluded that people infected with HIV make use of variety of coping strategies to sustain them during their HIV/AIDS illness process.

Since now-a-days people learn about their HIV positive status much earlier and also because there is rise in their life expectency due to advances in medicine so from the psychological point of view it is immensely important to enhance the quality of life and to alleviate adverse psychological consequences among the people living with HIV disease.

As is rightly said, *"health is not every thing but every thing without health is nothing"*. Therefore, every attempt should be in the direction of attaining good physical and mental health. Emerging evidence suggests that HIV patients who fare better on psyhosocial variables like social support, coping, etc. fare better in terms of disease progression and clinical status. Thus, the interventions should utilize a dual approach which includes a behaviour-modification and coping effectiveness training framework that is both gender-specific and culturally-appropriate. Because HIV infection typically occurs as a result of behaviour, these types of intervention programmes may be useful in teaching problem-solving skills, managing symptoms, and promoting adaptive coping strategies. People should be pursued to undergo counselling which in turn should be made so effective that the patients are motivated to come for the followup. Also, longitudinal studies will be essential in determining if coping effectiveness training increases coping efficacy and decreases psychological distress among HIV-infected. Individual differences are likely to play a pivotal role in coping with the stressful condition. Hence, understanding the role of personality in coping can broaden person centered change efforts to encompass simultaneous growth in personal resources and the development of more effective coping strategies. Though there is not much evidence in this regard but the present authors are exploring the possible relationship between coping and personality characteristcs of people living with HIV/AIDS. Lastly, it is well documented that there is a high level of stigma (in terms of social acceptance) associated with being HIV infected (Crandall, & Coleman,1992) which may prevent HIV infected people from accessing needed health services and may affect their functional health status and perceptions of disease severity. Hence it is all the more important to provide a congenial environment which will facilitate desensitization of community to remove stigma and discrimination associated with the disease and enables people living with HIV/AIDS in coping sucessfully with the disease which would further improve their quality of life .

REFERENCES

Brashers, D.E., Hass, S.M., Neidig, J.L. & Rintamaki, L.S. (2002). Social activism, self advocacy, and coping with HIV illness, *Journal of Social Science and Personal Relationships, 19,* 113-133.

Catz, S.L., Kelly, J.A., Bogart, L.M., Benotsch, E.G. & McAuliffe, T.L. (2000). Patterns, correlates, and barriers to medication adherence among persons prescribed new treatments for HIV disease, *Health Psychology, 19,* 124-133.

Chesney, M., Folkman, S., & Chambers, D. (1996). Coping effectiveness training for men living with HIV : preliminary findings, *International Journal of STD and AIDS, 2,* 75-82.

Chidwick, A., & Borill, J. (1996). Dealing with a life threatening diagnosis : The experience of people with the human immunodeficiency virus, *AIDS Care, 8,* 271-284.

Cotton, D.J. (1989). Improving survival in Acquired Immunodefeciency Syndrome : Is experience everything? *Journal of the American Medical Association, 261,* 3016-17.

Crandall, C.S., & Coleman, R. (1992). AIDS-related stigmatization and the disruption of social relationships, *Journal of Social and Personal Relationships, 9,* 163-177.

Fleishman, J.A. & Fogel, B. (1994). Coping and depressive symptoms among people with AIDS, *Health Psychology, 13,* 156-169.

Goodkin, K., Blaney, N.T., Feaster, D., Fletcher, M.A., Baum, M.K., Mantero-Atienza, E., Klimas, N.G., Millon, C. Szapocznik, J., & Eisendorfer, C. (1992). Active coping style is associated with natural killer cell cytotoxicity in asymptomatic HIV-1 seropositive homosexual males, *Journal of Psychosomatic Research, 36,* 635-650.

Hackl, K., Somlai, A., Kelly, J. & Kalichman, S. (1996). Women Living with HIV/AIDS : The Dual Challenges of Being a Medical Patient and a Primary Family Caregiver, *International Conference on AIDS*.

Hart, S., Gore, F.C., Maldonado, J., Lagana, L. & Blake M.J. (2000). The relationship between pain and coping styles among HIV positive men and women, *Psychology and Health, 15,* 869-879.

Haussman, K. (1983). Treating victims of AIDS poses challenge to psychiatrists, *Psychiatric News, Aug. 5.*

Lazarus, R.S. & Folkman, S. (1984). *Stress, appraisal, and coping*, New York : Springer.

Longini, I.M., Scott C.W., Byers, R.H., Ward, J.W., Darrow, W. M., Lemp, G.F. & Hethcote, H.W. (1989). Statistical analysis of the stages of HIV infection using a Markov model, *Statistics in Medicine, 8,* 831- 43.

Low-Beer, S., Chan, K., Yip, B., Wood, E., Montaner, J. S., O'Shaughnessy, M.V., & Hogg, R.S. (2000). Depressive symptoms decline among persons on HIV protease inhibitors, *Journal of Acquired Immune Deficiency Syndrome, 23,* 295-301.

Mayne, T., Vittinghoff, E., Chesney, M., Barrett, D.C., & Coates, T.J. (1996). Depressive affect and survival among gay and bisexual men infected with HIV, *Archives of International Medicine, 156,* 2233-2238.

Mc Kusick, L. (1992). In psychosocial issues related to death and dying, Website www.apa.org/in/aids/major.html.

Mc Kusick, L., Horstman, W. & Coates, T.J. (1985). AIDS and sexual behaviour reported by gay men in Francisco, *American Journal of Public Health, 75,* 493-496.

Morris, N.J. (1996). Depression and HIV+ disease : A critical review, *Journal of the American Psychiatric Nurses Association, 2,* 154-163.

Nichols, S.E. (1983). Psychiatric aspects of AIDS, *Psychosomatics, 24,* 1083-1089.

Nichols, S.E. (1985). Psychosocial reactions of persons with Acquired Immune Deficiency Syndrome, *Annals of Internal Medicine, 103,* 765-767.

Penzak, S.R., Reddy, Y.S. & Grimsley, S.R. (2000). Depression in patients with HIV infection, *American Journal of Health-System Pharmacy, 57,* 376-386.

Reeves, P.M., Merriam, S.B. & Courtenay, B.C. (1999). Adaptation to HIV infection : the development of coping strategies over time, *Qualitative Health Research, 9,* 344-361.

Siegal, K., & Krauss, B.J. (1991). Living with HIV infection : Adaptive tasks of seropositive gay men, *Journal of Health and Social Behaviour, 32,* 17-32.

Solomon, L., Gleghorn, A., Astemborski, J. & Vlahov, D. (I 993). Sex differences in coping and social support among HIV seropositive and seronegative injection drug users, *International Conference on AIDS, 9,* 822.

Taylor, S.E., Kemeny, M.E., Reed. G.M., Bower, J.E. & Gruenewald, T.L. (2000). Psychological resources, positive illusions, and health, *American Psychologist, 55,* 99-109.

Thoits, P.A. (1991). Gender differences in coping with emotional distress. In J. Eckenrode (Ed.), *The Social Context of Coping, pp. 107-138*, New York : Plenum.

Valente, S. & Saunders, J. (1997). Managing depression with people with HIV disease, *Journal of the Association of Nurses in AIDS Care, 8,* 51-67.

Walker, L. (1991). In psychosocial issues related to death and dying. website www.apa.org/pi/aids/major.html.

Weiss, R.S. (1976). Transitional states and other stressful situations : Their nature and programs for their management. In G. Caplan and M. Killilea (e.d.) Support systems and mutual help, New York : Grune and Stratton.

Woods, T.E., Antoni, M.H., Ironson, G.H. & Kling, D.W. (1999). Religiosity is associated with affective and immune status in symptomatic HIV infected gay men, *Journal of Psychosomatic Research, 46,* 165-176.

INDEX

M